Study Guide and Skills Performance Checklists

to Accompany

Canadian Fundamentals of Nursing

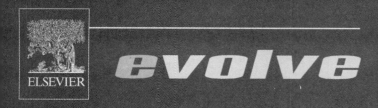

ELSEVIER

evolve

- **Student Learning Activities**
  Include crosswords, hangman puzzles, matching games, case studies, and short answer questions.

- **Review Questions**
  Include answers and rationales.

- **Concept Map Exercises**
  Challenge you to work with multiple nursing diagnoses and recognize their relationship to medical diagnoses.

- **Animations**
  Include exciting images related to various chapters in the textbook.

- **Critical Thinking Exercises**
  Challenge you to recognize how nursing process and critical thinking come together so that you can provide the best care for your clients.

- **Video Clips**
  Demonstrate important steps in a variety of nursing skills throughout the textbook.

- **WebLinks**
  Take you to hundreds of exciting websites carefully chosen to supplement the content of the textbook.

- **Content Updates**
  Include the latest information from the authors of the textbook to keep you current with recent developments in this area of study.

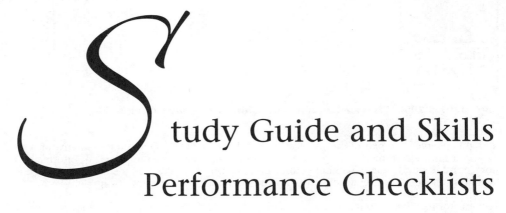

Study Guide and Skills Performance Checklists

to Accompany
POTTER • PERRY
Canadian Fundamentals of Nursing

3rd edition

Geralyn Ochs, RN, MSN, BC-ACNP, ANP
Assistant Professor in Adult Nursing
St. Louis University School of Nursing

Performance Checklists by
Patricia Castaldi, BSN, MSN
Director, Practical Nursing Program
Union County College
Plainfield, New Jersey

Canadian editors
Janet C. Ross-Kerr, RN, BScN, MS, PhD
Professor, Faculty of Nursing
University of Alberta
Edmonton, Alberta

Marilyn J. Wood, RN, BSN, MSN, DrPH
Professor, Faculty of Nursing
University of Alberta
Edmonton, Alberta

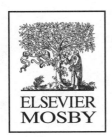

ELSEVIER
MOSBY

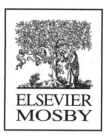

ELSEVIER MOSBY

Notice

Neither the Publisher not the Editors assume any responsibility for any loss or injury and/or damage to persons or property arising out of or related to any use of the material contained in this book. It is the responsibility of the treating practitioner, relying on independent expertise and knowledge of the patient, to determine the best treatment and method of application for the patient.

Library and Archives Canada Cataloguing in Publication

Potter, Patricia Ann
 Study guide to accompany Canadian fundamentals of nursing, third edition / Patricia Ann Potter, Anne Griffin Perry ; Canadian editors, Janet C. Ross-Kerr, Marilynn J. Wood.

ISBN 0-7796-9966-1

 1. Nursing–Problems, exercises, etc. I. Perry, Anne Griffin II. Kerr, Janet C., 1940-III. Wood, Marilynn J. IV. Title.

RT41.P68 2005 Suppl.   610.73   C2005-902797-5

Publisher: Ann Millar
Developmental Editors: Heather McWhinney and Joanne Sanche
Managing Developmental Editor: Martina van de Velde
Projects Manager: Liz Radojkovic
Production Editor: Marcel Chiera
Copy Editor: Shefali Mehta
Typesetting and Assembly: Kolam
Printing and Binding: Maple-Vail

Elsevier Canada
1 Goldthorne Ave., Toronto, ON, Canada M8Z 5S7
Phone: 1-866-896-3331
Fax: 1-866-359-9534

Printed in the United States of America

1 2 3 4 5 10 09 08 07 06

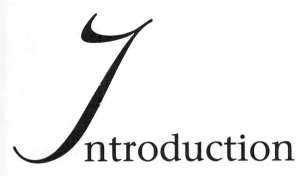

Introduction

The *Study Guide to accompany Canadian Fundamentals of Nursing*, third edition, has been developed to encourage independent learning for beginning nursing students. As you begin to read the text, you may note a difference in style and format from other books you've used in the past. The terms are new, and the focus of the content is different. You may be wondering, "How will I possibly learn all of the material in this chapter?" The essential objective of this study guide is to assist you in this endeavour—to help you learn *what* you need to know and then self-test with hundreds of review questions.

This study guide follows the text chapter for chapter. Whatever chapter your instructor assigns, you will use the same chapter number in this study guide. The outline format was designed to help you learn to read nursing content more effectively and with greater understanding. Each chapter of this study guide has the following sections to assist you to comprehend and recall.

The *Preliminary Reading* section is designed to teach pre-reading strategies. You need to become familiar with the chapter by first reading the chapter title, the key concepts and key terms (found at the end of each chapter), and all headings, as well as review all photographs, drawings, tables, and boxes. This can be done rather quickly and will give you an overall idea of the content of the chapter.

The *Comprehensive Understanding* section is next and is in outline format. This will prove to be a very valuable tool, not only as you first read the chapter but also as you review for tests. This outline identifies the topics and main ideas of each chapter as an aid to concentration, comprehension, and retaining textbook information. By completing this outline, you will learn to "pull-out" key information in the chapter. As you write the answers in the study guide, you will be reinforcing that content. Once completed, this outline will serve as a review tool for exams.

The Review Questions in each chapter provide a valuable means of testing and reinforcing your knowledge of the material read and the answers written in the outline. Each question is multiple choice. As a further aid for independent learning, each answer requires a rationale (the reason *why* the option you selected is correct). After you have completed the review questions, you can check the answers in the back of the study guide.

Chapters 22 to 26 and 32 to 45 include exercises based on the care plans found in the text. These exercises provide practice in synthesizing the nursing process and critical thinking as you, the nurse, care for clients. Taking one aspect of the nursing process, you will be asked to imagine you are the nurse in the case study and to think about what knowledge, experiences, standards, and attitudes might be used in caring for the client. Write your answers in the appropriate boxes and check them against the answer key.

When you finish answering the review questions and synthesis exercises, take a few minutes for self-evaluation. If you answered a question incorrectly, begin to analyze the thoughts that led you to the wrong answer:

- Did you miss the key word or phrase?
- Did you read into something that wasn't stated?
- Did you not understand the subject matter?
- Did you use an incorrect rationale for selecting your response?

Each incorrect response is an opportunity to learn. Go back to the text and re-read any content that is still unclear. In the long run, it will be a time-saving activity.

A performance checklist is provided for each of the skills presented in the text. The checklists may be used by instructors to evaluate your competence in performing the techniques. You may need to adapt these skills in order to meet a client's special needs or follow the particular policy of an institution.

The learning activities presented in this study guide will assist you in completing the semester with a firm understanding of nursing concepts and processes that you can rely on for all of your professional career.

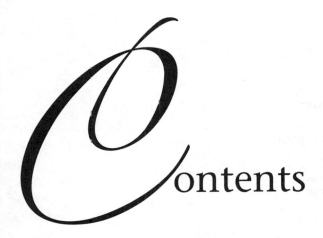

ontents

Skills Performance Checklists

1

$\mathcal{H}$ealth and Wellness

Adapted by Linda Reutter, RN, PhD, University of Alberta

$\mathcal{P}$reliminary Reading

Chapter 1, pp. 1-17

$\mathcal{C}$omprehensive Understanding

Conceptualizations of Health

- Compare and contrast three different conceptualizations of health.

  _____

  _____

  _____

Historical Approaches to Health in Canada

- Historically, there have been 3 different approaches to health in Canada: medical, behavioural, and socio-environmental. Identify the distinguishing features of each of these approaches.

  a. Medical: _____

  b. Behavioural: _____

  c. Socio-environmental: _____

- Identify the contributions of the following Canadian documents to the understanding of health and health determinants.

  a. *Lalonde Report* _____

  b. *Ottawa Charter* _____

c. *Epp Report* _____

_____

d. *Strategies for Population Health* _____

_____

e. *Toronto Charter* _____

_____

Determinants of Health

- Identify major determinants of health as outlined by Health Canada and the Ottawa Charter.

_____

_____

_____

- Why is it important for nurses to understand the concept of health determinants?

_____

_____

_____

Strategies to Influence Health Determinants

- The concepts of *health promotion* and *disease prevention* are distinct yet interrelated. Briefly explain each one.

  a. Health promotion: _____

  _____

  b. Disease prevention: _____

  _____

- Define the *three levels of prevention* and give an example of each.

  a. Primary prevention: _____

  _____

  b. Secondary prevention: _____

  _____

  c. Tertiary prevention: _____

  _____

- Define the *five health promotion strategies* contained in the Ottawa Charter and give examples of activities in each strategy.

  a. Strengthen community action: _____

  _____

  b. Build healthy public policy: _____

  _____

  c. Create supportive environments: _____

  _____

  d. Develop personal skills: _____

  _____

  e. Reorient health services: _____

  _____

Population Health Promotion Model

- What are the three elements of the Population Health Promotion Model?

  a. _____

  b. _____

  c. _____

- Provide an example of how you might use this model in your practice.

  _____

  _____

*R*eview Questions

The student should select the appropriate answer and cite the rationale for choosing that particular answer.

1. The "watershed" document that marked the shift *from* a lifestyle *to* a social approach to health was:
   a. Lalonde Report
   b. National Forum on Health
   c. Toronto Charter
   d. Ottawa Charter

   Answer: _____ Rationale: _____

   _____

   _____

2. The major determinants of health in a socio-environmental view of health are:
   a. Psychosocial risk factors and socio-environmental health conditions
   b. Physiological risk factors and behavioural risk factors
   c. Behavioural and psychosocial risk factors
   d. Behavioural and socio-environmental risk factors

Answer: _____ Rationale: _____
_____
_____

3. The main reason that intersectoral collaboration is a necessary strategy to reach the goal of Health for All is because:
   a. The determinants of health are broad
   b. Intersectoral collaboration is cost-effective
   c. Intersectoral collaboration encourages problem-solving at a local level
   d. Intersectoral collaboration is less likely to result in conflict

Answer: _____ Rationale: _____
_____
_____

4. Providing immunizations against measles is an example of:
   a. Health promotion
   b. Primary prevention
   c. Secondary prevention
   d. Tertiary prevention

Answer: _____ Rationale: _____
_____
_____

5. Which one of the following statements DOES NOT accurately characterize health promotion?
   a. Health promotion addresses health issues within the context of the social, economic, and political environment
   b. Health promotion emphasizes empowerment
   c. Health promotion strategies focus primarily on helping people to develop healthy behaviours
   d. Health promotion is political

Answer: _____ Rationale: _____
_____
_____

6. The belief that health is primarily an *individual* responsibility is most congruent with the _____ approach to health.
   a. Medical
   b. Behavioural
   c. Socio-environmental
   d. Public health

Answer: _____ Rationale: _____
_____
_____

7. All of the following statements accurately describe the Population Health Promotion Model, *except*:
   a. The model suggests that action can address the full range of health determinants.
   b. The model incorporates the health promotion strategies of the Ottawa Charter.
   c. The model focuses primarily on interventions at the society level.
   d. The model attempts to integrate the concepts of population health and health promotion.

Answer: _____ Rationale: _____
_____
_____

8. Which of the following is the most influential health determinant?
   a. Personal health practices
   b. Income and social status
   c. Health care services
   d. Physical environment

Answer: _____ Rationale: _____
_____
_____

9. A medical approach to health is to health services as a behavioural approach is to:
   a. Income and social status
   b. Employment and working conditions
   c. Physical environments
   d. Personal health practices

Answer: _____ Rationale: _____
_____
_____

4   Chapter 1: Health and Wellness

2

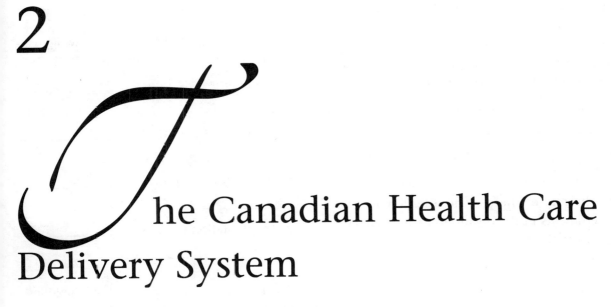

The Canadian Health Care Delivery System

Adapted by Ardene Robinson Vollman, RN, BScN, MA, PhD,
University of Calgary

Preliminary Reading

Chapter 2, pp. 18-33

Comprehensive Understanding

Evolution of the Canadian Health Care Delivery System

- Canada has constructed a social safety net for the protection of its citizens. Medicare is an important part of this safety net. Briefly explain the role of the following in the development of Medicare.

  a. The Depression: _____

  _____

  b. Tommy Douglas: _____

  _____

  c. *The Medical Care Act (1966):* _____

  _____

  d. *The Canada Health Act (1984):* _____

  _____

The Organization of Health Care

- Briefly explain:

  a. The four areas of health for which the federal jurisdiction is responsible:

  _____

  _____

  _____

  _____

  b. The role of the provincial/territorial governments in the organization and delivery of health care:

  _____

  _____

  _____

  c. The five principles enshrined in the *Canada Health Act:*

  _____

  _____

Right to Health Care

- Explain the role and influence of the *Canadian Charter of Rights and Freedoms* (1982) and the *Canada Health Act* in establishing health care as a right for all Canadians.

  _____

  _____

  _____

  _____

- Describe the four rights contained in the *Policy Statement on Consumers and Health* by the Consumers Association of Canada.

  a. _____

  b. _____

  c. _____

  d. _____

Settings for Health Care Delivery

- Explain the role of each of the following institutions in delivering health care.

  a. Hospitals: _____

  _____

  b. Long-term Care Facilities: _____

  _____

  c. Psychiatric Facilities: _____

  _____

  d. Rehabilitation Centres: _____

  _____

- Explain the role of each of each of the following in delivering health care in the community.

  a. Public Health: _____

  _____

  b. Physician Offices: _____

  _____

  c. Community Health Centres and Clinics:

  _____

  _____

  d. Assisted Living: _____

  _____

  e. Home Care: _____

  _____

  f. Adult Daycare Centres: _____

  _____

  g. Community and Voluntary Agencies:

  _____

  h. Occupational Health: _____

  _____

  i. Hospice/Palliative Care: _____

  _____

  j. Parish Nursing: _____

  _____

Levels of Care

- List and briefly describe five levels of health care.

  a. _____
  _____
  _____

  b. _____
  _____
  _____

  c. _____
  _____
  _____

  d. _____
  _____
  _____

  e. _____
  _____
  _____

- Explain primary care, secondary care, and tertiary care. _____
  _____
  _____
  _____

- Explain the difference between primary care and primary health care. _____
  _____
  _____

Health Care Spending

- In 2004, a Conference Board of Canada study compared Canada's spending on health care with 23 other industrialized countries. How did Canada compare in health spending and health status to these other countries? _____
  _____

Challenges to the Health Care System

- Describe four cost accelerators.

  a. _____
  b. _____
  c. _____
  d. _____

- Explain the principle of universality. _____
  _____

Trends and Reforms in Canada's Health Care System

- Describe the main recommendations of the Romanow and Kirby reports. _____
  _____
  _____
  _____

- Define primary health care. _____
  _____

- Explain the five principles associated with primary health care.

  a. _____
  b. _____
  c. _____
  d. _____
  e. _____

- Describe the benefits and potential drawbacks involved with increasing funding to primary health care and home care services. _____
  _____
  _____
  _____
  _____
  _____

Review Questions

The student should select the appropriate answer and cite the rationale for choosing that particular answer.

1. When the *Canada Health Act* of 1984 amalgamated the previous acts of 1957 and 1966, it added which principle to the existing four?
   a. Accessibility
   b. Comprehensiveness
   c. Portability
   d. Public administration

   Answer: _____ Rationale: _____
   _____
   _____

2. The amount of money Canada (public and private) spent on health care per capita is approximately:
   a. $1,820
   b. $3,839
   c. $2,950
   d. $2,440

   Answer: _____ Rationale: _____
   _____
   _____

3. A 16-year old sees a physician at a walk-in clinic to find out if she is pregnant. This service can be best described as an example of:
   a. Primary care
   b. Primary health care
   c. Tertiary care
   d. Secondary care

   Answer: _____ Rationale: _____
   _____
   _____

4. The 16-year old girl student attends a community program on prenatal health for teenage mothers. The program is taught by a nurse, a nutritionist, and a social worker. This service can best be described as an example of:
   a. Primary care
   b. Primary health care
   c. Tertiary care
   d. Secondary care

   Answer: _____ Rationale: _____
   _____
   _____

5. Which of the following is a false statement?
   a. There is a great deal of variety across the provinces and territories in the delivery of home care services.
   b. Home care is covered under the *Canada Health Act*.
   c. Home care accounts for 2% to 6% of provincial health budgets.
   d. All provinces and territories fund home care assessment and case management, nursing care, and support services for eligible clients.

   Answer: _____ Rationale: _____
   _____
   _____

3

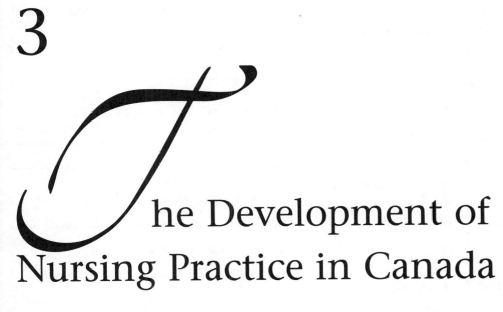

The Development of Nursing Practice in Canada

Adapted by Janet C. Ross-Kerr, RN, BScN, MS, PhD,
University of Alberta

Preliminary Reading

Chapter 3, pp. 34-50

Comprehensive Understanding

- Define *nursing* (according to the International Council of Nurses). _____

Early History of Nursing in Canada

The First Nurses and Hospitals in New France

- What was the contribution of Mme Hébert to health care in the new colony? _____
_____

- List five important milestones in the development of nursing in Canada.

    a. _____

    b. _____

    c. _____

    d. _____

    e. _____

Nursing During the British Regime

- How did British nursing compare with French nursing during the 18th Century? _____

  _____

  _____

- _____ carried by _____ and _____ spread rapidly in the British colonies. Established French-Canadian orders expanded their services and new English-speaking orders were founded to help the sick and the poor.

Nursing Education in Canada

- What was the main reason for establishing the first Canadian nursing schools? _____

  _____

- Describe the growth of hospital nursing schools in the late 19th Century. _____

  _____

  _____

The Impact of Nursing Organizations on Nursing Education

- How did the ICN influence the development of nursing organizations worldwide? _____

  _____

  _____

- How did the struggle for women's rights influence nursing? _____

  _____

  _____

- When and where was the first university program in nursing established? _____

  _____

From the Depression to the Post World War II Years

- The depression brought _____ and _____ to nurses.

- How did WWII affect health education? ____

  _____

  _____

Expansion in the 1950s and 1960s

- Describe the development of graduate programs during these years. _____

  _____

  _____

Nursing Education Today

- Where does the responsibility for monitoring standards of nursing education lie? _____

  _____

Post-Graduate Degrees

- A masters degree in nursing is necessary for

  _____

- Nurses with doctorates can _____

Continuing and In-Service Education

- Define continuing education: _____

Professional Roles and Responsibilities

- Briefly describe the following nursing roles.
  a. Advanced practice nurse: _____
  b. Clinical nurse specialist: _____
  c. Nurse practitioner: _____
  d. Nursing educator: _____
  e. Nursing administrator: _____
  f. Nursing researcher: _____

Professional Nursing Organizations

- What is the role of a professional organization? How does the CNA fulfill this role? ____
  _____
  _____

Unions

- How did the Supreme Court decision of 1973 change the situation for Canadian nursing? Within a decade, every province had both _____ and _____.

Standards of Nursing Practice

- Nursing is a self-regulating profession and sets its own standards of practice. Standards are developed and established based on _____ and _____.

- Briefly describe the responsibility of nurses under the Ontario Standards of Practice in the following areas:
  a. Professional service to the public: _____
  b. Knowledge: _____
  c. Application of knowledge: _____
  d. Ethics: _____
  e. Continued competence: _____

Nursing Best Practice Guidelines

- Define best practices. _____

- Describe what the RNAO has done to develop Best Practice Guidelines. _____
  _____
  _____

Ethical Standards of Practice

- The *Code of Ethics* provides nurses with direction for ethical decision making and practice in everyday situations.

Registration/Licensure

- In all provinces and territories, nursing registration acts regulate _____ and _____ of nursing. Legislation in each province outlines nursing scope of practice.

Certification

- Define certification: _____. In Canada, certification is offered by the CNA.

*R*eview Questions

The student should select the appropriate answer and cite the rationale for choosing that particular answer.

1. Hippocrates is considered the father of scientific medicine because
   a. He was the first to make observations of patients and develop treatments on the basis of symptoms
   b. He recognized the importance of fresh water and hygiene for public health
   c. He believed in a spiritual basis of illness
   d. He recognized the importance of nutrition in maintaining health

   Answer: _____ Rationale: _____
   _____
   _____

2. The first visiting nurses in Canada were
   a. Led by Jeanne Mance in 1642
   b. The first three Augustinian nuns in 1639
   c. Marie Rollet Hébert and her surgeon-apothecary husband in 1617
   d. The Grey Nuns under Margaret d'Youville in 1738

   Answer: _____ Rationale: _____
   _____
   _____

3. Which of the following is *not* attributed to Florence Nightingale?
   a. Dramatically reduced morbidity and mortality rates among the wounded
   b. Developed nursing as a profession independent from medicine
   c. Introduced nursing to the British army
   d. Made nursing an acceptable field of work for middle and upper class women outside the home

   Answer: _____ Rationale: _____
   _____
   _____

4. The first integrated basic undergraduate degree program in nursing in Canada was developed at:
   a. St. Francis Xavier University
   b. University of Toronto
   c. University of Alberta
   d. University of British Columbia

   Answer: _____ Rationale: _____
   _____
   _____

5. Best Practice Guidelines (BPGs) such as those developed by the Registered Nurses Association of Ontario are:
   a. Courses of action
   b. Ethical guidelines
   c. Minimum standards
   d. Guiding principles

   Answer: _____ Rationale: _____
   _____
   _____

12   Chapter 3: The Development of Nursing Practice in Canada

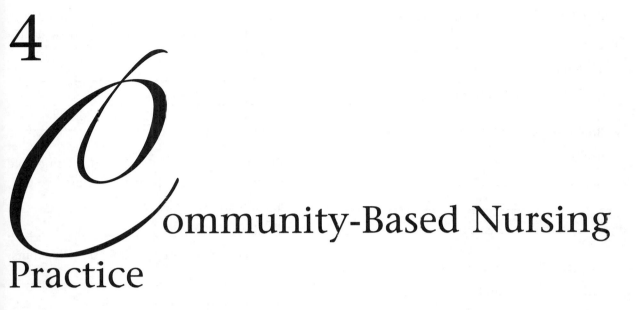

4 Community-Based Nursing Practice

Adapted by Kaysi Eastlick Kushner, RN, PhD, University of Alberta

Preliminary Reading

Chapter 4, pp. 51-65

Comprehensive Understanding

- Community nursing care involves: _____
  _____
  _____

Achieving Healthy Populations and Communities

- Distinguish between a *population* and a *community* and give an example of each. _____
  _____
  _____
  _____

- Give an example of each of the strategies identified in the framework for public health programs.
  a. Promote individual and family action: _____
  b. Provide direct care: _____
  c. Influence the environment: _____
  d. Build partnerships: _____

Community Nursing Practice

- Briefly describe the differences between:

  a. Public health focus: _____

  b. Community health nursing: _____

- Briefly explain the nursing focus in primary health care. _____

  _____

  _____

  _____

- Community based nursing involves the _____ and _____ care of individuals and families that enhance _____

- The philosophical foundation is: _____

  _____

- Briefly explain the focus of the community-based nurse. _____

  _____

  _____

The Changing Focus of Community Nursing Practice

- Vulnerable populations are: _____

  _____

  _____

- Explain how a nurse becomes culturally competent. _____

  _____

  _____

- List some of the reasons why vulnerable populations typically experience poorer health outcomes.

  _____

  _____

  _____

- Briefly describe the following vulnerable groups and identify their risk factors.

  a. Poor and homeless clients: _____

  b. Abused clients: _____

  c. Clients who engage in risk behaviours:

  _____

  d. Clients with chronic conditions: _____

  e. Gender: _____

  f. Age: _____

- A nurse in a community health practice must have a variety of skills and knowledge to assist individuals and families within the community, as well as communities broadly. Briefly explain the competencies the nurse needs in the following roles.

  a. Direct Care/Service Provider: _____

  b. Educator: _____

  c. Consultant: _____

  d. Facilitator: _____

  e. Communicator: _____

  f. Collaborator: _____

  g. Coordinator: _____

  h. Researcher: _____

  i. Social Marketer: _____

  j. Community Developer: _____

Community Assessment

- The community is viewed as having three components. Briefly explain each one.

  a. Structure: _____

  b. Population: _____

  c. Social system: _____

Promoting Clients' Health

- The challenge is how to promote and protect the client's health, whether the client is an individual or family within the context of the community, or the community itself. The most important theme to consider, in order to be an effective community health nurse, is to:

_____

_____

_____

_____

- Identify some factors that nurses must consider in community nursing practice. _____

_____

_____

_____

*R*eview Questions

The student should select the appropriate answer and cite the rationale for choosing that particular answer.

1. Which of the following would not typically be considered an example of primary health care?
   a. Lunch-time nutrition and activity program in an inner-city school run by nurses, nutritionists, social workers, and teachers
   b. A rehabilitation program in a hospital provided by physical therapists, physicians, nurses, and social workers for clients and families recovering from a stroke
   c. Activities provided by childcare workers in a daycare at a corporation
   d. A well-baby clinic conducted by nurses and nutritionists for new mothers at a neighbourhood health centre

   Answer: _____ Rationale: _____

   _____

   _____

2. Among the communication skills needed to provide nursing care to community clients is the ability to:
   a. Clarify client values and care expectations
   b. Follow medical prescriptions in many settings
   c. Manage generational interfamilial conflict
   d. Speak the client's language or dialects

   Answer: _____ Rationale: _____

   _____

   _____

3. Which of the following is not a known risk factor for abuse in families?
   a. Immigration to Canada within the past five years
   b. Mental health problems
   c. Substance abuse
   d. Socio-economic stressors

   Answer: _____ Rationale: _____

   _____

   _____

4. When the community health nurse refers clients to appropriate resources and monitors and coordinates the extent and adequacy of services to meet family health care needs, the nurse is functioning in the role of:
   a. Collaborator
   b. Educator
   c. Consultant
   d. Coordinator

   Answer: _____ Rationale: _____

   _____

   _____

5. Which of the following is not a trend in community health nursing?
   a. Closer contact with primary care team
   b. Increase in focus on at-risk populations
   c. Less care of young, disabled individuals at home
   d. More acute care in the community

Answer: _____ Rationale: _____

_____

_____

5

*T*heoretical Foundations of Nursing Practice

Adapted by Sally Thorne, RN, PhD, University of British Columbia

*P*reliminary Readings

Chapter 5, pp. 66-79

*C*omprehensive Understanding

- Define the terms "theory" and "nursing theory," and explain why knowledge of nursing theory can help nurses become better practitioners. _____

_____

_____

_____

_____

Early Nursing Practice and the Emergence of Theory

- Briefly describe how developments in science and technology affected the development of nursing as a science. _____

_____

_____

_____

- Explain the relationship between the development of nursing theory and the challenge of building curriculum for nursing education.

  _____

  _____

  _____

  _____

- Describe the purpose of nursing theory. _____

  _____

  _____

Nursing Process

- Describe the four basic steps of nursing process.
  a. Assessment: _____
  b. Planning: _____
  c. Intervention: _____
  d. Evaluation: _____

- The relationship between clinical judgment and nursing process is: _____

  _____

  _____

  _____

Conceptual Frameworks

- Briefly describe how systematic thinking using conceptual nursing models differs from linear reasoning processes. _____

  _____

  _____

  _____

Metaparadigm Concepts

- Explain the importance of each metaparadigm concept for the clinical reasoning process in nursing.
  a. Person: _____
  b. Environment: _____
  c. Health: _____
  d. Nursing: _____

- For each metaparadigm concept, identify at least two possible ways it might be defined for the purpose of guiding nursing practice.
  a. Person: _____

  _____

  b. Environment: _____

  _____

  c. Health: _____

  _____

  d. Nursing: _____

  _____

Philosophy of Nursing Science

- Kuhn's ideas about paradigms helped nursing understand its scientific basis not as simply theoretical propositions but as: _____

  _____

  _____

- Chaos theory provided nursing with a new way to think about: _____

  _____

Nursing's Ways of Knowing

- List five forms of knowledge identified by Carper that have contributed to excellent nursing practice:
  a. _____
  b. _____

c. _____

d. _____

e. _____

- The two distinct paradigms that have been associated with debates surrounding nursing's theoretical development are: _____

_____

_____

Nursing Diagnosis

- Identify advantages and disadvantages of adopting a fixed list of diagnostic categories for nursing care.

  a. Advantages: _____

  _____

  b. Disadvantages: _____

  _____

Major Theoretical Models

- Identify one characteristic of each of the following categories of theoretical models.

  a. Practice-Based Theories: _____

  b. Needs Theories: _____

  c. Interactionist Theories: _____

  d. Systems Theories: _____

  e. Simultaneity Theories: _____

- Name one theory/theorist as an example for each of these categories.

  a. _____

  b. _____

  c. _____

  d. _____

  e. _____

Review Questions

The student should select the appropriate answer and cite the rationale for choosing that particular answer.

1. Which of the following is *not* an intended outcome of a grand theory?
   a. To provide guidance for specific nursing interventions
   b. To provide a framework for broad ideas abut nursing
   c. To provide a structural framework within which smaller-range theories can be developed
   d. To stimulating critical thinking about nursing ideas

   Answer: _____ Rationale: _____

   _____

   _____

2. Which of the following is *not* an intended outcome of a prescriptive theory?
   a. To provide insight into general and broad phenomenon
   b. To be action-oriented
   c. To test validity
   d. To predict the consequence of a specific intervention

   Answer: _____ Rationale: _____

   _____

   _____

3. Which nursing theorist's model conceptualizes the person as an adaptive system?
   a. Virginia Henderson
   b. Rosemary Parse
   c. Hildegard Peplau
   d. Sr. Callista Roy

   Answer: _____ Rationale: _____

   _____

   _____

4. Which nursing theorist's model conceptualizes the person as an irreducible energy field, co-extensive with the universe?
   a. Adam's Interactionist Theory
   b. Orem's Self-Care Theory
   c. Rogers' Simultaneity Theory
   d. Watson's Transpersonal Theory

Answer: _____ Rationale: _____

_____

_____

5. Which of the following levels of abstraction is *not* part of Liaschenko's ideas about nursing knowledge?
   a. Knowing the case
   b. Knowing the client
   c. Knowing the disease
   d. Knowing the person

Answer: _____ Rationale: _____

_____

_____

6

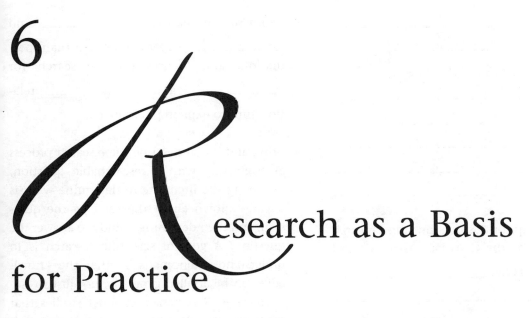

Research as a Basis for Practice

Adapted by Marilynn J. Wood, RN, BSN, MSN, DrPH,
University of Alberta

Preliminary Reading

Chapter 6, pp. 80-94

Comprehensive Understanding

- Nursing research involves: _____
  _____

- Briefly describe the relationship between research and theory. _____
  _____
  _____

The History of Nursing Research

- Briefly explain the significance of each of the following.

  a. Florence Nightingale: _____
     _____

  b. Goldmark report: _____
     _____

c. Weir report: _____

_____

d. 1952: _____

_____

e. 1969–70: _____

_____

f. 1999: _____

_____

- Identify the priorities for nursing research as identified by the Canadian Association of Schools of Nursing. _____

_____

_____

- Define *evidence-based practice*. _____

_____

Knowledge Development in Nursing

- Briefly describe Carper's four patterns of knowing in nursing. _____

_____

_____

_____

_____

The Development of Research in Nursing

The Scientific Paradigm

- The scientific paradigm gave rise to *the scientific method*, a _____ means of acquiring and testing knowledge, by which researchers try to _____, _____, and _____ or _____ nursing phenomenon.

- The dominant paradigm for most of the 19th and 20th centuries has been _____.

- *Positivism* emphasizes _____ and _____ experience, rather than speculation, and focuses on the search for _____ and _____ relationships to explain phenomena.

- Brink and Wood describe the research process as beginning with a researchable question, reviewing the literature to determine what is already known about the topic of the question, and then designing a study to answer the question. A goal of scientific research is to understand phenomena so that the knowledge can be applied generally, not just to isolated cases. Researchers conduct studies that contribute to the testing or development of theories thereby advancing knowledge that can be applied in practice.

The Qualitative Paradigm

- _____ is an alternative to positivism and promotes the idea that there are many truths depending on the perception of people in the situation. This philosophy leads to _____, which strives to understand the situation from the perspective of the participant, not the researcher.

Research Designs

- The two broad approaches to research are _____ and _____.

Nursing Research in the Scientific Paradigm

- Briefly describe the three requirements of a true experiment. _____

_____

_____

- A quasi-experiment is one in which groups are formed and the conditions are controlled, but _____.

- Surveys are designed to _____.

- Exploratory descriptive designs provide in-depth descriptions of populations or variables not previously studied.

Nursing Research in the Qualitative Paradigm

- Qualitative studies stem from questions that cannot be quantified and measured.

- Define the following designs that are used with qualitative research.

    a. Ethnography: _____

    _____

    b. Phenomenology: _____

    _____

    c. Grounded theory: _____

    _____

Conducting Nursing Research

- Who should conduct nursing research? _____

    _____

- Research mindedness means _____

    _____

Ethical Issues in Research

- Describe the purpose and responsibilities of a Research Ethics Board._____

    _____

    _____

- Informed consent means that research sub-jects: _____

    _____

- Briefly describe the eight guiding ethical principles for research in Canada:

    a. _____

    b. _____

    c. _____

    d. _____

    e. _____

    f. _____

g. _____

h. _____

Applying Research Findings to Nursing Practice

- To use findings in clinical practice, nurses must _____, _____, and _____.

Research Report Versus Clinical Article

- The typical research report has the following parts. Briefly explain each section.

    a. Introduction: _____

    b. Methods section: _____

    c. Results section: _____

    d. Discussion section: _____

    e. Reference list: _____

- Explain the difference between a primary and secondary source. _____

    _____

Locating Research Studies

- Describe where and how to find research studies in nursing.

    _____

    _____

    _____

Research Utilization

- A systematic review is _____.

    _____

- List the steps used in successful research utilization.

    a. _____

    b. _____

    c. _____

    d. _____

    e. _____

    f. _____

g. _____

h. _____

Evidence-Based Practice and Research

- Differentiate *research-based practice* from *evidence-based practice.* _____

_____

_____

Review Questions

The student should select the appropriate answer and cite the rationale for choosing that particular answer.

1. The researcher's refusal to disclose the names of subjects is:
   a. Respect for privacy and confidentiality
   b. Minimizing harm
   c. Informed consent
   d. Balancing harms and benefits

   Answer: _____ Rationale: _____

   _____

   _____

2. The purpose of a research ethics board is to:
   a. Ensure that federal funds are equitably appropriated
   b. Conduct research benefiting the public
   c. Determine the risk status of clients in research projects
   d. Ensure that ethical principles are being upheld

   Answer: _____ Rationale: _____

   _____

   _____

3. Research studies can most easily be identified by:
   a. Looking for the word "research" in the title of the report
   b. Looking for the study only in research journals

   c. Examining the contents of the report
   d. Reading the abstract and conclusion of the report

   Answer: _____ Rationale: _____

   _____

   _____

4. Which statement concerning research reports is accurate?
   a. Nursing textbooks are primary sources of information.
   b. Primary sources are those written by one of the researchers in the study.
   c. The fact that a report is a primary source guarantees its accuracy.
   d. Secondary sources are the best source of information about the research study.

   Answer: _____ Rationale: _____

   _____

   _____

5. A research report includes all of the following except:
   a. A summary of literature used to identify the research problem
   b. The researcher's interpretation of the study results
   c. A summary of other research studies with the same results
   d. A description of methods used to conduct the study

   Answer: _____ Rationale: _____

   _____

   _____

7

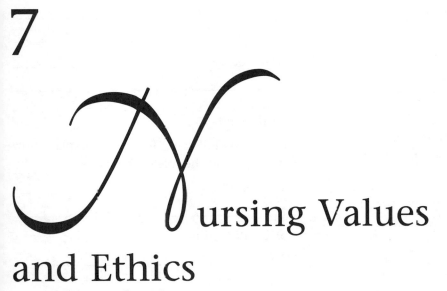

ursing Values
and Ethics

Adapted by Shelley Raffin Bouchal, RN, BScN, MN, PhD,
University of Calgary

Preliminary Reading

Chapter 7, pp. 95-111

Comprehensive Understanding

- A value is a _____

- *Ethics* is the study of _____
  _____

- The Canadian Nurses Association (CNA) publishes a _____ that outlines nurses' professional values and ethical commitment to their clients.

Values

- Value formation is _____

- Value conflict occurs when _____
  _____

- Value clarification is _____

- Identify and explain the three steps of value clarification.
  a. _____
  b. _____
  c. _____

- Identify and briefly describe the eight values that must be upheld by Canadian nurses according to the CNA.
  a. _____
  b. _____
  c. _____
  d. _____
  e. _____
  f. _____
  g. _____
  h. _____

Ethics

- Differentiate between the terms *ethics* and *morals*. _____
  _____
  _____

Professional Nursing and Ethics

- A *code of ethics* is _____.

- List and describe the four fundamental responsibilities of nurses as identified by the International Council of Nurses (ICU) Code of Ethics.
  1. _____
  2. _____
  3. _____
  4. _____

- Define the following terms, and explain how they apply to the role of the nurse.
  a. Responsibility: _____
  _____

  b. Accountability: _____
  _____

  c. Advocacy: _____
  _____

Ethical Theory

- Define the following terms, and explain how they apply to the role of the nurse.
  a. Deontology: _____
  _____

  b. Utilitarianism: _____
  _____

  c. Bioethics: _____
  _____

  d. Autonomy: _____
  _____

  e. Beneficence: _____
  _____

  f. Non-maleficence: _____
  _____

  g. Justice: _____
  _____

  h. Feminist ethics: _____
  _____

  i. Ethic of care: _____
  _____

  j. Relational ethics: _____
  _____

How to Process an Ethical Dilemma

- An ethical dilemma is _____.

- Briefly describe each of the seven steps in the processing of an ethical dilemma.
  a. Step 1: _____
  _____

  b. Step 2: _____
  _____

c. Step 3: _____

_____

d. Step 4: _____

_____

e. Step 5: _____

_____

f. Step 6: _____

_____

g. Step 7: _____

_____

Institutional Ethics Committees

• Identify the functions of ethics committees.

_____

_____

Ethical Issues in Nursing Practice

Client Care Issues

• Explain the following client care issues and how they apply to nursing:

a. Informed consent: _____

b. Advance directives: _____

c. Food and hydration: _____

Issues in the Work Environment

• Ethical issues in the work place are problematic when they compromise practice by preventing nurses from making effective decisions. Reporting the wrongdoing of a colleague can be distressful. Nurses need to examine relative risks and benefits and decide on appropriate action.

Emerging Societal Issues

• Explain the role of ethics in public debates on resource allocation for health care.

_____

_____

_____

Review Questions

The student should select the appropriate answer and cite the rationale for choosing that particular answer.

1. A health care issue often becomes an ethical dilemma because:
   a. A client's legal rights co-exist with a health care professional's obligations.
   b. Decisions must be made quickly, often under stressful conditions.
   c. Decisions must be made based on value systems.
   d. The choices involved do not appear to be clearly right or wrong.

   Answer: _____ Rationale: _____

   _____

   _____

2. A document that lists the medical treatment a person chooses to refuse if unable to make decisions is the:
   a. Durable power of attorney
   b. Informed consent
   c. Living will
   d. Advance directives

   Answer: _____ Rationale: _____

   _____

   _____

3. Which statement about an institutional ethics committee is correct?
   a. The ethics committee is an additional resource for clients and health care professionals.
   b. The ethics committee relieves health care professionals from dealing with ethical issues.
   c. The ethics committee would be the first option in addressing an ethical dilemma.
   d. The ethics committee replaces decision making by the client and health care providers.

Answer: _____ Rationale: _____

_____

_____

4. The nurse is working with parents of a seriously ill newborn. Surgery has been proposed for the infant, but the chances of success are unclear. In helping the parents resolve this ethical conflict, the nurse knows that the next step is:
   a. Exploring reasonable courses of action
   b. Collecting all available information about the situation
   c. Clarifying values related to the cause of the dilemma
   d. Identifying people who can solve the difficulty

Answer: _____ Rationale: _____

_____

_____

5. The goal of informed consent is to protect the client's right to:
   a. Autonomy
   b. Beneficence
   c. Ethic of care
   d. Advocacy

Answer: _____ Rationale: _____

_____

_____

8

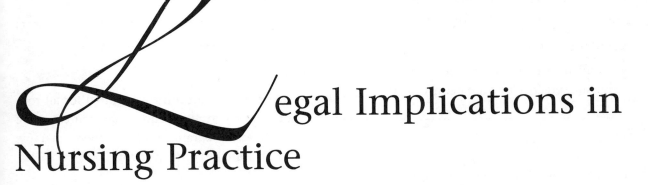

$\mathcal{L}$egal Implications in Nursing Practice

Adapted by Carla Shapiro, RN, MN, University of Winnipeg

$\mathcal{P}$reliminary Reading

Chapter 8, pp. 112-126

$\mathcal{C}$omprehensive Understanding

Legal Limits of Nursing

- Professional nurses must understand the legal limits influencing their daily practice.

Sources of Law

- The legal guidelines that nurses must follow are derived from the following. Briefly explain each one.

  a. Statute law: _____

  b. Nursing Practice Acts: _____

  c. Standards of Care: _____

  d. Common law: _____

- Define the following terms.

  a. Criminal law: _____

  _____

  b. Civil law: _____

  _____

Professional Regulation

- Nurses must be registered or licensed by the professional nursing association or college of the province or territory in which they practice.

- All provinces and territories (except Quebec) use the Canadian Registered Nurse Examination.

Standards of Care

- Standards of care are the legal guidelines for nursing practice and are defined by the: _____

  _____

  _____

- The nursing practice acts establish: _____

  _____

- In a negligence lawsuit, these standards are used to determine: _____

  _____

- All nurses should know the standards of care they are expected to meet within their specialty and work setting. Ignorance of the law or of standards of care is not a defense to negligence.

Legal Liability Issues in Nursing Practice

Intentional Torts

- Define the following.
  a. Tort: _____
  b. Assault: _____
  c. Battery: _____
  d. Invasion of privacy: _____
  e. False imprisonment: _____
  f. Negligence: _____

Unintentional Torts

Preventing Negligence

- Briefly explain how a nurse can avoid being liable for negligence. _____

  _____

  _____

Criminal Liability

- Describe the difference between the tort of negligence and criminal negligence charges.

  _____

  _____

  _____

  _____

Consent

- A signed consent form is required for all routine treatment, hazardous procedures, some treatment programs such as chemotherapy, and research involving clients.

- *Informed consent* is a person's agreement to:

  _____

  _____

- The following factors must be verified for consent to be valid.
  a. _____
  b. _____
  c. _____

- The nurse assumes the responsibility for witnessing the client's signature on the consent form but does not legally assume the duty of obtaining consent.

- The nurse's signature witnessing the consent means: _____

  _____

- Only a person who can understand the explanations provided and who can truly understand the decision they are making can provide informed consent.

- A client who refuses surgery or any other medical treatment must be informed of any harmful consequences.

- In emergency situations, if it is impossible to obtain consent from the client or an authorized person (proxy) the procedure required to save a life may be undertaken in accordance with the *emergency doctrine*.

- Clients with mental health problems and the frail elderly retain the right to consent to or refuse treatment unless a court deems them to be incompetent.

Nursing Students and Legal Liability

- If a client is harmed as a direct result of a nursing student's actions or lack of action, the liability for the incorrect action is generally shared by the student, instructor, hospital or health care facility, and university or educational institution.

- When students are employed as nursing assistants or nurse's aides when not attending classes, they should not perform tasks that do not appear in a job description for a nurses' aide or assistant.

- Briefly explain the term vicarious liability.

  _____

  _____

  _____

Abandonment, Assignment, and Contract Issues

Short Staffing

- Nursing supervisors should be informed when a nurse is assigned to care for more clients than is reasonable, and a written protest should be filed to document such an assignment.

- When staffing is inadequate, nurses should not walk out because charges of abandonment can be made.

Floating

- Nurses who float should inform the supervisor of experience they may lack caring for the type of clients on the nursing unit.

- A supervisor can be held liable if a staff nurse is given an assignment he or she cannot safely handle.

Physicians' Orders

- The physician is responsible for directing the medical treatment.

- Nurses are obligated to follow the physician's orders unless: _____

  _____

- A nurse should not perform a physician's order if it is foreseeable that harm will come to the client.

- If a verbal order is necessary, it should be written out and signed by the physician within 24 hours.

Legal Issues in Nursing Practice

Abortion

- Summarize the legal rights of women relative to abortion. _____

  _____

  _____

  _____

Drug Regulations and Nurses

- Describe the two federal acts that control the manufacture, distribution, and sale of food, drugs, and therapeutic devices in Canada.

  a. _____

  _____

  b. _____

  _____

- A competent nurse is expected to know the purpose and effects of any drug administered, as well as potential side-effects and contraindications.

Communicable Diseases

- Nurses have an ethical and legal obligation to provide care to all assigned clients.

- Nurses must be aware of any statutes in their jurisdiction that address the reporting of communicable diseases to the authorities.

- Whenever confidential health care information is requested by a third party, nurses must obtain a signed release from the client.

Death and Dying

- Explain the legal definition of *death*. _____
  _____
  _____

- Define the following terms and explain their legal status in Canada.
  a. Euthanasia: _____
     _____
  b. Assisted suicide: _____
     _____
  c. Withdrawing and withholding treatment:
     _____
     _____

Advance Directives and Health Care Surrogates

- Describe the function of an advance directive for health care. _____
  _____
  _____

- If the existence of an advance directive for health care (ADHC) is known, the instructions must be followed.

- If a physician ignores an advance directive for health care (ADHC), a nurse must document that it was brought to the physician's attention along with the physician's response to this information.

Organ Donation

- Every province and territory has human tissue legislation that provides for both live donor and cadaveric donation of tissues and organs.

Mental Health Issues

- Mental health legislation serves to protect client autonomy while recognizing that some individuals are unable to appreciate the consequences of their health condition.

- Clients admitted to a psychiatric unit on a voluntary basis should be treated no differently than any other client—they have the right to refuse treatment and may discharge themselves from hospital.

- If a client's history and medical records indicate suicidal tendencies, the client must be kept under close supervision.

- Documentation of precautions against suicide is essential.

Public Health Issues

- Briefly explain the purpose of public health legislation. _____
  _____
  _____

- Describe nurses' obligation when child abuse or neglect is witnessed or suspected. _____
  _____
  _____

Risk Management

- Risk management is: _____
  _____

- The steps involved in risk management include:
  a. _____
  b. _____
  c. _____
  d. _____

- A tool used by risk managers is the: _____
  _____

- Risk management includes documentation. It should be:
  a. _____
  b. _____
  c. _____

Professional Involvement

- Nurses must be involved in their professional organizations and on committees that define the standards of care for nursing practice.

- Nurses become more powerful and more effective as a profession when they are organized and cohesive.

Review Questions

The student should select the appropriate answer and cite the rationale for choosing that particular answer.

1. Nursing Practice Acts are an example of
   a. Statute law
   b. Common law
   c. Public law
   d. Criminal law

   Answer: _____ Rationale: _____
   _____
   _____

2. An example of an *unintentional tort* is:
   a. Assault
   b. Battery
   c. Invasion of privacy
   d. Negligence

   Answer: _____ Rationale: _____
   _____
   _____

3. What should you do if you doubt a client's capacity to give informed consent?
   a. Do not be concerned if the consent is already signed.
   b. Notify the physician and document your concerns.

   c. Send her for the procedure and discuss it afterwards.
   d. Ask a family member to give consent.

   Answer: _____ Rationale: _____
   _____
   _____

4. When a client is harmed as a result of a nursing student's actions or lack of action, the liability is generally held by:
   a. The student
   b. The student's instructor or preceptor
   c. The hospital or health care facility
   d. All of the above

   Answer: _____ Rationale: _____
   _____
   _____

5. A confused client who fell out of bed because side rails were not used is an example of which type of liability?
   a. False imprisonment
   b. Assault
   c. Battery
   d. Negligence

   Answer: _____ Rationale: _____
   _____
   _____

6. When the nurse stops to help in an emergency at the scene of an accident, if the injured party files suit and the nurse's employing institution's insurance does not cover the nurse, the nurse would probably be covered by:
   a. The nurse's automobile insurance
   b. The nurse's homeowner insurance
   c. The Patient Care partnership, which may grant immunity from suit if the injured party consents
   d. The Good Samaritan laws, which grant immunity from suit if there is no gross negligence

Answer: _____ Rationale: _____

_____

_____

7. Treating a client without the person's consent is considered
   a. Battery
   b. Negligence
   c. Implied consent
   d. Expressed consent

Answer: _____ Rationale: _____

_____

_____

8. Even though the nurse may obtain the client's signature on a form, obtaining informed consent is the responsibility of the
   a. Client
   b. Physician
   c. Student nurse
   d. Supervising nurse

Answer: _____ Rationale: _____

_____

_____

9. The nurse restrains a client without the client's permission and without a physician's order. The nurse may be guilty of
   a. Assault
   b. False imprisonment
   c. Invasion of privacy
   d. Neglect

Answer: _____ Rationale: _____

_____

_____

10. The nurse is obligated to follow a physician's order unless
   a. The order is a verbal order
   b. The physician's order is illegible
   c. The order has not been transcribed
   d. The order is in error, violates hospital policy, or would be detrimental to the client

Answer: _____ Rationale: _____

_____

_____

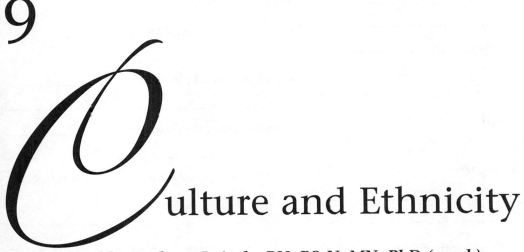

9

Culture and Ethnicity

Adapted by Barbara J. Astle, RN, BScN, MN, PhD (cand.),
University of Calgary

Preliminary Reading

Chapter 9, pp. 127-147

Comprehensive Understanding

- To provide culturally competent care, the nurse must understand cultural concepts. Briefly explain each of the following.

    a. Culture: _____

    _____

    b. Dominant culture: _____

    _____

    c. Subculture: _____

    _____

    d. Ethnicity: _____

    _____

    e. Race: _____

    _____

    f. Enculturation: _____

    _____

    g. Acculturation: _____

    _____

h. Assimilation: _____

_____

i. Multiculturalism:_____

_____

Cultural Concepts

Cultural Conflicts

- Define the following terms.

  a. Ethnocentrism: _____

  _____

  b. Discrimination: _____

  _____

  c. Cultural Imposition: _____

  _____

  d. Stereotypes: _____

  _____

Cultural Awareness

- Define *cultural awareness.* _____

  _____

- Briefly describe how a nurse can identify his or her personal beliefs and values. _____

  _____

  _____

- Drew (2004) describes a cultural awareness exercise that nurses can use to begin to identify their own beliefs and values. List four things to help you become more culturally aware.

  a. _____

  b. _____

  c. _____

  d. _____

Transcultural Nursing

- Define *transcultural nursing.* _____

  _____

- Define *culturally congruent care.* _____

  _____

- Define *culturally competent care.* _____

  _____

- Cultural competence has five interlocking components. Briefly explain each one.

  a. _____

  b. _____

  c. _____

  d. _____

  e. _____

Cultural Context of Health and Caring

- Culture is the context by which groups interpret and define their experiences relevant to life transitions.

- Culture is the framework used in defining social phenomena.

- Briefly explain the difference between western and non-western cultures. _____

  _____

  _____

  _____

Cultural Healing Modalities and Healers

- Health care systems have evolved into the following. Explain each one.

  a. Externalizing systems: _____

  _____

  b. Internalizing systems: _____

  _____

- Foster identified two distinct categories of cross-cultural healers. Explain each one.

  a. Naturalistic practitioners: _____

  _____

  b. Personalistic practioners: _____

  _____

Cultural Assessment

- The goal of a *cultural assessment* is: _____

  _____

- Briefly explain the six cultural phenomena used in the Giger and Davidhizar's Transcultural Assessment Model.

  a. Communication: _____

  _____

  b. Space: _____

  _____

  c. Social Organization: _____

  _____

  d. Time: _____

  _____

  e. Environmental Control: _____

  _____

  f. Biological Variations: _____

  _____

- Briefly explain how using Giger and Davidhizar's Transcultural Assessment Model with a client with a varied background can assist with providing culturally competent care. _____

  _____

  _____

Review Questions

The student should select the appropriate answer and cite the rationale for choosing that particular answer.

1. When providing care to clients with varied cultural backgrounds, it is imperative for the nurse to recognize that:
   a. Cultural consideration must be put aside if basic needs are in jeopardy.
   b. Generalizations about the behaviour of a particular group may be inaccurate.
   c. Current health standards should determine the acceptability of cultural practices.
   d. Similar reactions to stress will occur when individuals have the same cultural background.

   Answer: _____ Rationale: _____

   _____

   _____

2. To be effective in meeting various ethnic needs, the nurse should:
   a. Treat all clients alike.
   b. Be aware of clients' cultural differences.
   c. Act as if he or she is comfortable with the client's behaviour.
   d. Avoid asking questions about the client's cultural background.

   Answer: _____ Rationale: _____

   _____

   _____

3. To provide culturally competent nursing care, the nurse should:
   a. Identify his or her values, attitudes, beliefs and practices.
   b. Make decisions based solely upon his or her own assessment of the client.
   c. Not be overly concerned with using knowledge from conceptual or theoretical models.
   d. Acknowledge that a client's response to his or her health is similar among various ethnic groups.

   Answer: _____ Rationale: _____
   _____
   _____

4. To respect a client's personal space and territoriality, the nurse:
   a. Avoids the use of touch.
   b. Explains nursing care and procedures.
   c. Keeps the curtains pulled around the client's bed.
   d. Stands 2.5 metres away from the bed, if possible.

   Answer: _____ Rationale: _____
   _____
   _____

5. Which of the following is not included in providing culturally competent care to a client?
   a. Being sensitive and open to a client's cultural beliefs.
   b. Providing opportunities for a client to discuss their view to the nurse.
   c. Ensuring a client's traditional health care practice is handled separately from current health approaches.
   d. Working collaboratively with a client in making health care decisions.

   Answer: _____ Rationale: _____
   _____
   _____

10

Client Care: Leadership, Delegation, and Quality Management

Adapted by Marlene Smadu, RN, BScN, MAdEd, ED,
University of Saskatchewan

Preliminary Reading

Chapter 10, pp. 148-164

Comprehensive Understanding

Building a Nursing Team

- Building an empowered nursing team begins with the nurse executive.

- Define *philosophy of care*. _____

_____

_____

Nursing Care Delivery Models

- Care delivery must be effective in helping nurses achieve desirable outcomes for their clients.

- Briefly explain the following delivery systems.

  a. Functional nursing: _____

_____

b. Team nursing: _____

_____

c. Total patient care: _____

_____

d. Primary nursing: _____

_____

e. Case management: _____

_____

Decentralized Decision Making

- Briefly explain the following management structures.

    a. Centralized management: _____

    _____

    b. Decentralized management: _____

    _____

    c. Matrix: _____

    _____

- Identify the responsibilities of a nurse manager.

    _____

    _____

    _____

- The following are key elements in empowering staff and establishing decentralized decision making. Briefly explain each one.

    a. Responsibility: _____

    _____

    b. Autonomy: _____

    _____

    c. Authority: _____

    _____

    d. Accountability: _____

    _____

- The nurse manager nurtures and supports staff involvement through the following approaches. Briefly explain each.

    a. Shared governance: _____

    _____

    b. Nurse/physician collaborative practice: _____

    _____

    c. Interdisciplinary collaboration: _____

    _____

    d. Staff communication: _____

    _____

    e. Staff education: _____

    _____

Leadership Skills for Nursing Students

- Summarize each of the following leadership skills a student nurse may develop.

    a. Clinical care coordination: _____

    _____

    b. Clinical decision making: _____

    _____

    c. Priority setting: _____

    _____

    d. Organizational skills: _____

    _____

    e. Use of resources: _____

    _____

    f. Time management: _____

    _____

    g. Evaluation: _____

    _____

- Summarize the following principles of time management.

  a. Goal setting: _____

  _____

  b. Priority setting: _____

  _____

  c. Organizational skills: _____

  _____

  d. Use of resources: _____

  _____

  e. Time management: _____

  _____

  f. Evaluation: _____

  _____

- Give an example of team communication.

  _____

  _____

  _____

- *Delegation* is defined as: _____

  _____

- Identify the five rights of delegation.

  a. _____

  b. _____

  c. _____

  d. _____

  e. _____

- Identify the purposes of delegation. _____

  _____

- Summarize the requirements for appropriate delegation.

  a. _____

  b. _____

  c. _____

  d. _____

  e. _____

- List some ways that professional nurses build on their existing knowledge base.

  _____

  _____

  _____

Quality Improvement

- *Quality improvement* is defined as: _____

  _____

Quality in Nursing Practice

- The quality of nursing practice is defined by each of the following.

  a. Professional standards: _____

  _____

  b. Care guidelines: _____

  _____

  c. Outcomes: _____

  _____

- Differentiate between the two types of outcomes.

  a. Professional outcomes: _____

  b. Client outcomes: _____

- Differentiate between the two different types of quality improvement teams.

  a. Organization-wide: _____

  b. Unit-based: _____

- Identify models for process improvement.

  _____

  _____

  _____

  _____

- Identify who is responsible for the QI program. _____
  _____

- A unit's scope of service includes: _____
  _____

- Some key aspects of service include: _____
  _____

- A *quality indicator* is defined as: _____
  _____

- Explain the following three types of quality indicators.
  a. Structure: _____
     _____
  b. Process: _____
     _____
  c. Outcome: _____
     _____

- List some processes and related outcomes that may be in need of improvement.
  _____
  _____
  _____

- *Threshold* is defined as: _____
  _____

- When QI is an ongoing process, staff continuously work to improve outcomes or performance by raising thresholds.

- Explain the purpose of data collection and analysis. _____
  _____
  _____

- After evaluating quality problems, the staff needs to do the following. Explain each.
  a. Resolve problems: _____
     _____
  b. Evaluate improvement: _____
     _____
  c. Communicate results: _____
     _____

Review Questions

The student should select the appropriate answer and cite the rationale for choosing that particular answer.

1. Primary nursing refers to:
   a. Nurses who work with physicians in primary care
   b. Nurses who hold management positions
   c. Placing RNs at the bedside
   d. Nursing carried out in primary health care

   Answer: _____ Rationale: _____
   _____
   _____

2. A student nurse practising primary leadership skills would demonstrate all of the following, *except*:
   a. Being sensitive to the group's feelings
   b. Recognizing others for their contribution
   c. Assuming primary responsibility for planning, implementation, follow-up, and evaluation
   d. Developing listening skills and being aware of personal motivation

   Answer: _____ Rationale: _____
   _____
   _____

3. Decentralized management is best described as
   a. Care decisions being made by a manager in another location
   b. Situations in which there is lack of coordination of care
   c. Situations when staff overrule the decisions made by managers
   d. Situations in which decision making occurs at the staff level

Answer: _____ Rationale: _____
_____
_____

4. Autonomy is best described as:
   a. The duties and activities that an individual is employed to perform
   b. The right to act in areas where an individual has been given and accepts responsibility
   c. The freedom to decide and act
   d. Being answerable for one's actions

Answer: _____ Rationale: _____
_____
_____

5. Which of the following is *not* a purpose for delegation?
   a. Improves efficiency
   b. Provides job enrichment
   c. Transfers accountability for client care
   d. Improves utilization of health care providers

Answer: _____ Rationale: _____
_____
_____

11

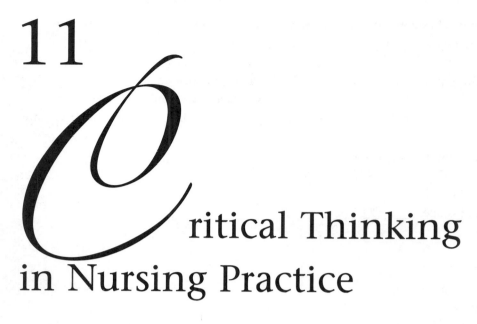

Critical Thinking in Nursing Practice

Adapted by Donna M. Romyn, RN, PhD, Athabasca University

Preliminary Reading

Chapter 12, pp. 165-181

Comprehensive Understanding

Critical Decisions in Nursing Practice

- Critical decision making separates professional nurses from technical or ancillary personnel.

- Describe the process of critical thinking in nursing. _____
  _____
  _____

- To think critically, the nurse must be able to:

  a. _____

  b. _____

  c. _____

  d. _____

  e. _____

Critical Thinking Defined

- Define *critical thinking*. _____
  _____

- Identify the core critical thinking skills that apply to nursing.
  a. _____
  b. _____
  c. _____
  d. _____
  e. _____

- Learning to think critically helps a nurse to care for clients as their advocate and to make better informed choices about their care.

Reflection

- Define *reflection*. _____
  _____

- Briefly summarize seven tips to facilitate critical thinking.
  a. _____
  b. _____
  c. _____
  d. _____
  e. _____
  f. _____
  g. _____

- Provide some examples of how a nurse can use reflection. _____
  _____

- Identify a common approach to reflection that a student nurse may use. _____
  _____

Language

- To become a critical thinker, a nurse must be able to use language precisely and clearly. It is important not only to communicate clearly with clients and families, but to be able to communicate findings clearly to other health professionals.

Intuition

- Define *intuition*. _____
  _____

- Cite some examples of how a nurse gains intuitive knowledge. _____
  _____
  _____

Levels of Critical Thinking in Nursing

- Three levels of critical thinking in nursing have been identified. Briefly describe each.
  a. Basic: _____
     _____
  b. Complex: _____
     _____
  c. Commitment: _____
     _____

Critical Thinking Competencies

- Critical thinking competencies are the cognitive processes a nurse uses to make judgments.

General Critical Thinking Competencies

Applying the Scientific Method

- Define *scientific method*._____
  _____

- List the steps of the scientific method.

  a. _____

  b. _____

  c. _____

  d. _____

  e. _____

Problem Solving

- Define *problem solving*. _____

  _____

- Solving a problem in one situation allows the nurse to apply the knowledge to future client situations.

Decision Making

- Define *decision making*. _____

  _____

- Explain the process that an individual needs to go through to make a decision.

  _____

  _____

  _____

Specific Critical Thinking Competencies

Diagnostic Reasoning and Inferences

- Explain the process of diagnostic reasoning.

  _____

  _____

  _____

Clinical Decision Making

- The clinical decision making process requires

  _____.

- List the criteria for decision making (Strader, 1992).

  a. _____

  b. _____

  c. _____

- After determining a client's priorities, a nurse selects therapies most likely to solve each problem.

- Cite some examples of how nurses make decisions about their clients. _____

  _____

  _____

Specific Clinical Thinking in Nursing

Applying the Nursing Process

- The nursing process is a systematic and comprehensive approach for nursing care. List the five steps of the nursing process.

  a. _____

  b. _____

  c. _____

  d. _____

  e. _____

Critical Thinking Model

- Summarize the critical thinking model and list its five components. _____

  _____

  _____

Specific Knowledge Base

- Identify what constitutes a nurse's knowledge base. _____

  _____

Experience

- Identify the ways that critical thinking is developed through experience. _____

  _____

Attitudes for Critical Thinking

- The following attributes are important for critical thinking. Briefly explain each of them.

  a. Confidence: _____

  _____

  b. Thinking independently: _____

  _____

  c. Fairness: _____

  _____

  d. Responsibility and accountability: _____

  _____

  e. Risk taking: _____

  _____

  f. Discipline: _____

  _____

  g. Perseverance: _____

  _____

  h. Creativity: _____

  _____

  i. Curiosity: _____

  _____

  j. Integrity: _____

  _____

  k. Humility: _____

  _____

Standards for Critical Thinking

- The fifth component of critical thinking includes _____ and

  _____.

- Intellectual standards refer to _____.

- Professional standards refer to _____.

Critical Thinking Synthesis

- *Critical thinking* is defined as: _____

  _____

- The nursing process is the traditional critical thinking competency that allows nurses to make clinical judgments and take actions based on reason.

- Briefly explain how the nursing process and the critical thinking model work together.

  _____

  _____

  _____

*R*eview Questions

The student should select the appropriate answer and cite the rationale for choosing that particular answer.

1. Clinical decision making requires the nurse to:
   a. Improve a client's health
   b. Establish and weigh criteria in deciding the best choice of therapy for a client
   c. Follow the physician's orders for client care
   d. Standardize care for the client

   Answer: _____ Rationale: _____

   _____

   _____

2. Which of the following is *not* one of the five steps of the nursing process?
   a. Planning
   b. Evaluation
   c. Hypothesis testing
   d. Assessment

   Answer: _____ Rationale: _____

   _____

   _____

3. Gathering, verifying, and communicating data about the client to establish a database is an example of which component of the nursing process?
   a. Assessment
   b. Planning
   c. Evaluation
   d. Nursing diagnosis
   e. Implementation

Answer: _____ Rationale: _____

_____

_____

4. Completing nursing actions necessary for accomplishing a care plan is an example of which component of the nursing process?
   a. Assessment
   b. Planning
   c. Evaluation
   d. Nursing diagnosis
   e. Implementation

Answer: _____ Rationale: _____

_____

_____

12

The Nursing Process

*Adapted by Marilynn J. Wood, RN, BSN, MSN, DrPH,
University of Alberta*
Janet C. Ross-Kerr, RN, BScN, MS, PhD, University of Alberta
Julie A. Gilbert, RN, BScN, MN, University of Alberta
Tracey Stephen, RN, BScN, MN, University of Alberta
Rene A. Day, RN, PhD, University of Alberta

Preliminary Reading

Chapter 12, pp. 182-232

Comprehensive Understanding

- The nursing process is used to _____, _____, and _____ human responses to _____ and _____.

Step 1: Nursing Assessment

- Nursing assessment is the systematic process of _____, _____, and _____.

- Identify the purpose of the assessment.

  _____

- As the nurse initiates the assessment component for a specific client, the nurse is also synthesizing critical knowledge, experience, standards, and attitudes simultaneously.

- A comprehensive database includes: _____
  _____

Organization of Data Gathering

- Accurate assessment makes it possible to develop appropriate nursing diagnoses and to devise appropriate goals and strategies.

- It is important for the nurse's assessment to first consider the _____.

- Identify some non-verbal behaviour that a nurse may observe during an assessment.
  _____

  _____

- Whichever approach is used, the nurse must cluster cues of information and identify emerging patterns and potential problems.

Data Collection

- Assessment data must be _____, _____, and _____.

- The collection of inaccurate, incomplete, or inappropriate data leads to incorrect identification of the client's health care needs and subsequent inaccurate, incomplete, or inappropriate nursing diagnoses.

Types of Data

- Define each of the following.

  a. Subjective data: _____
     _____

  b. Objective data: _____
     _____

Sources of Data

- Each source provides information about the client's level of wellness, anticipated prognosis, risk factors, health practices and goals, and patterns of health and illness.

The Client

- Identify the types of information a client can provide.

  a. _____

  b. _____

  c. _____

  d. _____

  e. _____

Families and Significant Others

- Families can be an important secondary source of information about the client's health status. Give an example. _____
  _____

  _____

Health Care Team Members

- Identify the ways that health care team members identify data.

  a. _____

  b. _____

  c. _____

Medical Records

- By reviewing medical records, the nurse can _____, _____, and _____.

Other Records

- Identify records that may contain pertinent health care information._____
  _____

Literature Review

- Reviewing nursing, medical, and pharmacological literature about an illness helps the nurse complete the database.

Nurse's Experience

- A nurse's ability to make an assessment will improve as he or she uses _____, applies _____, and focuses _____.

Methods of Data Collection

Interview

- During an interview nurses have the opportunity to:

  a. _____

  b. _____

  c. _____

  d. _____

  e. _____

  f. _____

- Define *nurse-client relationship*. _____
  _____

- Describe the phases of the interview.

  a. _____

  b. _____

  c. _____

- The nurse uses various types of interview techniques. Describe some of the information obtained in an interview. _____
  _____
  _____

Nursing Health History

- The nursing health history is data collected about:

  a. _____

  b. _____

  c. _____

  d. _____

  e. _____

- Briefly describe the elements of a health
  history. _____
  _____
  _____

Physical Examination

- During the physical examination _____, and _____ are taken and _____.

Formulating Nursing Judgments

- Through a process of inferential reasoning and judgment, the nurse decides what information has meaning in relation to the client's health status.

Data Clustering

- After collecting and validating subjective and objective data and interpreting the data, the nurse organizes the information into meaningful clusters. This depends on recognizing
  _____.

- During data clustering, the nurse organizes data and focuses attention on client functions needing support and assistance for recovery.

Data Documentation

- Identify the two essential reasons for thoroughness in data documentation.

  a. _____

  b. _____

Step 2: Nursing Diagnosis

- Define *nursing diagnosis*. _____
  _____

- Define *medical diagnosis*. _____
  _____

Evolution of Nursing Diagnosis

- Briefly summarize the evolution of nursing
  diagnosis. _____
  _____
  _____
  _____

- Explain the purpose of NANDA. _____

  _____

  _____

- Explain the purpose of using nursing diagnoses. _____

  _____

  _____

Critical Thinking and the Nursing Diagnostic Process

- The diagnostic reasoning process includes:

  _____

  _____

Analysis and Interpretation of Data

- Data analysis involves recognizing
  _____, comparing _____,
  and making_____.

- Defining characteristics are: _____

- Defining characteristics that are beyond
  healthy norms form the basis for problem
  identification.

Formulation of the Nursing Diagnosis

- NANDA has identified three types of nursing
  diagnoses. Briefly explain each one.

  a. _____

  b. _____

  c. _____

- An actual nursing diagnosis describes: _____

  _____

- An at risk nursing diagnosis describes: _____

  _____

- A wellness nursing diagnosis describes: _____

  _____

Components of a Nursing Diagnosis

- Nursing diagnoses are stated in a two-part
  format: the _____ followed by a
  _____.

- The diagnostic label of the nursing diagnosis
  is: _____

  _____

- The related factors of the nursing diagnosis are

  _____

  _____

- The etiology of the nursing diagnosis is: _____

  _____

- NANDA approves a definition for each diagnosis following clinical use and testing.

- Risk factors are: _____

  _____

- Nursing assessment data must support the
  diagnostic label, and the related factors must
  support the etiology.

Diagnostic Errors

- Identify 11 ways nurses can avoid making
  common diagnostic errors:

  a. _____

  b. _____

  c. _____

  d. _____

  e. _____

  f. _____

  g. _____

  h. _____

  i. _____

  j. _____

  k. _____

Step 3: Planning Nursing Care

Establishing Priorities

- Priority setting involves ranking nursing diagnoses in order of importance.

- Priorities are classified as high, immediate, or low. Give an example of each.

  High: _____

  Immediate: _____

  Low: _____

Critical Thinking in Establishing Goals and Expected Outcomes

- Once a nursing diagnosis is identified for a client, the nursing process consists of finding the best approach to address and resolve the problem.

- Goals and expected outcomes are specific statements of client _____ or _____ that the nurse sets to achieve problem resolution.

- Identify the two purposes for writing goals and expected outcomes.

  a. _____

  b. _____

Goals of Care

- Define the following.

  a. Client-centred goal: _____

  _____

  b. Short-term goal: _____

  _____

  c. Long-term goal: _____

  _____

Expected Outcomes

- Define *expected outcomes*. _____

  _____

- Outcomes are desired responses of the client's condition in the _____, _____, _____, _____, or _____ dimensions.

- The expected outcomes should be written in measurable behavioral terms sequentially, with time frames.

- Identify the functions of an expected outcome.

  a. _____

  b. _____

  c. _____

  d. _____

Guidelines for Writing Goals and Expected Outcomes

- There are seven guidelines to follow when writing goals and expected outcomes. Define and give an example of each.

  a. Client-centred factors: _____

  _____

  b. Singular factors: _____

  _____

  c. Observable factors: _____

  _____

  d. Measurable factors: _____

  _____

  e. Time-limited factors: _____

  _____

  f. Mutual factors: _____

  _____

  g. Realistic factors: _____

  _____

Critical Thinking in Planning Nursing Interventions

- Nursing interventions are those actions designed to assist the client in moving from the present level of health to that described in the expected outcome.

Types of Interventions

- There are three categories of interventions, and category selection is based on the client's needs. Define and give an example of each.

    a. Nurse-initiated: _____

    _____

    b. Physician-initiated: _____

    _____

    c. Collaborative: _____

    _____

Selection of Interventions

- Identify the six factors the nurse uses to select nursing interventions for a specific client.

    a. _____

    b. _____

    c. _____

    d. _____

    e. _____

    f. _____

- Define *collaboration*. _____

    _____

- The advantages of the taxonomy of nursing interventions are:

    a. _____

    b. _____

    c. _____

    d. _____

Developing a Plan of Care

- Define *nursing care plan*. _____

    _____

Purpose of Care Plans

- Briefly explain the purpose of a nursing care plan in relation to the following.

    a. Communication: _____

    _____

    b. Identification and coordination of resources: _____

    _____

    c. Continuity of care: _____

    _____

    d. Change-of-shift reports: _____

    _____

    e. Long-term needs of client: _____

    _____

    f. Expected outcome criteria: _____

    _____

- The complete care plan is the blueprint for nursing action. It provides direction for implementation of the plan and a framework for evaluation of the client's response to nursing actions.

- Briefly explain each of the following.

    a. Institutional care plans: _____

    _____

    b. Standardized care plans: _____

    _____

    c. Care plans for community-based settings:

    _____

    _____

    d. Critical pathways or CareMaps: _____

    _____

    e. Concept maps: _____

    _____

Consulting Other Health Care Professionals

- Consultation is a process in which _____

    _____.

- Consultation is based on the problem-solving approach, and the consultant is the stimulus for change.

- The need to consult occurs when the nurse has identified a problem that cannot be solved using personal knowledge, skills, and resources.

Step 4: Implementing Nursing Care

- Implementation describes: _____ _____

- A nursing intervention is: _____ _____

- Define each.
  a. Direct care interventions: _____ _____

  b. Indirect care interventions: _____ _____

Protocols and Standing Orders

- Nursing interventions can be based on protocols and standings orders. Briefly explain each and provide an example of where they are commonly used.
  a. Protocols: _____ _____

  b. Standing orders: _____ _____

Critical Thinking in Implementation

- Identify the factors that should be considered when choosing interventions.
  a. _____
  b. _____
  c. _____
  d. _____
  e. _____
  f. _____

- When making decisions about implementing care, the nurse needs to consider the following:
  a. _____
  b. _____
  c. _____
  d. _____

Implementation Process

Reassessing the Client

- When new data are obtained and a new need is identified, the nurse modifies nursing care.

Reviewing and Revising the Existing Nursing Care Plan

- If the client's status has changed and the nursing diagnosis and related nursing interventions are no longer appropriate, the nursing care plan needs to be modified.

- Modification of the existing care plan includes several steps. Identify them.
  a. _____
  b. _____
  c. _____
  d. _____

Organizing Resources and Care Delivery

- Before implementing care, the nurse evaluates the plan to determine the need for assistance and the type of assistance required.

- Describe how each of the following contributes to the preparation of care delivered:
  a. Equipment: _____ _____

  b. Personnel: _____ _____

  c. Environment: _____ _____

  d. Client: _____ _____

Anticipating and Preventing Complications

- Risks to clients arise from illness, conditions, and treatment.

- Nurses must identify need for additional assistance and/or nursing skills.

Direct Care
Activities of Daily Living

- Define *activities of daily living* (ADLs). _____

  _____

- Conditions that result in the need for assistance with ADLs can be temporary, permanent, or rehabilitative.

Instrumental Activities of Daily Living (IADLs)

- IADLs include: _____

  _____

- A *life-saving measure* is: _____

  _____

Counselling

- *Counselling* is defined as: _____.

- Identify some areas in which clients or families may need counselling.

  a. _____

  b. _____

  c. _____

Teaching

- Define the following.

  a. Teaching: _____

  _____

  b. Teaching-learning process: _____

  _____

Observing for Adverse Reactions

- What is an adverse reaction? _____

  _____

- How do nurses control for adverse reactions?

  _____

  _____

Indirect Care
Communicating Nursing Interventions

- Nursing interventions are written (via the nursing care plan and medical record) or communicated orally (one nurse to another or to another health care professional).

- Define *interdisciplinary plan*. _____

  _____

Delegating, Supervising, and Evaluating Others' Work

- Give examples of tasks you could delegate to anther member of the health care team.

  _____

  _____

Step 5: Evaluating Nursing Care
Critical Thinking and Evaluation

- Evaluation of care requires the nurse to reflect on the client's responses to nursing interventions and to determine their effectiveness in promoting the client's well-being.

- Evaluation is the step in the nursing process whereby the nurse continually redirects nursing care to meet client needs.

- Explain the two types of evaluations.

  a. Positive: _____

  b. Negative: _____

- A client whose health status changes continuously requires frequent evaluation.

The Evaluation Process

- Identify the five elements of the evaluation process.

  a. _____

  b. _____

  c. _____

  d. _____

  e. _____

- A goal specifies: _____

  _____

- Expected outcomes are: _____

  _____

- The purposes of the Nursing Outcomes Classification (NOC) are:

  a. _____

  b. _____

  c. _____

Collecting Evaluative Data

- Identify the two aspects of care that need to be identified.

  a. _____

  b. _____

- The primary source of data for evaluation is:

  _____

  _____

  _____

Interpreting and Summarizing Findings

- To objectively evaluate the success in achieving a goal, the nurse should use the following steps.

  a. _____

  b. _____

  c. _____

  d. _____

  e. _____

- When documenting the client's response to interventions, the nurse always includes the same evaluative measures gathered during assessment.

Care Plan Revision and Critical Thinking

- Accurate evaluation leads to the appropriate revision of ineffective care plans and discontinuation of therapy that has been successful.

Discontinuing a Care Plan

- After determining that expected outcomes and goals have been achieved, the nurse confirms this evaluation with the client and discontinues that care plan.

Modifying a Care Plan

- When goals are not met, the nurse identifies the factors that interfered with goal achievement.

- Lack of goal achievement may also result from an error in nursing judgment or failure to follow each step of the nursing process.

- When there is failure to achieve a goal, the entire _____ sequence is repeated to discover changes that need to be made to _____ or _____ the client's health.

- A complete reassessment of all client factors relating to the nursing diagnosis and etiology is the first step in reevaluating the nursing process. Briefly explain the following.

  a. Reassessment: _____

  b. Nursing diagnosis: _____

  c. Goals and expected outcomes: _____

  d. Interventions: _____

  e. Evaluation: _____

  f. Client outcomes: _____

Review Questions

The student should select the appropriate answer and cite the rationale for choosing that particular answer.

1. In most circumstances, the best source of information for nursing assessment of the adult client is the:
   a. Nursing literature
   b. Physician
   c. Client
   d. Medical record

   Answer: _____ Rationale: _____
   _____
   _____

2. Measuring the client's response to nursing interventions and his or her progress toward achieving goals occurs during which phase of the nursing process?
   a. Planning
   b. Nursing diagnosis
   c. Evaluation
   d. Assessment

   Answer: _____ Rationale: _____
   _____
   _____

3. Evaluation is:
   a. Begun immediately before the client's discharge
   b. Only necessary if the physician orders it
   c. An integrated, ongoing nursing care activity
   d. Performed primarily by nurses in the quality assurance department

   Answer: _____ Rationale: _____
   _____
   _____

4. The primary source of data for evaluation is the:
   a. Physician
   b. Client
   c. Nurse
   d. Medical record

   Answer: _____ Rationale: _____
   _____
   _____

5. The nursing care plan calls for the client, a 136 kg woman, to be turned every 2 hours. The client is unable to assist with turning. The nurse knows that she may hurt her back if she attempts to turn the client by herself. The nurse should:
   a. Rewrite the care plan to eliminate the need for turning
   b. Ignore the intervention related to turning in the care plan
   c. Turn the client by herself
   d. Ask another nurse to help her turn the client

   Answer: _____ Rationale: _____
   _____
   _____

6. Mary Benoit is a newly diagnosed diabetic patient. The nurse shows Mary how to administer an injection. This intervention activity is:
   a. Counselling
   b. Communicating
   c. Teaching
   d. Managing

   Answer: _____ Rationale: _____
   _____
   _____

7. A nursing diagnosis:
    a. Is a statement of a client response to a health problem that requires nursing intervention
    b. Identifies nursing problems
    c. Is derived from the physician's history and physical examination
    d. Is not changed during the course of a client's hospitalization

Answer: _____ Rationale: _____

_____

_____

8. Mr. Margauz, a 52-year-old business executive, is admitted to the coronary care unit. During his admission interview he denies chest pain or shortness of breath. His pulse and blood pressure are normal. He appears tense and does not want the nurse to leave his bedside. When questioned, he states that he is very nervous. At this moment, which nursing diagnosis is most appropriate?
    a. Alteration in comfort, chest pain
    b. Alteration in bowel elimination related to restricted mobility
    c. High risk for altered cardiac output related to heart attack
    d. Anxiety related to intensive care unit admission

Answer: _____ Rationale: _____

_____

_____

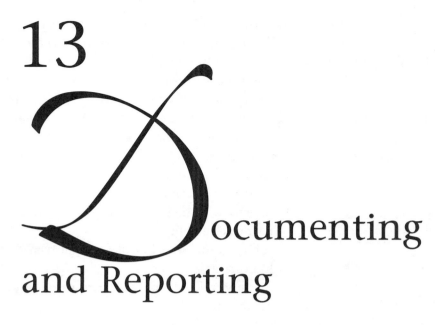

13

$\mathcal{D}$ocumenting and Reporting

Adapted by Maureen Barry, BScN, MScN, University of Toronto

$\mathcal{P}$reliminary Reading

Chapter 13, pp. 233-257

$\mathcal{C}$omprehensive Understanding

- What is documentation? _____

_____

Confidentiality

- Explain two reasons why nurses are obligated to keep information about clients confidential.

    a. _____

    _____

    b. _____

    _____

Multidisciplinary Communication Within the Health Care Team

- Caregivers use a variety of ways to exchange information about clients. Briefly explain the following.

    a. Client record or chart: _____

    _____

b. Reports: _____

_____

Purposes of Records

- Briefly explain the following purposes of a record.

  a. Communication and care planning: _____

  b. Legal documentation: _____

  c. Education: _____

  d. Research: _____

  e. Quality review: _____

Guidelines for Quality Documentation and Reporting

- Six important guidelines must be followed to ensure quality documentation and reporting. Explain each one.

  a. Factual: _____

  _____

  b. Accurate: _____

  _____

  c. Complete: _____

  _____

  d. Current: _____

  _____

  e. Organized: _____

  _____

  f. Complies with standards: _____

  _____

Common Documentation Systems

- Narrative documentation is a story-like format that documents information specific to client conditions and nursing care. The disadvantages of this style are:

  a. _____

  b. _____

  c. _____

- Problem-oriented medical records (POMR) place emphasis on the client's problems. The method corresponds to the nursing process and facilitates communication of client needs. Explain the following major sections of the POMR.

  a. Database: _____

  _____

  b. Problem list: _____

  _____

  c. Care plan: _____

  _____

  d. Progress notes: _____

  _____

- Briefly explain the POMR forms of documentation.

  a. SOAP or SOAPIE notes: _____

  b. PIE format: _____

  c. Focus charting or DAR: _____

- Briefly explain these forms of documentation.

  a. Source records: _____

  _____

  b. Charting by exception (CBE): _____

  _____

  c. Critical pathways or care maps: _____

  _____

Common Record-Keeping Forms

- Briefly explain the following formats used for record keeping.

  a. Admission nursing history forms: _____

  _____

  b. Flow sheets and graphic records: _____

  _____

  c. Client care summary or Kardex: _____

  _____

d. Acuity records or workload measurement systems: _____

_____

e. Standardized care plans: _____

_____

f. Discharge summary forms: _____

_____

Home Health Care Documentation

- Documentation in the home health care system has different implications than it does in other areas of nursing. The primary difference is: _____

_____

_____

- The nurse is the pivotal person in the documentation of home health care delivery.

Long-Term Health Care Documentation

- Because residents are stable, document is done using _____ and assessment may be done only _____.

Computerized Documentation and the Electronic Health Record

- Explain the many benefits of computerized documentation. _____

_____

_____

- What is an Electronic Health Record (EHR)?

_____

_____

Reporting

- Nurses communicate information about clients so that all members of the health care team can make informed decisions about the client and his or her care.

Change-of-Shift Reports

- Identify the eight major areas to include in a change-of-shift report.

a. _____

b. _____

c. _____

d. _____

e. _____

f. _____

g. _____

h. _____

Telephone Reports

- It is important that information in a telephone report be clear, accurate, and concise.

Transfer Reports

- List the nine major information areas in a transfer report.

a. _____

b. _____

c. _____

d. _____

e. _____

f. _____

g. _____

h. _____

i. _____

Incident Reports

- Define the purpose of an incident report.

_____

_____

Telephone or Verbal Orders

- List the guidelines the nurse should follow when receiving telephone orders from physicians.

  a. _____

  b. _____

  c. _____

  d. _____

  e. _____

  f. _____

Review Questions

The student should select the appropriate answer and cite the rationale for choosing that particular answer.

1. What is the primary purpose of a client's medical record?
   a. To satisfy requirements of accreditation agencies
   b. To communicate accurate, timely information about the client
   c. To provide validation for hospital charges
   d. To provide the nurse with a defense against malpractice

   Answer: _____ Rationale: _____

   _____

   _____

2. Which of the following is charted according to the six guidelines for quality recording?
   a. "Respirations rapid; lung sounds clear."
   b. "Was depressed today."
   c. "Crying. States she doesn't want visitors to see her like this."
   d. "Had a good day. Up and about in room."

   Answer: _____ Rationale: _____

   _____

   _____

3. Which of the following best describes a change-of-shift report?
   a. Two or more nurses always visit all clients to review their plan of care.
   b. Nurses should exchange judgments they have made about client attitudes.
   c. The nurse should identify nursing diagnoses and clarify client priorities.
   d. Client information is communicated from a nurse on a sending unit to a nurse on a receiving unit.

   Answer: _____ Rationale: _____

   _____

   _____

4. What is an incident report?
   a. A legal claim against a nurse for negligent nursing care
   b. A summary report of all falls occurring on a nursing unit
   c. A report of an event inconsistent with the routine care of a client
   d. A report of a nurse's behaviour submitted to the hospital administration

   Answer: _____ Rationale: _____

   _____

   _____

5. If an error is made while recording, what should the nurse do?
   a. Erase it or scratch it out
   b. Obtain a new nurse's note and rewrite the entries
   c. Leave a blank space in the note
   d. Draw a single line through the error and initial it

   Answer: _____ Rationale: _____

   _____

   _____

14

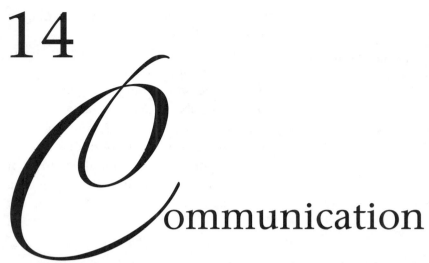

Communication

Adapted by Nancy C. Goddard, RN, BScN, MN, PhD,
University of Alberta & Red Deer College

Preliminary Reading

Chapter 14, pp. 258-281

Comprehensive Understanding

- Communication is a lifelong process. This process allows: _____
  _____

- Competency in communication helps the nurse maintain effective relationships with the entire sphere of professional practice and helps meet legal, ethical, and clinical standards of care.

Communication and Interpersonal Relationships

- Communication is the means to establishing helping-healing relationships.

- Communication is essential to the nurse-client relationship because:
  a. _____
  b. _____

- Nurses with expertise in communication can express caring by: _____
  _____
  _____

- The nurse's ability to relate to others is: _____
  _____
  _____

Developing Communication Skills

- Briefly explain the qualities of critical thinking in relation to the communication process.
  _____
  _____

- Critical thinking can help the nurse overcome perceptual biases.

- Nurses use communication skills to gather, analyze, and transmit information and to accomplish the work of each phase.

Levels of Communication

- Summarize the following communication interactions.
  a. Intrapersonal: _____
  b. Interpersonal: _____
  c. Transpersonal: _____
  d. Small-group: _____
  e. Public: _____

Basic Elements of the Communication Process

- Briefly summarize the following elements of communication.
  a. Referent: _____
  b. Sender: _____
  c. Receiver: _____
  d. Message: _____
  e. Channels: _____
  f. Feedback: _____
  g. Interpersonal variables: _____
  h. Environment: _____

Forms of Communication

- Messages are conveyed verbally and nonverbally, concretely and symbolically.

Verbal Communication

- Verbal communication involves spoken or written words. Verbal language is a code that conveys specific meaning as words are combined.

- Briefly explain the important aspects of verbal communication listed below.
  a. Vocabulary: _____
  _____
  b. Denotative and connotative meaning: ____
  _____
  _____
  c. Pacing: _____
  _____
  d. Intonation: _____
  _____
  e. Clarity: _____
  _____
  f. Brevity: _____
  _____
  g. Timing and relevance: _____
  _____

Non-Verbal Communication

- Non-verbal communication includes: _____
  _____
  _____

- Non-verbal communication is much more powerful than verbal communication.

- Becoming an astute observer of nonverbal behaviour takes practice, concentration, and sensitivity to others. Briefly explain the following non-verbal behaviours.

   a. Personal appearance: _____

   _____

   b. Posture and gait: _____

   _____

   c. Facial expression: _____

   _____

   d. Eye contact: _____

   _____

   e. Gestures: _____

   _____

   f. Sounds: _____

   _____

   g. Territoriality and personal space: _____

   _____

- Identify the zones of personal space. _____

   _____

   _____

   _____

- Identify the zones of touch. _____

   _____

   _____

   _____

Symbolic Communication

- Summarize symbolic communication. _____

   _____

   _____

Metacommunication

- Define *metacommunication*. _____

   _____

Professional Nursing Relationships

- Professional relationships are created through _____, _____, and _____.

Nurse-Client Helping Relationships

- The relationship is therapeutic, promoting a psychological climate that facilitates positive change and growth.

- Acceptance conveys a: _____

   _____

- The nurse-client relationship is characterized by four goal-directed phases. Explain the phases.

   a. Pre-interaction phase: _____

   b. Orientation phase: _____

   c. Working phase: _____

   d. Termination phase: _____

- Nurses often encourage clients to share personal stories. This is called _____.

Nurse-Family Relationships

- Summarize the principles related to nurse-family relationships. _____

   _____

   _____

Nurse-Health Team Relationships

- Communication in nurse-health team relationships is geared by: _____

   _____

   _____

Nurse-Community Relationships

- Communication within the community occurs through channels such as: _____

   _____

Elements of Professional Communication

- Briefly explain the following elements of professional communication.

  a. Courtesy: _____

  b. Use of names: _____

  c. Privacy and confidentiality: _____

  d. Trustworthiness: _____

  e. Autonomy and responsibility: _____

  f. Assertiveness: _____

Communication Within the Nursing Process

𝒩𝒫 Assessment

- Assessment of a client's ability to communicate includes gathering data about the many contextual factors that influence communication.

- List the contextual factors that influence communication.

  a. _____

  b. _____

  c. _____

  d. _____

  e. _____

- Identify the psycho-physiological factors that influence communication. _____
  _____

- Physical barriers cause _____,
  _____, or _____.

- Explain how developmental factors influence communication. _____
  _____
  _____

- Summarize how socio-cultural factors influence communication. _____
  _____
  _____

Gender influences communication. Explain how communication differs in regard to gender.

  a. Male: _____

  b. Female: _____

𝒩𝒫 Nursing Diagnosis

- List three nursing diagnoses appropriate for a client with alterations in communication.

  a. _____

  b. _____

  c. _____

𝒩𝒫 Planning

- List three goals for effective interpersonal communication.

  a. _____

  b. _____

  c. _____

𝒩𝒫 Implementation

- Therapeutic communication techniques are specific responses that encourage the expression of feelings and ideas and convey the nurse's acceptance and respect. Briefly explain the following techniques.

  a. Active listening: _____
  _____

  b. Sharing observations: _____
  _____

  c. Sharing empathy: _____
  _____

  d. Sharing hope: _____
  _____

e. Sharing humour: _____
_____

f. Sharing feelings: _____
_____

g. Using touch: _____
_____

h. Using silence: _____
_____

i. Providing information: _____
_____

j. Clarifying: _____
_____

k. Focusing: _____
_____

l. Paraphrasing: _____
_____

m. Asking relevant questions: _____
_____

n. Summarizing: _____
_____

o. Self-disclosing: _____
_____

p. Confronting: _____
_____

- Certain communication techniques can hinder or damage professional relationships. These techniques are referred to as *non-therapeutic*. Briefly explain the following non-therapeutic techniques.

  a. Asking personal questions: _____
  _____

  b. Giving personal opinions: _____
  _____

  c. Changing the subject: _____
  _____

  d. Automatic responses: _____
  _____

  e. False reassurance: _____
  _____

f. Sympathy: _____
_____

g. Asking for explanations: _____
_____

h. Approval or disapproval: _____
_____

i. Defensive responses: _____
_____

j. Passive or aggressive responses: _____
_____

k. Arguing: _____
_____

- Briefly identify the communication techniques to use with the client with special needs.

  a. Clients who cannot speak clearly: _____
  _____

  b. Clients who are cognitively impaired: _____
  _____

  c. Clients who are unresponsive: _____
  _____

  d. Clients who do not speak English: _____
  _____

Evaluation

- List four expected outcomes for the client with impaired communication.

  a. _____
  b. _____
  c. _____
  d. _____

Review Questions

The student should select the appropriate answer and cite the rationale for choosing that particular answer.

1. Transpersonal communication is:
   a. Interaction that occurs within a person's spiritual domain
   b. One-to-one interaction between the nurse and client
   c. Communication within groups
   d. Self-talk

   Answer: _____ Rationale: _____

   _____

   _____

2. In demonstrating the method for deep-breathing exercises, the nurse places his or her hands on the client's abdomen to explain diaphragmatic movement. This technique involves the use of which communication element?
   a. Feedback
   b. Tactile channel
   c. Referent
   d. Message

   Answer: _____ Rationale: _____

   _____

   _____

3. Which statement about non-verbal communication is correct?
   a. It is easy for a nurse to judge the meaning of a client's facial expression.
   b. The nurse's verbal messages should be reinforced by non-verbal cues.
   c. The physical appearance of the nurse rarely influences nurse-client interaction.
   d. Words convey meanings that are usually more significant than non-verbal communication.

   Answer: _____ Rationale: _____

   _____

   _____

4. The term referring to the sender's attitude toward the self, the message, and the listener is:
   a. Non-verbal communication
   b. Metacommunication
   c. Connotative meaning
   d. Denotative meaning

   Answer: _____ Rationale: _____

   _____

   _____

5. The referent in the communication process is:
   a. That which motivates the communication
   b. The means of conveying messages
   c. Information shared by the sender
   d. The person who initiates the communication

   Answer: _____ Rationale: _____

   _____

   _____

15

$\mathscr{C}$aring in Nursing Practice

Adapted by Cheryl Sams, RN, BScN, MSN,
York University & Seneca College

Preliminary Reading

Chapter 15, pp. 282-294

Comprehensive Understanding

- _____ and _____ should be a natural part of every client encounter.

Theoretical Views on Caring

- Caring in nursing has been studied from a variety of philosophical and ethical perspectives.

Caring Is Primary

- *Holism* is a concept that means _____. A nurse cares for a whole person who has

   _____, _____, _____, _____, _____, and

   _____ dimensions.

- Dr. Patricia Benner does not try to predict or control phenomena but attempts to give nurses a rich,

   holistic understanding of nursing practice and caring through the interpretation of _____.

- Briefly summarize how Benner describes the relationship among health, illness, and disease.

   _____

   _____

   _____

Caring Is Universal

- Explain Leininger's concept of care from a transcultural perspective. _____
  _____
  _____

- Define *acts of caring* according to Leininger.
  _____
  _____
  _____

- Caring, according to Leininger, is a universal phenomenon, but the expressions, processes, and patterns of caring vary among cultures.

Caring Is Transformative

- Summarize Watson's transpersonal caring theory (transformative model). _____
  _____
  _____
  _____

Caring Is Nurturing

- Swanson's theory of caring consists of five categories. Explain each.

  a. Knowing: _____
  _____

  b. Being with: _____
  _____

  c. Doing for: _____
  _____

  d. Enabling: _____
  _____

  e. Maintaining belief: _____
  _____

Summary of Theoretical Views

- Identify the common themes among the many nursing theorists. _____
  _____
  _____

Clients' Perceptions of Caring

- Establishing a _____,
  _____, and _____ are recurrent caring behaviours that researchers have identified.

- When clients sense that health care providers are interested in them as people, clients will be more willing to follow recommendations and therapeutic plans.

- The nurse needs to consider how clients perceive caring and the best approaches to providing care.

Ethic of Care

- Caring is interpreted by many as being a moral imperative.

- In any client encounter, a nurse must know what behaviour is ethically appropriate.

- Define *ethic of care*. _____
  _____
  _____

Caring in Nursing Practice

- As nurses deal with health and illness in their practice, they grow in their ability to care.

- Nurse behaviours that have been shown to be related to caring include: _____
  _____
  _____

Providing Presence

- Summarize the concept of *presence*. _____
  _____

- Identify ways a nurse can establish presence with his or her clients. _____
  _____

Touch

- The use of touch is one comforting approach whereby the nurse reaches out to clients to communicate concern and support.

- Give some examples of protective and task-oriented touch. _____
  _____
  _____

Listening

- Listening conveys the nurse's full attention and interest. Listening to the meaning of what a client says helps create a mutual relationship.

- A nurse must be able to give clients his or her full, focused attention as their stories are told.

- When an ill person chooses to tell his or her story, it involves reaching out to another human being.

- Briefly summarize Frank's view of the clinical relationship the nurse and client share. _____
  _____
  _____

- Describe what listening involves. _____
  _____
  _____
  _____

Knowing the Client

- To know a client means that the nurse _____, _____, and _____.

- Knowing the client is at the core of the process by which nurses make clinical decisions. By establishing a caring relationship, the mutuality that develops helps the nurse to better know the client as an individual and to then choose the most appropriate and efficacious nursing therapies.

- Describe the following nurses and how they differ in knowing their clients.
  a. Expert nurse: _____
     _____
  b. Novice nurse: _____
     _____

Spiritual Caring

- Spiritual health is achieved when: _____
  _____

- Spirituality offers a sense of _____,
  _____, and _____.

- When a caring relationship is established, the client and nurse come to know one another so that both move toward a healing relationship by:
  a. _____
  b. _____
  c. _____

Family Care

- Success with nursing interventions often depends on the family's willingness to_____
  _____
  _____, _____,
  _____, and _____.

- List the 10 caring behaviours that are perceived as most hopeful by families of cancer clients.
  a. _____
  b. _____
  c. _____
  d. _____
  e. _____
  f. _____
  g. _____

h. _____

i. _____

j. _____

The Challenge of Caring

- Nursing professionals can care for and assist people without medical diagnoses or new technologies and treatments.

- Caring motivates people to become nurses, and it becomes a source of satisfaction when they know they have made a difference in their clients' lives.

- Summarize the challenges facing nursing in today's health care system. _____

_____

_____

_____

ℛeview Questions

The student should select the appropriate answer and cite the rationale for choosing that particular answer.

1. Leininger's care theory states that the client's caring values and behaviours are derived largely from:
   a. Experience
   b. Gender
   c. Culture
   d. Religious beliefs

Answer: _____ Rationale: _____

_____

_____

2. The central common theme of the caring theories is:
   a. Pathophysiology and self-care abilities
   b. Compensation for client disabilities
   c. The nurse-client relationship and psychosocial aspects of care
   d. Maintenance of client homeostasis

Answer: _____ Rationale: _____

_____

_____

3. In order for the nurse to effectively listen to the client, he or she needs to:
   a. Sit with the legs crossed
   b. Lean back in the chair
   c. Respond quickly with appropriate answers to the client
   d. Maintain good eye contact

Answer: _____ Rationale: _____

_____

_____

4. The nurse demonstrates caring by:
   a. Helping family members become active participants in the care of the client
   b. Doing all the necessary tasks for the client
   c. Following all of the physician's orders accurately
   d. Maintaining a professional distance at all times

Answer: _____ Rationale: _____

_____

_____

5. Illness is best described as:
   a. A disease state that manifests as an abnormality at the cellular, tissue, or organ level
   b. An abnormal condition at the cellular, tissue, or organ level that can be acute or chronic
   c. The client's personal experience of sickness
   d. The physical experience of disease and disability

Answer: _____ Rationale: _____

_____

_____

16

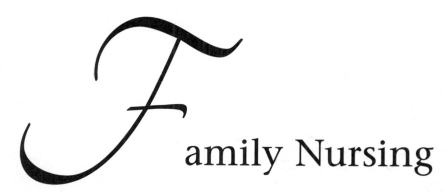

Family Nursing

Adapted by Janet C. Ross-Kerr, RN, BScN, MS, PhD, University of Alberta
Marilynn J. Wood, RN, BSN, MSN, DrPH, University of Alberta

Preliminary Reading

Chapter 16, pp. 295-314

Comprehensive Understanding

- Define the concept of family nursing. _____
  _____
  _____

- Describe the *goal* of family nursing. _____
  _____
  _____

- Define the two important attributes that characterize healthy families.
  a. Hardiness: _____
  b. Resiliency: _____

What Is a Family?

- The family can be defined as _____, or as a _____.

- To effectively provide care, nurses must understand that individual attitudes about family are deeply ingrained and deserve respect.

- To provide individualized care, the nurse must understand that families take many forms and have diverse cultural and ethnic orientations.

Current Trends in the Canadian Family

- Summarize the various family forms.

  a. Nuclear family: _____

  _____

  b. Extended family: _____

  _____

  c. Step family: _____

  _____

  d. Blended family: _____

  _____

  e. Lone-parent family: _____

  _____

  f. Other family forms: _____

  _____

- Identify at least three current trends that challenge the family.

  a. _____

  b. _____

  c. _____

- Explain the following trends and social factors that impact the structure and function of the family.

  a. Marital roles: _____

  b. Economic status: _____

  c. Family caregivers: _____

The Family and Health

- The health of the family is influenced by many factors, such as:

  a. _____

  b. _____

  c. _____

- The family's beliefs, values, and practices influence the health-promoting behaviours of its members. In turn, the health status of each individual influences how the family unit functions and its ability to achieve goals.

- Family environment is crucial because health behaviour reinforced in early life has a strong influence on later health practices.

Attributes of Healthy Families

- The crisis-proof or effective family is able to integrate the need for stability with the need for growth and change. Explain. _____

  _____

  _____

- Define *family hardiness*. _____

  _____

- Define *family resiliency*. _____

  _____

Family Nursing

- List the three things that nurses should examine when they consider how a health problem or illness affects a family and how a family affects a health problem or illness:

  a. _____

  b. _____

  c. _____

- Identify the two focuses proposed for family nursing practice. Briefly explain each.

  a. Family as context: _____

  _____

  b. Family as client: _____

  _____

Assessing the Needs of the Family: The Calgary Family Assessment Model (CFAM)

- Summarize the following three major categories of family life that the Calgary Family Assessment Model (CFAM) offers as a framework for nurses to follow when conducting family assessments.

    a. The structural dimension: _____

    b. The developmental dimension: _____

    c. The functional dimension: _____

Structural Assessment

- Explain these terms.

    a. Internal structure: _____

    b. External structure: _____

    c. Context: _____

- Explain the purpose of a genogram. _____
_____

- Explain the purpose of an ecomap. _____
_____

Developmental Assessment

- Listed below are Carter and McGoldrick's family life cycle stages. Describe the emotional process of transition associated with each stage.

    a. Between families: _____
    _____

    b. Joining of families: _____
    _____

    c. Family with young children: _____
    _____

    d. Family with adolescents: _____
    _____

    e. Launching children and moving on: _____
    _____

    f. Family in later life: _____
    _____

- What does Carter and McGoldrick's model *not* address? _____
_____

Functional Assessment

- A functional assessment focuses mainly on how family members interact and behave toward each other.

- Describe the two subcategories of family functioning.

    a. Instrumental functioning: _____
    _____

    b. Expressive functioning: _____
    _____

Family Intervention: The Calgary Family Intervention Model (CFIM)

- Describe the goal of family intervention. _____
_____

- Name the three domains of family functioning that the Calgary Family Intervention Model (CFIM) focuses on promoting and improving.

    a. _____

    b. _____

    c. _____

Asking Interventive Questions

- The practice of asking questions leads the family to reflect on their situation, clarify their opinions and ideas, and understand how they are affected by their family member's illness or condition.

- Describe the two types of interventive questions.

    a. Linear questions: _____
    _____

    b. Circular questions: _____
    _____

Offering Commendations

- Describe the meaning of a commendation and why it is important for nurses to make commendations to families. _____

  _____

  _____

- List five common family strengths.

  a. _____

  b. _____

  c. _____

  d. _____

  e. _____

Providing Information

- One of the roles nurses need to adopt is that of educator.

- Family and client needs for information may be recognized through direct questioning, but they are generally _____.

- When the nurse assumes a humble position instead of coming across as an authority on the subject, this attitude often decreases the client's _____ and invites the client to listen without feeling _____.

Validating or Normalizing Emotional Responses

- What is the purpose of validating emotional responses? _____

  _____

Encouraging Illness Narratives

- Describe an illness narrative: _____

  _____

Encouraging Family Support

- Nurses can enhance family functioning by encouraging and assisting family members to listen to each other's _____ and

  _____.

Supporting Family Caregivers

- Describe the concept of reciprocity. _____

- What are some of the benefits to reciprocity?

  _____

Encouraging Respite

- List five community resources that may be beneficial to caregivers.

  a. _____

  b. _____

  c. _____

  d. _____

  e. _____

Interviewing the Family

- When interviewing the family, the nurse must display keen perceptual, conceptual, and executive skills. Describe each of these skills in the space provided below.

  a. Perceptual skills: _____

  _____

  b. Conceptual skills: _____

  _____

  c. Executive skills: _____

  _____

- Describe the four stages of family interviewing skills for nurses using the CFAM and the CFIM.

  Stage 1: _____

  Stage 2: _____

  Stage 3: _____

  Stage 4: _____

*R*eview Questions

The student should select the appropriate answer and cite the rationale for choosing that particular answer.

1. Family functioning can best be described as:
   a. The processes that a family uses to meet its goal
   b. The way the family members communicate with each other
   c. Interrelated with family structure
   d. Adaptive behaviours that foster health

   Answer: _____ Rationale: _____
   _____
   _____

2. Family structure can best be described as:
   a. A basic pattern of predictable stages
   b. Flexible patterns that contribute to adequate functioning
   c. The pattern of relationships and ongoing membership
   d. A complex set of relationships

   Answer: _____ Rationale: _____
   _____
   _____

3. These family forms—"skip-generation" families (grandparents caring for grandchildren), "non-families" (adults living alone), and homosexual couples (with or without children)—are considered:
   a. Other family forms
   b. Blended families
   c. Extended families
   d. Step-families

   Answer: _____ Rationale: _____
   _____
   _____

4. The majority of families today:
   a. Consist of a mother, father, and one or more children
   b. Include step-children
   c. Include a mother who works outside the home
   d. Are very similar to families of the past

   Answer: _____ Rationale: _____
   _____
   _____

5. When planning care for a client and using the concept of family as client, the nurse:
   a. Considers the developmental stage of the client and not the family
   b. Realizes that cultural background is an important variable when assessing the family
   c. Includes only the client and his or her significant other
   d. Understands that the client's family will always be a help to the client's health goals

   Answer: _____ Rationale: _____
   _____
   _____

6. Interventions recommended by the Calgary Family Intervention Model include:
   a. Providing solutions for problems as they arise
   b. Validating emotional responses, encouraging illness narratives, and encouraging the client to request help from his or her family
   c. Asking interventive questions, offering commendations, providing information, and encouraging respite
   d. Administering nursing care in a manner that provides opportunity for change

   Answer: _____ Rationale: _____
   _____
   _____

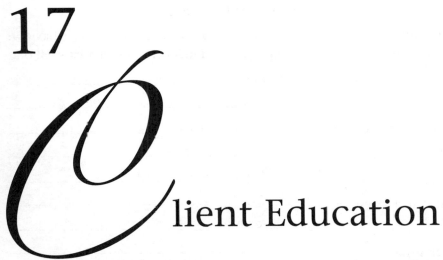

17

Client Education

Adapted by Janet C. Ross-Kerr, RN, BScN, MS, PhD,
University of Alberta

Preliminary Reading

Chapter 17, pp. 315-335

Comprehensive Understanding

Goals of Client Education

- Comprehensive client education includes which three important goals?

  a. _____

  b. _____

  c. _____

Maintaining and Promoting Health and Illness Prevention

- The nurse is a visible, competent resource for clients who are intent on improving their physical and psychological well-being. In the school, home, clinic, or workplace, the nurse provides information and skills that will allow clients to practise healthier behaviours.

- Promoting healthy behaviours through education increases self-esteem by allowing clients to assume more responsibility for their health. Greater knowledge can result in better health maintenance habits.

Restoring Health

- Injured or ill clients need information and skills that will help them regain or maintain their levels of health.

- The family is a vital part of a client's return to health, and family members may need as much information as the client.

- The nurse should not assume that the family should be involved and must first assess the client-family relationship.

Coping With Impaired Functioning

- In the case of a serious disability, the client's family role may change, making understanding and acceptance by family members necessary.

- The family's ability to provide support can result from education, which begins as soon as the client's needs are identified and the family displays a willingness to help.

Teaching and Learning

Role of the Nurse in Teaching and Learning

- The nurse has an ethical responsibility to teach his or her clients.

- The nurse clarifies information provided by physicians and may become the primary source of information for adjusting to health problems.

Teaching as Communication

- The teaching process closely parallels the communication process.

Domains of Learning

- Learning occurs in cognitive (understandings), affective (attitudes), and psychomotor (motor skills) domains.

- The characteristics of learning within each domain affect the teaching and evaluation methods used.

Cognitive Learning

- Bloom (1956) classifies cognitive behaviours in an ordered hierarchy. Summarize each one.

  a. Knowledge: _____

  _____

  b. Comprehension: _____

  _____

  c. Application: _____

  _____

  d. Analysis: _____

  _____

  e. Synthesis: _____

  _____

  f. Evaluation: _____

  _____

Affective Learning

- Affective learning deals with the expression of feelings and the acceptance of attitudes, opinions, and values.

- Summarize the following hierarchy behaviours.

  a. Receiving: _____

  _____

  b. Responding: _____

  _____

  c. Valuing: _____

  _____

  d. Organizing: _____

  _____

  e. Characterizing: _____

  _____

Psychomotor Learning

- Psychomotor learning involves acquiring skills that require the integration of mental and muscular activity.

- Summarize the following hierarchy behaviours.

  a. Perception: _____

  _____

  b. Set: _____

  _____

  c. Guided response: _____

  _____

  d. Mechanism: _____

  _____

  e. Complex overt response: _____

  _____

  f. Adaptation: _____

  _____

  g. Origination: _____

  _____

Basic Learning Principles

- Learning depends on the learning environment, the ability to learn, learning style and preferences, and the motivation to learn.

Learning Environment

- Factors in the physical environment where teaching takes place can make learning pleasant or difficult. List five factors to consider when selecting the learning setting.

  a. _____

  _____

  b. _____

  _____

  c. _____

  _____

  d. _____

  _____

  e. _____

  _____

Ability to Learn

- Summarize how each of the following influences the ability to learn.

  a. Developmental capability: _____

  _____

  b. Learning in children: _____

  _____

  c. Adult learning: _____

  _____

  d. Physical capability: _____

  _____

Learning Style and Preferences

- Everyone has different learning preferences and styles. The nurse should ask clients their preferred method for learning. In a group, the nurse should: _____

  _____

Motivation to Learn

- An *attentional set* is: _____

  _____

- Briefly explain how the following distractions influence the ability to learn.

  a. Physical discomfort: _____

  _____

  b. Anxiety: _____

  _____

  c. Environment: _____

  _____

- *Motivation* is: _____

  _____

- Briefly explain how the following can affect motivation.

  a. Social mastery: _____

  _____

  b. Task mastery: _____

  _____

  c. Physical mastery: _____

  _____

- *Compliance* is: _____

  _____

- *Self-efficacy* is: _____

  _____

Integrating the Nursing and Teaching Processes

- The nurse sets specific learning objectives and implements the teaching plan using teaching and learning principles to ensure: _____

  _____

  _____

- The nursing and teaching processes are not the same. The nursing process requires: _____

  _____

  _____

- The teaching process focuses on: _____

  _____

  _____

𝒩𝒫 Assessment

- The client requires the nurse to assess the following factors. Summarize each one.

Learning Needs

a. _____

b. _____

c. _____

d. _____

Ability to Learn

a. _____

b. _____

c. _____

Motivation to Learn

a. _____

b. _____

c. _____

d. _____

e. _____

f. _____

g. _____

h. _____

i. _____

Teaching Environment

a. _____

b. _____

c. _____

Resources for Learning

a. _____

b. _____

c. _____

d. _____

e. _____

𝒩𝒫 Nursing Diagnosis

- Classifying diagnoses by the three learning domains helps the nurse focus specifically on subject matter and teaching methods.

𝒩𝒫 Planning

- After determining the nursing diagnoses that identify a client's learning needs, the nurse develops a teaching plan, determines goals and expected outcomes, and involves the client in selecting learning experiences. Expected outcomes guide the: _____

_____

_____

- A learning objective identifies the _____ of a planned learning experience and helps _____ for learning.

- A learning objective includes the same criteria as goals or outcomes in a nursing care plan. These are:

  a. _____

  b. _____

  c. _____

  d. _____

- The principles of teaching are techniques that incorporate the principles of learning. Explain the following principles.

  a. Setting priorities: _____

  _____

  b. Timing: _____

  _____

  c. Organizing teaching material: _____

  _____

  d. Maintaining learning attention and participation: _____

  _____

  e. Building on existing knowledge: _____

  _____

  f. Selecting teaching methods: _____

  _____

  g. Selecting teaching resources: _____

  _____

  h. Writing teaching plans: _____

_____

𝒩𝒫 Implementation

- Briefly explain the following teaching approaches.

  a. Telling: _____

  _____

  b. Selling: _____

  _____

  c. Participating: _____

  _____

  d. Entrusting: _____

  _____

  e. Reinforcing: _____

  _____

- Summarize the following instructional methods.

  a. One-to-one discussion: _____

  _____

  b. Group instruction: _____

  _____

  c. Preparatory instruction: _____

  _____

  d. Demonstrations: _____

  _____

  e. Analogies: _____

  _____

  f. Role playing: _____

  _____

  g. Discovery: _____

  _____

- Identify some teaching tools to be used with the following.

  a. Functional disability: _____

  _____

Chapter 17: Client Education   83

b. Illiteracy: _____

_____

c. Cultural diversity: _____

_____

d. Children's needs: _____

_____

e. Older adults: _____

_____

Evaluation

- Evaluation reinforces correct behaviour by the learner, helps learners realize how they should change incorrect behaviour, and helps the teacher determine the adequacy of teaching.

- Identify some evaluation measures. _____

_____

_____

- List the three areas to be included when documenting client teaching.

a. _____

b. _____

c. _____

Review Questions

The student should select the appropriate answer and cite the rationale for choosing that particular answer.

1. An internal impulse that causes a person to take action is:
   a. Anxiety
   b. Motivation
   c. Compliance
   d. Adaptation

Answer: _____ Rationale: _____

_____

_____

2. Demonstration of the principles of body mechanics used when transferring clients from bed to chair would be classified under which domain of learning?
   a. Cognitive
   b. Social
   c. Psychomotor
   d. Affective

Answer: _____ Rationale: _____

_____

_____

3. Which of the following clients is most ready to begin a client-teaching session?
   a. Ms. Benoit, who is unwilling to accept that her back injury may result in permanent paralysis
   b. Mr. Chang, a newly diagnosed diabetic, who is complaining that he was awake all night because of his noisy roommate
   c. Mrs. Ho, a client with irritable bowel syndrome, who has just returned from a morning of testing in the GI lab
   d. Mr. Cinelli, a client who had a heart attack 4 days ago and now seems somewhat anxious about how this will affect his future

Answer: _____ Rationale: _____

_____

_____

4. The nurse works with pediatric clients who have diabetes. Which is the youngest age group to which the nurse can effectively teach psychomotor skills such as insulin administration?
   a. Toddler
   b. Adolescent
   c. School-age
   d. Preschool

Answer: _____ Rationale: _____

_____

_____

84   Chapter 17: Client Education

5. Which of the following is an appropriately stated learning objective for Mr. Chang, who has just been diagnosed with Type 2 Diabetes?
   a. Mr. Chang will be taught self-administration of insulin by 5/2.
   b. Mr. Chang will perform blood glucose monitoring with the EZ-Check Monitor by the time of discharge.
   c. Mr. Chang will know the signs and symptoms of low blood sugar by 5/5.

Answer: _____ Rationale: _____

_____

_____

18

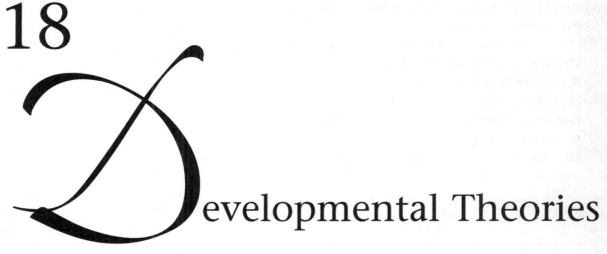

Developmental Theories

Adapted by Jane Drummond, RN, PhD, University of Alberta
Lenora Marcellus, RN, PhD (candidate), University of Victoria

Preliminary Reading

Chapter 18, pp. 336-355

Comprehensive Understanding

Growth and Development

- Define *growth*. *a measurable aspect of person life*

- Define *development*. *progression + continually change*

Factors Influencing Growth and Development

- Identify the major factors influencing growth and development.

  a. *genetic*
  b. *environment*
  c. *interaction*

Traditions of Developmental Theories

- Explain briefly the five traditions of developmental theories.
  a. Organicism: _____
  _____
  b. Psychoanalytic/psychosocial: _____
  _____
  c. Mechanistic: _____
  _____
  d. Contextualism: _____
  _____
  e. Dialecticism: _____
  _____

Biophysical Developmental Theories

- Briefly summarize Gesell's theory. _____
  _____

- Identify and describe the mechanisms of Gesell's theory.
  a. _____
  b. _____

- Briefly describe Chess and Thomas's theory of temperament development._____
  _____

- Identify and describe the three categories of temperament in Chess and Thomas's theory.
  a. _____
  _____
  b. _____
  _____
  c. _____
  _____

- Identify and describe the mechanisms of Thomas and Chess's theory. _____
  _____

Cognitive Developmental Theories

- Briefly summarize Piaget's theory of cognitive development._____
  _____

- Identify and describe the mechanisms of Piaget's theory.
  a. _____
  b. _____

- Explain the four stages of Piaget's theory of cognitive development.
  a. Sensorimotor: _____
  _____
  b. Preoperational: _____
  _____
  c. Concrete operations:_____
  _____
  d. Formal operations:_____
  _____

Moral Developmental Theories

- Moral developmental theories try to explain
  _____

- Explain the three stages of Piaget's moral development theory.
  a. Premoral stage: _____
  _____
  b. Conventional stage: _____
  _____
  c. Autonomous stage: _____
  _____

- Explain the following six stages of Kohlberg's moral development theory:

Level I: Pre-conventional level

Stage 1: _____

Stage 2: _____

Level II: Conventional level

Stage 3: _____

Stage 4: _____

Level III: Post-conventional level

Stage 5: _____

Stage 6: _____

- Identify the limitations to Kohlberg's research.

_____

_____

- Briefly explain Gilligan's argument against Kohlberg's theory._____

_____

Psychoanalytic/Psychosocial Tradition

- Briefly summarize Freud's theory of psychoanalytic development. _____

_____

- Identify and describe the mechanisms of Freud's theory.

  a. _____

  b. _____

  c. _____

- Explain the five stages of Freud's theory.

  a. _____

  b. _____

  c. _____

  d. _____

  e. _____

- Briefly summarize Erikson's theory of psychosocial development. _____

_____

_____

- Identify and describe the mechanisms of Erikson's theory.

  a. _____

  b. _____

- Explain the following eight stages of Erikson's theory.

  a. Trust versus mistrust: _____

  _____

  b. Autonomy versus shame and doubt: _____

  _____

  c. Initiative versus guilt: _____

  _____

  d. Industry versus inferiority: _____

  _____

  e. Identity versus role confusion: _____

  _____

  f. Intimacy versus isolation: _____

  _____

  g. Generativity versus stagnation: _____

  _____

  h. Integrity versus despair: _____

  _____

- Briefly summarize Havighurst's theory of development. _____

_____

_____

- Explain the following three stages of Havighurst's theory.

  a. Early adulthood: _____

  _____

  b. Middle age: _____

  _____

  c. Later maturity: _____

  _____

- Identify a limitation to Havighurst's theory.

  _____

  _____

  _____

- Havighurst defined a series of essential tasks that arise from predictable and external pressures. These pressures include _____, _____, and _____.

- Briefly summarize Gould's five themes of Adult Development.

  a. _____
  b. _____
  c. _____
  d. _____
  e. _____

Contextualism

Urie Bronfenbrenner

- Briefly summarize Bronfenbrenner's theory of bioecological development. _____

  _____

  _____

- Identify and describe the mechanisms of Bronfenbrenner's theory. _____

  _____

- Explain the four layers of environment in Bronfenbrenner's theory.

  a. _____
  b. _____
  c. _____
  d. _____

Dialecticism

Keating and Hertzman's Population Health Theory

- Briefly summarize Keating and Hertzman's population health approach. _____

  _____

  _____

- Identify and describe the mechanisms of Keating and Hertzman's theory.

  a. _____
  b. _____
  c. _____

Resilience Theory

- Briefly describe the resilience approach to development. _____

  _____

  _____

- Identify and describe the mechanisms of resilience theory.

  a. _____
  b. _____

$\mathcal{R}$eview Questions

The student should select the appropriate answer and cite the rationale for choosing that particular answer.

1. According to Piaget, the school-age child is in the third stage of cognitive development, which is characterized by:
   a. Conventional thought
   b. Concrete operations
   c. Identity versus role diffusion
   d. Post-conventional thought

   Answer: _____ Rationale: _____
   _____
   _____

2. According to Bronfenbrenner's developmental theory, the individual and their environment are seen as mutually influential. Development of a national child care policy is an example of an intervention at which level?
   a. Microsystem
   b. Mesosystem
   c. Exosystem
   d. Macrosystem

   Answer: _____ Rationale: _____
   _____
   _____

3. According to Erikson's developmental theory, the primary developmental task of the middle years is to:
   a. Achieve generativity
   b. Achieve intimacy
   c. Establish a set of personal values
   d. Establish a sense of personal identity

   Answer: _____ Rationale: _____
   _____
   _____

4. Which of the following behaviours is most characteristic of the concrete operations stage of cognitive development?
   a. Progression from reflex activity to imitative behaviour
   b. Inability to put oneself in another's place
   c. Thought processes become increasingly logical and coherent
   d. Ability to think in abstract terms and draw logical conclusions

   Answer: _____ Rationale: _____
   _____
   _____

5. According to Kohlberg, children develop moral reasoning as they mature. Which of the following is most characteristic of a preschooler's stage of moral development?
   a. Obeying the rules of correct behaviour
   b. Showing respect for authority is important behaviour
   c. Behaviour that pleases others is considered good
   d. Actions are determined as good or bad in terms of their consequences

   Answer: _____ Rationale: _____
   _____
   _____

19

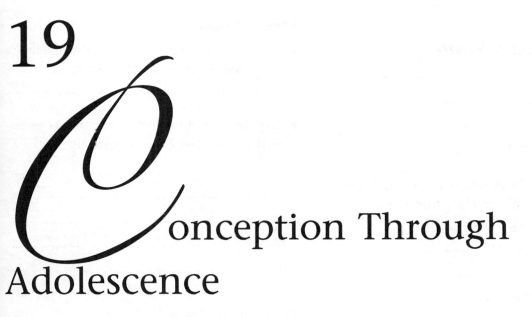

Conception Through Adolescence

Adapted by Shirley Solberg, BN, MN, PhD, Memorial University of Newfoundland

Preliminary Reading

Chapter 19, pp. 356-396

Comprehensive Understanding

- Human growth and development are continuous, intricate, and complex processes that are often divided into stages organized by age groups.

- Providing nursing care that is developmentally appropriate is easier when planning on a theoretical framework.

- A developmental approach encourages organized care directed at the child's current level of functioning to motivate self-direction and health promotion.

Conception

Intrauterine Life

- Define the following terms/events.
  a. Nagele's rule: _Count 3 months back + 7 days from period._
  b. Fertilization: _Sperm penatrates the ovum + unite_

c. Zygote: _diploid (diploid cell)_

d. Morula: _Solid mass of cells (32 cells)_

e. Blastocyst: _Center cavity of morula_

f. Embryo: _____

g. Placenta: _____

h. Implantation: _____

- Explain the development process and health concerns for the following trimesters.

  a. *First trimester*

  Physical changes: _____

  _____

  Health promotion: _____

  _____

  Teratogens: _____

  _____

  b. *Second trimester*

  Physical changes: _____

  _____

  Health promotion: _____

  _____

  c. *Third trimester*

  Physical changes: _____

  _____

  Health promotion: _____

  _____

  Cognitive changes: _____

  _____

  Psychosocial changes: _____

  _____

Transition From Intrauterine to Extrauterine Life

- _____, _____, and _____ influence adjustment to the external environment.

Physical Changes

- An immediate assessment of the neonate's condition is performed because the first concern is the _____

- List the five physiological parameters evaluated through the Apgar assessment.

  a. _____

  b. _____

  c. _____

  d. _____

  e. _____

Psychosocial Changes

- Which two factors are most important in promoting closeness of the parents and neonate?

  a. _____

  b. _____

- Define *bonding*. _____

  _____

Health Risks

- Briefly explain the three most important physical needs of the newborn.

  a. Airway: _____

  b. Temperature: _____

  c. Prevention of infection: _____

Newborn

- The *neonatal period* is defined as: _____

  _____

Physical Changes

- Identify the normal characteristics of the newborn.

  a. Height: _____

  b. Weight: _____

  c. Head circumference: _____

92   Chapter 19: Conception Through Adolescence

d. Vital signs: _____

e. Physical characteristics: _____

f. Neurological function: _____

g. Behavioural characteristics: _____

Cognitive Changes

- Early cognitive development begins with innate behaviour, reflexes, and sensory functions.

- Identify the sensory functions that contribute to cognitive development in the newborn. _____
_____

Psychosocial Changes

- Explain the interactions that foster deep attachment between the infant and parents. _____
_____

Health Risks

- Define *hyperbilirubinemia*. _jandise_

Health Concerns

- Screening for inborn errors of metabolism applies to: _____
_____

- Circumcision is a common and controversial procedure. Identify the risks and benefits of this procedure.

a. Risks: _____
_____

b. Benefits: _____
_____

Infant

- Infancy is the period from _____ to
_____.

Physical Changes

- Summarize the normal characteristics of the infant.

a. Physical growth: _____

b. Vital signs: _____

c. Gross motor skills: _____

d. Fine motor skills: _____

Cognitive Changes

- Summarize the cognitive development of an infant. _____
_____

Psychosocial Changes

- During the first year, infants begin to differentiate themselves from others as separate beings capable of acting on their own.

- Erikson describes the psychosocial developmental crisis for the infant as trust versus mistrust.

- Define *play*. _____
_____

- Identify activities appropriate at this stage of development. _____
_____

Health Risks

- Identify the common types of injury and possible prevention strategies. _____
_____

- Child maltreatment includes: _____
_____

Health Concerns

- The foundation for children's perceptions of their health status is laid early in life.

- Internal body sensations and experiences with the outside world affect self-perceptions.

- The quality of nutrition influences the infant's growth and development.

- Identify the feeding alternatives for an infant.

  _____

  _____

- Identify some supplementation needs of an infant. _____

  _____

- Briefly explain health concerns related to the following.

  a. Dentition: _____

  b. Immunizations: _____

  c. Sleep: _____

  d. Overfeeding: _____

Toddler

- Toddlerhood ranges from _____ to _____.

Physical Changes

- Summarize the normal characteristics of the toddler.

  a. Self-care activities: _____

  b. Motor skills: _____

  c. Vital signs: _____

  d. Head circumference: _____

  e. Weight: _____

  f. Height: _____

  g. Physiological anorexia: _____

Cognitive Changes

- Summarize Piaget's preoperational thought stage. _____

  _____

- Describe language ability at this stage. _____

  _____

Psychosocial Changes

- Identify Erikson's psychosocial development stage. _____

  _____

- Explain the parental implications of the following developmental states.

  a. Independence: _____

  b. Social interactions: _____

  c. Play: _____

Health Risks

- Describe some developmental abilities for this age period. _____

  _____

- Identify injury prevention strategies. _____

  _____

Health Concerns

- Children increasingly recognize internal body sensations but have difficulty pinpointing their location.

- Children who deviate radically from their usual patterns of eating, sleeping, or playing require assessment to determine whether these alterations result from illness.

- Children begin to internalize the labels that parents or health care professionals give to the somatic stages.

- Briefly explain the nutrition requirements for this age group. _____

  _____

Preschooler

- The preschool period refers to _____.

Physical Changes

- Summarize the normal characteristics of the preschooler.

  a. Vital signs: _____

  b. Weight: _____

  c. Height: _____

  d. Coordination: _____

Cognitive Changes

- Preschoolers continue to master the preoperational stage of cognition.

- The first phase of this period (2 to 4 years) is characterized by _____.

- Define *artificialism*. _____
  _____

- Define *animism*. _____
  _____

- Summarize the intuitive phase of preconceptional thought (4 years). _____
  _____

- The greatest fear of this age-group is: _____
  _____

- Summarize this group's moral development.
  _____
  _____

- Describe the language ability for this age group. _____
  _____

Psychosocial Changes

- The preschooler's world expands beyond the family into the neighbourhood where they meet other children and adults.

- Identify some dependent behaviours that preschoolers may revert to during stress or illness. _____

- Summarize the pattern of play for the preschooler. _____
  _____

Health Risks

- Guidelines for injury prevention in the toddler also apply to the preschooler. _____ and _____ are the top priorities for this age group.

Health Concerns

- Parental beliefs about health, children's bodily sensations, and the ability to perform daily activities help children develop attitudes about their health.

- Explain health concerns related to the following for this group.

  a. Nutrition: _____

  b. Sleep: _____

  c. Vision: _____

School-Age Child

- The school-age years range from _____ to _____.

- _____ signals the end of middle childhood.

- The school and home influence growth and development, and adjustments by the parents and child are required.

- Parents must learn to allow their child to make decisions, accept responsibility, and learn from life's experiences.

Physical Changes

- Summarize the normal characteristics of the school-age child.

  a. Weight: _____

  b. Height: _____

  c. Cardiovascular functioning: _____

  d. Neuromuscular functioning: _____

  e. Skeletal growth: _____

Cognitive Changes

- Cognitive changes provide the school-age child with the ability to think in a logical manner about the here and now. They are not yet capable of abstract thinking.

- Define the cognitive skills that are developing in this group. _____ _____

- Describe the language development during middle childhood. _____ _____

Psychosocial Changes

- The developmental task for school-age children is _____ versus _____ .

- Summarize psychosocial development in relation to the following.

  a. Moral development: _____

  b. Peer relationships: _____

  c. Sexual identity: _____

Health Risks

- _____ and _____ are the leading causes of death or injury.

- Infections account for the majority of all childhood illnesses; respiratory infections are the most prevalent.

- Identify the specific health concerns of children living in poverty. _____ _____

Health Concerns

- Perception of wellness is based on _____ .

- Identify five critical functions of a school-based health promotion program.

  a. _____

  b. _____

  c. _____

  d. _____

  e. _____

- Accidents are the leading cause of death and injury in the school-age period. Children should be encouraged to take responsibility for their own safety.

- Identify at least five health promotion activities that are appropriate for the school-age child.

  a. _____

  b. _____

  c. _____

  d. _____

  e. _____

- Identify the nutritional requirements for the school-age child. _____ _____

Adolescent

- Adolescence is the period of development _____

- Define *puberty*, and explain the changes that occur at this time. _____ _____

Physical Changes

- List the four major physical changes associated with sexual maturation.

  a. _____

  b. _____

  c. _____

  d. _____

- Summarize the weight and skeletal changes that occur during adolescence. _____
  _____

- The hormones responsible for the development of secondary sex characteristics are
  _____ and _____.

- Explain the effects of physical changes on peer interactions. _____
  _____

Cognitive Changes

- Changes that occur within the mind and the widening social environment of the adolescent result in _____, the highest level of intellectual development.

- During this period of cognitive development, the adolescent develops the ability to solve problems through logical operations.

- For the first time, the young person can move beyond the physical or concrete properties of a situation and use reasoning powers to understand the abstract.

- Briefly explain the cognitive abilities of this group. _____
  _____

- Describe the language skills of the adolescent.
  _____
  _____

Psychosocial Changes

- The search for _____ is the major task of adolescent psychosocial development.

- Teenagers must establish close peer relationships or remain socially isolated.

- Explain identity versus role confusion Erikson.

- Behaviours indicating negative resolution are
  _____ and _____.

- Explain the following components of total identity.

  a. Sexual identity: _____

  b. Group identity: _____

  c. Family identity: _____

  d. Vocational identity: _____

  e. Health identity: _____

  f. Moral identity: _____

Health Risks

- Identify the leading cause of death and its sources among adolescents. _____
  _____

- _____ is the second leading cause of death.

- Suicide is the third leading cause of death among adolescents. List the six warning signs of suicide for this group.

  a. _____

  b. _____

  c. _____

  d. _____

  e. _____

  f. _____

- Substance abuse is a major concern. Adolescents at risk are _____.

- In forming healthy habits of daily living, emphasis is on exercise, sleep, nutrition, and stress reduction.

- Define the two eating disorders that follow.

    a. *Anorexia nervosa:* _____

    _____

    b. *Bulimia nervosa:* _____

    _____

- _____

    _____ and _____ expectations contribute to early heterosexual and homosexual relations.

- Briefly explain the two prominent consequences of adolescent sexual activity.

    a. Sexually transmitted infection (STI): _____

    _____

    b. Pregnancy: _____

    _____

- Identify health promotion interventions for the adolescent in regard to the following.

    a. Unintentional injuries: _____

    b. Substance abuse: _____

    c. Sexual activity: _____

Health Concerns

- Identify the health concerns of the following.

    a. Rural adolescents: _____

    b. Minority adolescents: _____

    c. Aboriginal adolescents: _____

Review Questions

The student should select the appropriate answer and cite the rationale for choosing that particular answer.

1. Which statement about human growth and development is accurate?
    a. Growth and development processes are unpredictable.
    b. Growth and development begins with birth and ends after adolescence.
    c. All individuals progress through the same phases of growth and development.
    d. All individuals accomplish developmental tasks at the same pace.

Answer: _____ Rationale: _____

_____

_____

2. The mother of a 2-year-old expresses concern that her son's appetite has diminished and that he seems to prefer milk to other solid foods. Which response by the nurse reflects knowledge of principles of communication and nutrition?
    a. "Oh, I wouldn't be too worried; children tend to eat when they're hungry. I just wouldn't give him dessert unless he eats his meal."
    b. "That is not uncommon in toddlers. You might consider increasing his milk to 2 litres per day to be sure he gets enough nutrients."
    c. "Have you considered feeding him when he doesn't seem interested in feeding himself?"
    d. "A toddler's rate of growth normally slows down. It's common to see a toddler's appetite diminish in response to decreased calorie needs."

Answer: _____ Rationale: _____

_____

_____

3. Which neonatal assessment finding would be considered abnormal?
   a. Cyanosis of the hands and feet during activity
   b. Palpable anterior and posterior fontanels
   c. Soft, protuberant abdomen
   d. Absence of the rooting, grasping, and sucking reflexes

Answer: _____ Rationale: _____

_____

_____

4. To stimulate cognitive and psychosocial development of the toddler, it is important for parents to:
   a. Set firm and consistent limits
   b. Foster sharing of toys with playmates and siblings
   c. Provide clarification about what is right and wrong
   d. Limit confusion by restricting exploration of the environment

Answer: _____ Rationale: _____

_____

_____

5. Which of the following is true of the developmental behaviours of school-age children?
   a. Formal and informal peer group membership is the key in forming self-esteem.
   b. Fears centre on the loss of self-control.
   c. Positive feedback from parents and teachers is crucial to development.
   d. A full range of defence mechanisms is used including rationalization and intellectualization.

Answer: _____ Rationale: _____

_____

_____

6. Adolescents have mastered age-appropriate sexuality when they feel comfortable with their sexual:
   a. Behaviours
   b. Choices
   c. Relationships
   d. All of the above

Answer: _____ Rationale: _____

_____

_____

20

Young to Middle Adult

Adapted by Marion Clauson, RN, MSN, PNC(C),
University of British Columbia

Preliminary Reading

Chapter 20, pp. 397-412

Comprehensive Understanding

- Young adulthood is the period from _____ to _____.

- Individuals in young adulthood _____, _____, and _____.

- Middle age occurs from _____ to _____.

- Transition into middle age may include changes in _____, _____, and _____.

- Briefly describe the characteristics of the mature adult. _____
  _____

Young Adult

Physical Changes

- The young adult has completed physical growth by the age of 20, with the exception of _____ or _____.

- Identify the main components of a personal lifestyle assessment of a young adult. _____ _____

Cognitive Changes

- Briefly explain the cognitive development of young adults in relation to educational, life, and occupational experiences. _____ _____

Psychosocial Changes

- The emotional health of the young adult is related to the individual's ability to address and resolve personal and social tasks. Explain the patterns of change that are common in the following age groups:

    a. 23 to 28 years: _____

    b. 29 to 34 years: _____

    c. 35 to 43 years: _____

- Briefly explain the types of decisions that a young adult needs to make in the following areas.

    a. Lifestyle: _____

    b. Career: _____

    c. Sexuality: _____

    d. Marriage: _____

    e. Childbearing: _____

- Identify five tasks to be completed by a couple prior to marriage.

    a. _____

    b. _____

    c. _____

    d. _____

    e. _____

- Identify six major tasks of adulthoood.

    a. _____

    b. _____

    c. _____

    d. _____

    e. _____

    f. _____

- Identify the changing norms and values in Canada related to alternative family structures. _____ _____

- Identify the aspects of emotional health that would be included in a psychosocial assessment of the young adult. _____ _____

Health Risk

- Briefly explain the risk factors for young adults in regard to the following.

    a. Family history: _____

    b. Accidental death and injury: _____

    c. Substance abuse: _____

    d. Unplanned pregnancies: _____

    e. Sexually transmitted diseases: _____

    f. Environmental and occupational risks: _____

Health Concerns

- Give examples of nursing assessment and interventions for young adults related to the following areas of health.

    a. Health promotion: _____

    b. Exercise: _____

    c. Infertility: _____

    d. Routine health screening: _____

- The psychosocial concerns of the young adult are often related to stress. Briefly explain each of the following sources of stress.

    a. Job stress: _____

    b. Family stress: _____

Pregnancy

- Explain the health practices that the nurse would discuss with a woman anticipating pregnancy. _____

  _____

  _____

  _____

- Prenatal care is _____

- Explain the physiological changes that occur during pregnancy, and the puerperium.

  a. First trimester: _____

  b. Second trimester: _____

  c. Third trimester: _____

  d. Puerperium: _____

- Explain each of the following changes occurring during pregnancy.

  a. Sensory perception: _____

  b. Psychosocial changes: _____

- Describe the educational needs of childbearing families. _____

  _____

- Provide examples of when acute care might be required for young adults. _____

  _____

- Describe the effect of chronic illness and disability on the young adult. _____

  _____

Middle Adult

- Briefly explain the characteristics of the middle adult years. _____

  _____

Physical Changes

- Briefly explain the major physiological changes that occur between 30 and 65 years of age.

  _____

  _____

- Define *menopause*. _____

  _____

Psychosocial Changes

- Summarize the psychosocial development of the middle adult in the following areas.

  a. Career transition: _____

  _____

  b. Sexuality: _____

  _____

  c. Singlehood: _____

  _____

  d. Marital changes: _____

  _____

  e. Family transitions: _____

  _____

  f. Care of aging parents: _____

  _____

- Define *sandwich generation*. _____

  _____

Health Concerns

- Briefly explain each of the following physiological concerns for the middle adult, and suggest appropriate nursing assessment and interventions.

  a. Stress: _____

  _____

  b. Health habits: _____

  _____

  c. Obesity: _____

  _____

- Summarize two psychosocial concerns of the middle adult and provide the appropriate nursing assessment and interventions.

  a. Anxiety: _____

  _____

  b. Depression: _____

  _____

- Community health programs for the middle adults are designed to _____,
  _____ and _____.

Acute Care

- Identify examples of acute illnesses and injuries that occur in middle adulthood. _____

  _____

Restorative and Continuing Care

- Identify some chronic illnesses and/or issues that occur in middle adulthood. _____

  _____

Review Questions

The student should select the appropriate answer and cite the rationale for choosing that particular answer.

1. The greatest cause of illness and death in the young adult population is:
   a. Sexually transmitted infection
   b. Accidents
   c. Cardiovascular disease
   d. Substance abuse

   Answer: _____ Rationale: _____

   _____

   _____

2. Psychosocial changes of pregnancy commonly involve all of the following areas except:
   a. Altered body image
   b. Anxiety and depression
   c. Ambivalence about becoming a parent
   d. Changes in sexual desire

   Answer: _____ Rationale: _____

   _____

   _____

3. Which physiological change would be a normal assessment finding in a middle adult?
   a. Increased breast size
   b. Abdominal tenderness
   c. Increased thoracic diameter
   d. Reduced auditory acuity

   Answer: _____ Rationale: _____

   _____

   _____

4. Which of the following is most likely to affect the overall level of health of a client in middle adulthood?
   a. Stress due to life changes
   b. Decreased visual acuity
   c. Declining sexual interest
   d. Onset of menopause

   Answer: _____ Rationale: _____

   _____

   _____

5. In planning client education for Mrs. Higuchi, a 45-year-old woman who had an ovarian cyst removed, which of the following facts is true about the sexuality of the middle-aged adult?
   a. Menstruation ceases after menopause.
   b. Estrogen is produced after menopause.
   c. Her middle-aged husband is unable to produce fertile sperm.
   d. With removal of the ovarian cyst, pregnancy cannot occur.

   Answer: _____ Rationale: _____

   _____

   _____

21

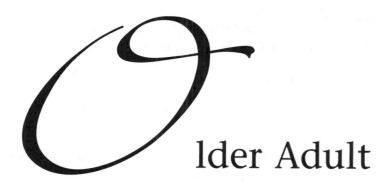

$\mathcal{O}$lder Adult

Adapted by Wendy Duggleby, DSN, RN, AOCN,
University of Saskatchewan

$\mathcal{P}$reliminary Reading

Chapter 21, pp. 413-438

$\mathcal{C}$omprehensive Understanding

- Briefly summarize demographic trends of older Canadians. _____
  _____

Variability Among Older Adults

- Briefly explain the challenges of the older adult.
  - a. Physiological: _____
  - b. Cognitive: _____
  - c. Psychosocial: _____

- Explain the following terminology:
  - a. Geriatrics: _____
  - b. Gerontology: _____
  - c. Gerontological nursing: _____
  - d. Gerotonic nursing: _____

Myths and Stereotypes

- Identify at least five myths and/or stereotypes regarding the older adult. _____

  _____

  _____

  _____

- Define *ageism*. _____

  _____

Nurses' Attitudes Toward Older Adults

- The attitude of the nurse toward older adults comes in part from _____,

  _____, _____, and

  _____.

Theories of Aging

- Give a brief description of the following biological theories.

  a. Stochastic theories: _____

  _____

  b. Non-stochastic theories: _____

  _____

- Describe the three classic psychosocial theories of aging. _____

  _____

  _____

  _____

Developmental Tasks for Older Adults

- List the seven developmental tasks of the older adult.

  a. _____

  b. _____

  c. _____

d. _____

e. _____

f. _____

g. _____

Community-Based and Institutional Health Care Services

- Briefly describe the following health services that are used by the older population.

  a. Retirement communities: _____

  _____

  b. Home care: _____

  _____

  c. Day care: _____

  _____

  d. Respite care: _____

  _____

  e. Long-term care: _____

  _____

Assessing the Needs of Older Adults

- Nurses need to take into account five key points to ensure an age-specific approach.

  a. _____

  b. _____

  c. _____

  d. _____

  e. _____

- List some techniques to use for the older adult with visual impairments.

  a. _____

  b. _____

  c. _____

- List some techniques to use with the older adult with hearing impairment.

  a. _____

  b. _____

  c. _____

  d. _____

Physiological Changes

- Identify the physiological changes that occur in the older adult with regard to the following.

  a. General survey: _____

  b. Integumentary system: _____

  c. Head and neck: _____

  d. Thorax and lungs: _____

  e. Heart and vascular system: _____

  f. Breasts: _____

  g. Gastrointestinal system and abdomen:

  _____

  h. Reproductive system: _____

  i. Urinary system: _____

  j. Musculoskeletal system: _____

  k. Neurological system: _____

Cognitive Changes

- The structural and physiological changes that occur in the brain during aging do not necessarily affect adaptive and functional abilities.

- Define:

  a. Dementia: _____

  b. Delirium: _____

  c. Depression: _____

- Describe major differences between dementia, delirium, and depression. _____

  _____

  _____

- Identify the characteristic progressive symptoms of Alzheimer's disease.

  a. _____

  b. _____

  c. _____

Psychosocial Changes

- Identify at least five areas that should be addressed when counselling an older adult about retirement.

  a. _____

  b. _____

  c. _____

  d. _____

  e. _____

- Briefly explain some of the reasons older adults experience social isolation. _____

  _____

- Briefly describe the sexual changes that occur in the older adult. _____

  _____

- List four factors to assess when assisting older adults with housing needs.

  a. _____

  b. _____

  c. _____

  d. _____

- A common misconception is that the death of an older adult is a blessing and the culmination of a full life.

- Many dying older adults still have goals and are not emotionally prepared to die.

Addressing the Health Concerns of Older Adults

- The three most common causes of death in the older adult are _____, _____, and _____.

- Health Canada's National Advisory Committee on Aging lists 10 factors to improve the health of older Canadians.

  a. _____
  b. _____
  c. _____
  d. _____
  e. _____
  f. _____
  g. _____
  h. _____
  i. _____
  j. _____

Health Promotion and Maintenance: Physiological Concerns

- Summarize the physiological health concerns related to each of the following.

  a. Heart disease: _____
  b. Cancer: _____
  c. Stroke: _____
  d. Smoking: _____
  e. Alcohol abuse: _____
  f. Nutrition: _____
  g. Dental problems: _____
  h. Exercise: _____
  i. Arthritis: _____
  j. Falls: _____
  k. Sensory impairments: _____
  l. Pain: _____
  m. Medication use: _____

- Briefly explain the age-related changes affecting drug therapy in adults over the age of 65.

  _____
  _____

Health Promotion and Maintenance: Psychosocial Health Concerns

- Briefly describe the interventions used to maintain the psychosocial health of the older adult.

  a. Therapeutic communication: _____
  b. Touch: _____
  c. Reality orientation: _____
  d. Validation therapy: _____
  e. Reminiscence: _____
  f. Body-image interventions: _____

Older Adults and the Acute Care Setting

- Older adults in the acute care setting are at increased risk for adverse events such as:

  _____, _____, _____, _____, _____, and _____.

- Explain why the older adult is at risk for each of the following.

  a. Delirium: _____
  b. Dehydration: _____
  c. Malnutrition: _____
  d. Nosocomial infections: _____
  e. Urinary incontinence: _____
  f. Falls: _____

Older Adults and Restorative Care

- Summarize the two types of ongoing care for the older adult and identify the focus of each.

  _____
  _____

Review Questions

The student should select the appropriate answer and cite the rationale for choosing that particular answer.

1. Which statement about older adults is accurate?
   a. Older adults are institutionalized.
   b. Most older adults live on a fixed income.
   c. Most older adults cannot learn to care for themselves.
   d. Most older adults have no sexual desire.

   Answer: _____ Rationale: _____
   _____
   _____

2. Which statement describing *delirium* is correct?
   a. Persons with delirium may experience delusions and hallucinations.
   b. The onset of delirium is slow and insidious.
   c. Symptoms of delirium are stable and unchanging.
   d. Symptoms of delirium are irreversible.

   Answer: _____ Rationale: _____
   _____
   _____

3. Nutritional needs of the older adult:
   a. Are exactly the same as those of young and middle adults
   b. Include increased amounts of vitamin C, vitamin A, and calcium
   c. Include increased kilocalories to support metabolism and activity
   d. Include increased proteins and carbohydrates

   Answer: _____ Rationale: _____
   _____
   _____

4. Ms. Dale states that she does not need the TV turned on because she cannot see very well. Normal visual changes in older adults include all of the following *except:*
   a. Decreased visual acuity
   b. Decreased accommodation to darkness
   c. Double vision
   d. Sensitivity to glare

   Answer: _____ Rationale: _____
   _____
   _____

5. Mr. DeLonghi states that he is worried about his parents' plans to retire. All of the following would be appropriate responses regarding retirement of the older adult, *except:*
   a. Positive adjustment is often related to how much a person planned for the retirement.
   b. Retirement for most persons represents a sudden shock that is irreversibly damaging to self-image and self-esteem.
   c. Reactions to retirement are influenced by the importance that has been attached to the work role.
   d. Retirement may affect an individual's physical and psychological functioning.

   Answer: _____ Rationale: _____
   _____
   _____

22

*S*elf-Concept

Adapted by Judee E. Onyskiw, RN, PhD,
University of New Brunswick

*P*reliminary Reading

Chapter 22, pp. 439-461

*C*omprehensive Understanding

Scientific Knowledge Base

- Each stage of development has specific activities that assist the client in developing a positive self-concept. Identify some activities for each stage.

    a. 0 to 1 year: _____

    b. 1 to 3 years: _____

    c. 3 to 6 years: _____

    d. 6 to 12 years: _____

    e. 12 to 20 years: _____

    f. Mid-20s to mid-40s: _____

    g. Mid-40s to mid-60s: _____

    h. Late 60s on: _____

Nursing Knowledge Base

Development of Self-Concept

- The four components of self-concept are _____, _____, _____, and

    _____.

- Self-concept is a dynamic perception that is based on the following:

  a. _____

  b. _____

  c. _____

  d. _____

  e. _____

  f. _____

  g. _____

  h. _____

  i. _____

  j. _____

  k. _____

  l. _____

- A healthy self-concept has a high degree of stability and generates positive or negative feelings toward the self.

Components and Interrelated Terms of Self-Concept

- Briefly explain the four significant components of self-concept.

  a. Identity: _____

  b. Body image: _____

  c. Self-esteem: _____

  d. Role performance: _____

- List the processes through which a child learns appropriate behaviours.

  a. _____

  b. _____

  c. _____

  d. _____

  e. _____

Stressors Affecting Self-Concept

- Stressors challenge a person's adaptive capacities.

- A self-concept stressor is any _____
  _____.

- Being able to adapt to stressors is likely to lead to a positive sense of self, whereas failure to adapt often leads to a negative sense of self.

- Any change in health can be a stressor that affects self-concept.

- A physical change in the body leads to an altered body image. Identity and self-esteem can also be affected.

- A crisis occurs when a person cannot overcome obstacles with the usual methods of problem solving and adapting.

- *Identity* is defined as: _____

- Stressors throughout life affect identity. Give an example of a stressor for each developmental stage.

  a. Adolescence: _____

  b. Adulthood: _____

  c. Retirement: _____

- Changes in the appearance, structure, or function of a body part will require change in body image. Identify at least five stressors that affect body image.

  a. _____

  b. _____

  c. _____

  d. _____

  e. _____

- Transitions within one's roles may lead to the following. Explain:

  a. Role conflict: _____
  _____

  b. Role ambiguity: _____
  _____

c. Role strain: _____

_____

d. Role overload: _____

_____

Family Effect on Self-Concept Development

- The family plays a key role in creating and maintaining its members' self-concepts.

- Children learn from their parents and siblings a basic sense of who they are and how they are expected to live.

The Nurse's Effect on the Client's Self-Concept

- A nurse's acceptance of a client with an altered self-concept helps stimulate positive rehabilitation.

- List five areas the nurses must clarify and assess about themselves in order to promote a positive self-concept in clients.

  a. _____

  b. _____

  c. _____

  d. _____

  e. _____

Self-Concept and the Nursing Process

𝒩𝒫 Assessment

- In assessing self-concept, the nurse should focus on each component of self-concept; behaviours suggestive of _____; actual and potential self-concept _____; and _____ patterns.

- Much of the data regarding self-concept are most effectively gathered through observation of a client's non-verbal behaviour and by paying attention to the content of the client's conversation rather than through direct questioning.

- The nursing assessment should include consideration of previous coping behaviours: the _____, _____, and _____ of the stressors; and the client's _____ and _____ resources.

- As the nurse identifies previous coping patterns, it is useful to consider if these patterns have contributed to healthy functioning or created more problems.

- Exploring resources and strengths, such as helpful significant others or prior use of community resources, can be important in formulating a realistic and effective plan.

- Asking the client how he or she believes interventions will make a difference in the problem can provide useful information regarding the client's expectations and can provide an opportunity to discuss the client's goals. Give an example. _____

_____

_____

𝒩𝒫 Nursing Diagnosis

- Accurate development of a nursing diagnosis requires discussing the problem with the client and the family.

𝒩𝒫 Planning

- The nurse, client, and family need to plan care directed at helping the client regain or maintain a healthy self-concept.

- Interventions focus on helping the client and on coping methods.

- The nurse looks for strengths in both the individual and the family and provides resources and education to turn limitations into strengths.

- Before involving the family, the nurse needs to consider the _____ and _____.

Implementation

Health Promotion

- List some healthy lifestyle measures that contribute to a healthy self-concept. _____
_____
_____
_____

Acute Care

- In acute care, the nurse is likely to encounter clients who are experiencing _____ to their self-concept due to the nature of the treatment and diagnostic procedure.

- Identify ways a nurse can assist a client in the adjustment to a change in physical appearance.
_____
_____
_____

Restorative Care

- Identify goals to help a client attain a more positive self-concept.
  a. _____
  b. _____
  c. _____
  d. _____
  e. _____

- Identify seven nursing interventions for the client to engage in self-exploration.
  a. _____
  b. _____
  c. _____
  d. _____
  e. _____
  f. _____
  g. _____

Evaluation

- Client care evaluates the actual care delivered by the health team based on expected outcomes. Briefly explain the expected outcomes for a self-concept disturbance. _____
_____
_____

- Client expectations evaluate care from the client's perspective. Give an example. _____
_____
_____

Review Questions

The student should select the appropriate answer and cite the rationale for choosing that particular answer.

1. Which developmental stage is particularly crucial for identity development?
   a. Infancy
   b. Preschool age
   c. Adolescence
   d. Young adult

Answer: _____   Rationale: _____
_____
_____

2. Which of the following statements about body image is correct?
   a. Physical changes are quickly incorporated into a person's body image.
   b. Body image refers only to the external appearance of a person's body.
   c. Body image involves attitudes related to the body, including physical appearance, structure, or function.
   d. Perceptions by other persons have no influence on a person's body image.

Answer: _____ Rationale: _____
_____
_____

3. Sandeep, who is 2 years old, is praised for using his potty instead of wetting his pants. This is an example of learning a behaviour by:
   a. Identification
   b. Imitation
   c. Substitution
   d. Reinforcement-extinction

Answer: _____ Rationale: _____
_____
_____

4. Mrs. Watson has just undergone a radical mastectomy. The nurse is aware that Mrs. Watson will probably have considerable anxiety over:
   a. Role performance
   b. Self-identity
   c. Body image
   d. Self-esteem

Answer: _____ Rationale: _____
_____
_____

5. Which of the following statements demonstrates that the nurse's self-concept is positively affecting the client?
   a. "You've got to take a more active part in caring for your ostomy."
   b. "I know your ostomy is difficult to look at, but you will get used to it in time."
   c. (While grimacing) "Ostomy care isn't so bad."
   d. "Let me show you how to place the bag on your stoma."

Answer: _____ Rationale: _____
_____
_____

Critical Thinking Model for Nursing Care Plan for Disturbed Body Image

Imagine that you are the student nurse, Miss Carr, in the Care Plan on page 454 of your text. Complete the *assessment phase* of the critical thinking model by writing in the appropriate boxes on the model shown. Think about the following:

- In developing Mrs. Johnson's plan of care, what knowledge did Miss Carr apply?

- In what way might Miss Carr's previous experience apply in this case?

- What intellectual or professional standards were applied to Mrs. Johnson?

- What critical thinking attitudes were used in assessing Mr. Johnson?

- As you review your assessment, what key areas did you cover?

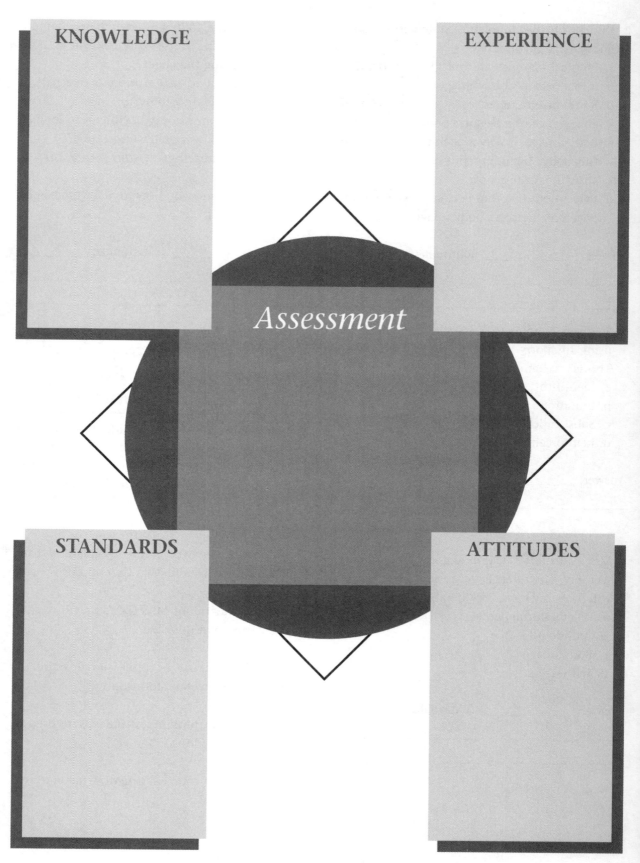

KNOWLEDGE

EXPERIENCE

Assessment

STANDARDS

ATTITUDES

CHAPTER 22   Critical Thinking Model for Nursing Care Plan for *Disturbed Body Image*

See answers on page 586.

23

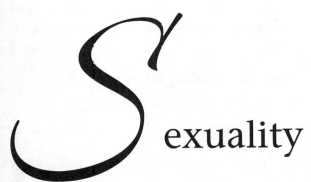exuality

Adapted by Anne Katz, RN, PhD, CancerCare Manitoba

Preliminary Reading

Chapter 23, pp. 462-485

Comprehensive Understanding

Scientific Knowledge Base

Sexual and Gender Identity

- Define the following.

  a. Sexual identity: _____

  b. Gender identity: _____

  c. Transsexuality: _____

Sexual Orientation

- *Sexual orientation* is defined as: _____

  _____

- *Heterosexuality* is defined as: _____

- *Homosexuality* is defined as: _____

- *Bisexuality* is defined as: _____

- Nurses must not assume that they know their clients' gender identity or sexual orientation.

- If nurses learn of their client's sexual orientation, they should not assume that they may tell anyone else or include it in the medical record without the client's knowledge.

- *Homophobia* is defined as: _____

- The nurse who is non-judgmental and equipped with an appropriate knowledge base can help to address the problems of homophobia and provide nursing care that does not discriminate against the client's sexual orientation.

Sexual Development

- Each stage of development brings changes in sexual functioning and the role of sexuality in relationships. Explain each stage.

    a. Infancy and childhood: _____

    _____

    b. Puberty/adolescence: _____

    _____

    c. Adulthood: _____

    _____

    d. Older adulthood: _____

    _____

Sexual Response Cycle

- The four phases of the sexual response cycle are _____, _____, _____, and _____.

- These phases are the result of vasocongestion and myotonia. Explain each of these physiological responses.

    a. Female: _____

    _____

    b. Male: _____

    _____

Sexual Behaviour

- Sexual behaviour comprises the broad array of sexual activities people participate in. It is difficult to say what is "normal" or "abnormal" because what is unusual or atypical varies between cultures and from one period to another.

High-Risk Sexual Behaviour

- *Safer sex* is defined as: _____

    _____.

- List three examples of unsafe sex practices.

    a. _____

    b. _____

    c. _____

Sexually Transmitted Infections

- A major problem in dealing with STIs is: _____

    _____

- List the prevalent STIs.

    a. _____

    b. _____

    c. _____

    d. _____

    e. _____

    f. _____

- People most likely to be infected with an STI are those who:

    a. _____

    b. _____

    c. _____

- The predominant routes of infection for HIV are _____, _____, and _____.

116   Chapter 23: Sexuality

Contraception

- There are numerous contraceptive options available. Briefly list the options available under the following categories.

  a. Non-prescriptive methods: _____

  _____

  b. Methods requiring a health care provider:

  _____

  _____

- *Emergency contraception pills (ECPs)* are most effective up to _____ days following intercourse, and are recommended to women when _____,

  _____, or _____.

Abortion

- Since 1988, Canada has been one of the few countries without any criminal law restricting abortion.

- Two-thirds of abortions are performed in hospitals; the remaining one-third are done in abortion clinics and health centres.

- Health care providers must reflect on personal values related to abortion. The health care provider is entitled to personal views and should not be forced to participate in counselling or procedures contrary to his/her beliefs or values.

Nursing Knowledge Base

Socio-Cultural Dimensions of Sexuality

- Global cultural diversity creates considerable variability in sexual norms and represents a wide spectrum of beliefs and values.

- Common areas of diversity include the following:

  a. _____

  b. _____

  c. _____

  d. _____

  e. _____

  f. _____

Discussing Sexual Issues

- Identify the issues regarding the difficulty the nurse has in discussing sexuality with clients.

  a. _____

  b. _____

  c. _____

  d. _____

Alterations in Sexual Health

- Explain the following issues.

  a. Infertility: _____

  b. Sexual Abuse: _____

  c. Sexual dysfunction: _____

Clients With Particular Sexual Concerns

- Describe the possible sexual concerns that should be considered for each of the following clients.

  a. Pregnant and postpartum women: _____

  _____

  b. Clients recovering from surgery: _____

  _____

  c. Clients with illness or disability: _____

  _____

Sexuality and the Nursing Process

- A person's sexuality has physical, psychological, social, and cultural elements.

𝒩𝓅 Assessment

- Briefly explain the following factors that affect sexuality.

  a. Physical: _____

  b. Self-concept: _____

  c. Relationship: _____

  d. Self-esteem: _____

- List the questions a nurse may use to elicit a brief sexual history from an adult.

  a. _____

  b. _____

  c. _____

  d. _____

- Explain how the nurse is able to anticipate when a client is at risk for sexual dysfunction.

  _____

  _____

  _____

- Briefly explain the physical assessment in evaluating the cause of sexual concerns or problems.

  a. Female: _____

  b. Male: _____

𝒩𝓅 Nursing Diagnosis

- Identify clues that may signal risk for or an actual nursing diagnosis related to sexuality.

  a. _____

  b. _____

  c. _____

  d. _____

  e. _____

𝒩𝓅 Planning

- The PLISSIT model developed by Annon (1974) guides the planning phases. Explain each of the following.

  a. P: _____

  _____

  b. LI: _____

  _____

  c. SS: _____

  _____

  d. IT: _____

  _____

𝒩𝓅 Implementation

Health Promotion

- Topics of education vary depending on the defining characteristics and related factors. Describe some situations. _____

  _____

Acute Care

- Nursing interventions that address alterations in sexuality are aimed at _____,

  _____, and/or _____.

- The client should be encouraged to investigate and acknowledge social and ethical values and analyze the role of sexuality in his or her self-concept.

- Identify situational and developmental crises that prompt education. _____

_____

Restorative Care

- In the home it is important to assist individuals in creating an environment comfortable for sexual activity.

- In the long-term care setting, facilities should make proper arrangements for privacy during resident's sexual experiences.

Evaluation

- Client care evaluates the actual care delivered by the health care team based on the expected outcomes.

- Client or spouse verbalizations determine if goals and outcomes have been achieved.

- Sexuality is felt more than observed, and sexual expression requires an intimacy not amenable to observation.

- All people involved may need to be reminded of the individual nature of sexual expression and the multiple factors that affect perceptions and responses.

- Client expectations evaluate care from the client's perspective. Briefly explain the client's perspective.

Review Questions

The student should select the appropriate answer and cite the rationale for choosing that particular answer.

1. At what developmental stage is it particularly important for children reared in single-parent families to be exposed to same-sex adults?
   a. Infancy
   b. Toddlerhood and preschool years
   c. School age
   d. Adolescence

   Answer: _____ Rationale: _____

   _____

   _____

2. In the school-age child, learning and reinforcement of gender-appropriate behaviours are most commonly derived from:
   a. Parents
   b. Teachers
   c. Siblings
   d. Peers

   Answer: _____ Rationale: _____

   _____

   _____

3. Why is it often more difficult to discuss sexuality issues with older patients?
   a. Older people are less likely to be sexually active.
   b. They are more likely to have complex causes for sexual problems.
   c. They may have more difficulty discussing intimate issues.
   d. They are frequently deaf and it is difficult to talk about this in a loud voice.

   Answer: _____ Rationale: _____

   _____

   _____

4. The least effective means of preventing pregnancy is:
   a. Coitus interruptus
   b. Calendar (rhythm) method
   c. Body temperature method
   d. Mucus method

Answer: _____ Rationale: _____
_____
_____

5. The only 100% effective method to avoid contracting a disease through sex is:
   a. Using condoms
   b. Avoiding sex with partners at risk
   c. Knowing the sexual partner's health history
   d. Abstinence

Answer: _____ Rationale: _____
_____
_____

Critical Thinking Model for Nursing Care Plan for Sexual Dysfunction

Imagine that you are Jack, the nurse in the Care Plan on page 479 of your text. Complete the *assessment phase* of the critical thinking model by writing your answers in the appropriate boxes of the model shown. Think about the following:

- In developing Mr. Clements' plan of care, what knowledge did Jack apply?

- In what way might Jack's previous experience assist in this case?

- What intellectual or professional standards were applied to Mr. Clements?

- What critical thinking attitudes did you utilize in assessing Mr. Clements?

- As you review your assessment, what key areas did you cover?

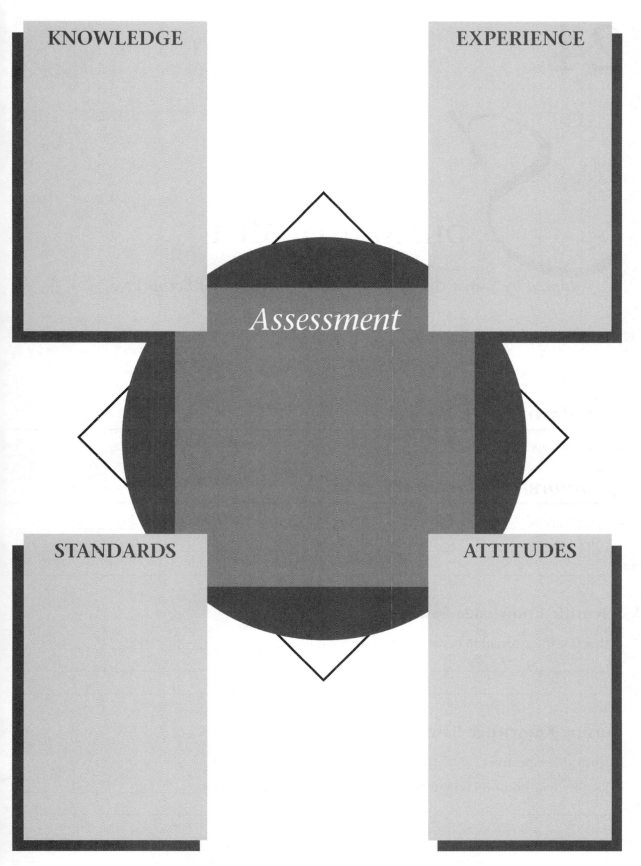

KNOWLEDGE

EXPERIENCE

Assessment

STANDARDS

ATTITUDES

CHAPTER 23   Critical Thinking Model for Nursing Care Plan for *Sexual Dysfunction*

See answers on page 587.

24

$\mathcal{S}$piritual Health

Adapted by Sonya Grypma, RN, PhD, University of Lethbridge

$\mathcal{P}$reliminary Reading

Chapter 24, pp. 486-509

$\mathcal{C}$omprehensive Understanding

- Spirituality is: _____
  _____
  _____

Scientific Knowledge Base

- Describe the association between spirituality and health. _____
  _____
  _____

Nursing Knowledge Base

Historical Perspectives

- Identify four historical milestones related to spirituality and nursing. _____
  _____
  _____
  _____

Theoretical Perspectives

- Describe spiritual care according to two nursing theories.

  a. Theory of Human Caring: _____

  _____

  b. Systems Model: _____

  _____

Traditional Concepts in Spiritual Health

- The concepts of _____,

  _____, _____, and

  _____ give direction in understanding the views each individual has of life and its value.

- Individuals' definitions of spirituality are influenced by their own _____,

  _____, _____,

  _____, and _____.

- Identify the central characteristic of spirituality in nursing._____

  _____

- Briefly describe spiritual care. _____

  _____

- Explain how the following view spirituality.

  a. Atheists: _____

  b. Agnostics:_____

- Explain the concept of faith. _____

  _____

- The belief that comes with faith involves

  _____, or an awareness of that which one cannot see or know in ordinary ways.

- Define *religion*. _____

  _____

- Religion serves different purposes in people's lives.

- Explain the differences between the terms *spirituality* and *religion*. _____

  _____

- Summarize the concept of hope. _____

  _____

Spiritual Challenges

- Spiritual distress is:_____

  _____

- Briefly explain each of the following causes of spiritual distress.

  a. Acute illness:_____

  _____

  b. Chronic illness: _____

  _____

  c. Terminal illness: _____

  _____

  d. Near-death experience: _____

  _____

Spiritual Health and the Nursing Process

- Spiritual care goes beyond assessing a client's

  _____

- Briefly explain shared community and compassion. _____

  _____

- It is important for nurses to sort out value judgments about other people's belief systems.

- The nurse must be willing to share and discover another person's meaning and purpose in life, sickness, and health.

𝒩𝒫 Assessment

- The assessment should focus on aspects of spirituality most likely to be influenced by life experiences, events, and questions in the case of illness and hospitalization.

- The JAREL spirituality well-being scale provides nurses and other health care professionals with a tool for assessing client's spiritual well-being. Briefly summarize the three dimensions.

    a. Faith/belief dimension: _____

    _____

    b. Life/self-responsibility: _____

    _____

    c. Life-satisfaction: _____

    _____

- Explain how the following can affect a client's spiritual health.

    a. Fellowship and community: _____

    _____

    b. Ritual and practice: _____

    _____

    c. Vocation: _____

    _____

𝒩𝒫 Nursing Diagnosis

- When reviewing a spiritual assessment and integrating the information into an appropriate nursing diagnosis, the nurse should consider the client's current health status from a holistic perspective, with spirituality as the unifying principle.

- State the defining characteristics for the following two diagnoses.

    a. Spiritual well-being: _____

    _____

    b. Spiritual distress: _____

    _____

𝒩𝒫 Planning

- In order to develop an individualized plan of care, the nurse integrates knowledge gathered from the assessment with knowledge relating to resources and therapies available for spiritual care.

- Identify three examples of goals and outcomes for spiritual care-giving.

    a. _____

    b. _____

    c. _____

𝒩𝒫 Implementation

Health Promotion

- Spiritual care should be a central theme in promoting an individual's overall well-being.

- Briefly explain the following interventions and how they are helpful in maintaining or promoting a client's spiritual health.

    a. Establishing presence: _____

    _____

    b. Supporting a healing relationship: _____

    _____

Acute Care

- Within acute care settings, clients experience multiple stressors that threaten to overwhelm their coping resources.

- Explain how the following interventions are helpful in the client's therapeutic plan.

    a. Support systems: _____

    _____

    b. Diet therapies: _____

    _____

    c. Supporting rituals: _____

    _____

d. Prayer: _____

_____

e. Supporting grief work: _____

_____

Evaluation

Client Care

- Client care evaluates the actual care delivered by the health team based on the expected outcomes. Give some examples. _____

_____

Client Expectations

- A client's expectation evaluates care from the client perspective. Give some examples.

_____

_____

Review Questions

The student should select the appropriate answer and cite the rationale for choosing that particular answer.

1. When planning care to include spiritual needs for a client of the Muslim faith, the religious practices the nurse should understand include all of the following, *except*:
   a. A priest must be present to conduct rituals.
   b. Strength is gained through group prayer.
   c. Family members are a source of comfort.
   d. Faith healing provides psychological support.

Answer: _____ Rationale: _____

_____

_____

2. When consulting with the dietary department regarding meals for a client of the Hindu religion, which of the following dietary items would not be included on the meal trays?
   a. Meats
   b. Dairy products
   c. Vegetable entrees
   d. Fruits

Answer: _____ Rationale: _____

_____

_____

3. If an Orthodox Jewish woman gives birth, the nurse should be aware of what religious practice?
   a. Sabbath observance might include having the nurse diaper or bathe the newborn.
   b. The husband is not allowed physical contact with wife during labour.
   c. Soy formula is not allowed.
   d. The newborn will be circumcised on the seventh day.

Answer: _____ Rationale: _____

_____

_____

4. If a nurse were to use a nursing diagnosis to relate concerns about spiritual health, which of the following would be used?
   a. Spiritual distress
   b. Inability to adjust
   c. Lack of faith
   d. Religious dilemma

Answer: _____ Rationale: _____

_____

_____

5. Mr. Lanois was recently diagnosed with a malignant tumour. The staff had observed him crying on several occasions, and now he cries as he reads from his Bible. Interventions to help Mr. Lanois cope with his illness would include:

a. Asking the parish nurse from his congregation to visit him
b. Engaging Mr. Lanois in diversional activities to reduce feelings of hopelessness
c. Sitting at Mr. Lanois bedside and listening to him with an encouraging yet realistic attitude.
d. Praying with Mr. Lanois as often as possible

Answer: _____ Rationale: _____

_____

_____

Critical Thinking Model for Nursing Care Plan for Spiritual Distress

Imagine that you are Leah, the nurse in the Care Plan on page 501 of your text. Complete the *planning phase* of the critical thinking model by writing your answers in the appropriate boxes of the model shown. Think about the following.

- In developing James's plan of care, what knowledge did Leah apply?

- In what way might Leah's previous experience assist in developing a plan of care for James?

- When developing a plan of care, what intellectual and professional standards were applied?

- What critical thinking attitudes might have been applied when developing James' plan?

- How will Leah accomplish the goals?

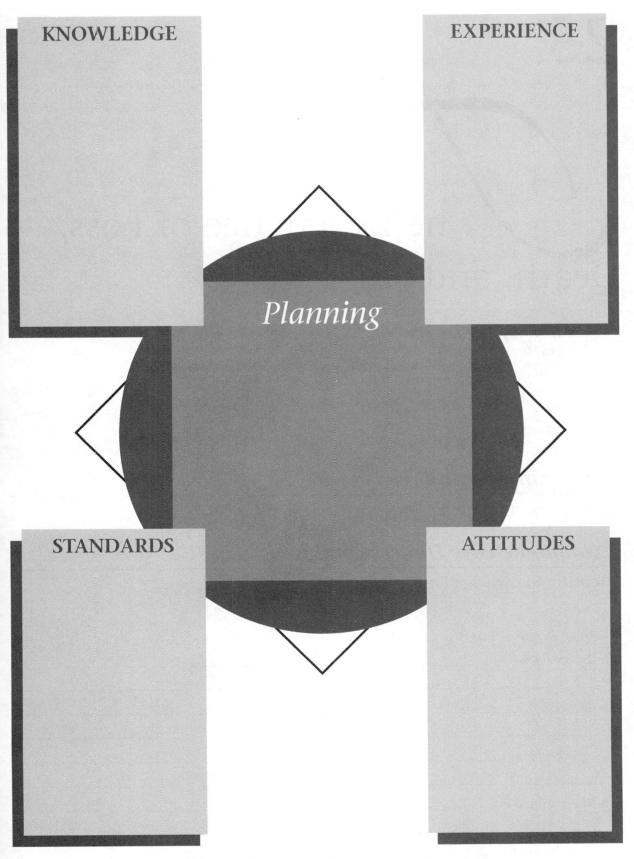

KNOWLEDGE

EXPERIENCE

Planning

STANDARDS

ATTITUDES

CHAPTER 24 Critical Thinking Model for Nursing Care Plan for *Spiritual Distress*

See answers on page 588.

25

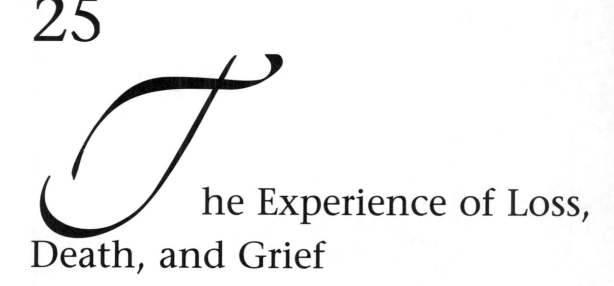

The Experience of Loss, Death, and Grief

Adapted by Barbara Brown, RN, BA, BScN, MScN, McMaster University

Preliminary Reading

Chapter 25, pp. 510-538

Comprehensive Understanding

Scientific Knowledge Base

Loss

- Give an example of the five categories of loss.

  a. Necessary loss: _____

  _____

  b. Actual loss: _____

  _____

  c. Perceived loss: _____

  _____

  d. Maturational loss: _____

  _____

  e. Situational loss: _____

  _____

Grief

- Describe the following terms.

  a. Grief: _____

  b. Bereavement: _____

Theories of Grief

- List the phases of the grieving process proposed by each of the theorists listed below.

Kübler-Ross's Stages of Dying

a. _____

b. _____

c. _____

d. _____

e. _____

Bowlby's Phases of Mourning

a. _____

b. _____

c. _____

d. _____

Worden's Four Tasks of Mourning

a. _____

b. _____

c. _____

d. _____

- Briefly describe the following types of grief.

  a. Normal grief: _____

  _____

  b. Anticipatory grief: _____

  _____

  c. Complicated grief: _____

  _____

  d. Disenfranchised grief: _____

  _____

Nursing Knowledge Base

- Briefly explain the factors that influence loss and grief.

  a. Human development: _____

  b. Psychosocial perspectives: _____

  c. Socio-economic status: _____

  d. Personal relationships: _____

  e. Nature of the loss: _____

  f. Culture and ethnicity: _____

  g. Spiritual beliefs: _____

- Explain how the mechanism of hope is used to cope with grief and loss. _____

  _____

The Nursing Process and Grief

Assessment

- The nurse should avoid assuming that a particular behaviour indicates grief; rather, the nurse should allow clients to share what is happening in their own ways.

- It is important for the nurse to assess how a client is reacting rather than how the client *should be* reacting. A single behaviour can represent various types of grief. Therefore, the identification of the type and stage of grief should be used only to guide the nurse's assessment and not to judge the outcomes of the grieving process.

- Identify some symptoms of normal grief feelings. _____

  _____

- Briefly explain end-of-life decisions. _____

  _____

- Assess your own experience with grief. _____

  _____

Nursing Diagnosis

- List four possible nursing diagnoses for clients or families experiencing grief.

  a. _____

  b. _____

  c. _____

  d. _____

Planning

- When caring for the dying client, it is important to devise a plan that helps a client to die with dignity and offers family members the assurance that their loved one is cared for with care and compassion.

- List three goals appropriate for a client dealing with loss.

  a. _____

  b. _____

  c. _____

- Briefly explain how to prioritize the needs of the grieving client. _____

  _____

  _____

Implementation

Health Promotion

- Nurses help clients and families to deal with loss, make decisions about the client's health care, and adjust to any disappointment, frustration, and anxiety created by their loss.

- Describe five therapeutic communication strategies the nurse can use to help clients discuss and work through their loss.

  a. _____

  b. _____

  c. _____

  d. _____

  e. _____

- Give an example of a nursing strategy to promote hope for each dimension.

  a. Affective dimension: _____

  b. Cognitive dimension: _____

  c. Behavioural dimension: _____

  d. Affiliative dimension: _____

  e. Temporal dimension: _____

  f. Contextual dimension: _____

- Identify the nursing strategies to facilitate mourning for the client.

  a. _____

  b. _____

  c. _____

  d. _____

  e. _____

  f. _____

  g. _____

Acute Care

- According to the World Health Organization, when health care providers deliver palliative care, they do the following:

  a. _____

  b. _____

  c. _____

  d. _____

  e. _____

  f. _____

  g. _____

- Give examples of how the following contribute to comfort for the dying client.

  a. Symptom control: _____

  _____

  b. Maintaining dignity and self-esteem: ____

  _____

  c. Preventing abandonment and isolation:

  _____

  _____

d. Providing a comfortable and peaceful environment: _____

_____

Hospice Care

- Identify the components of hospice care. _____

_____

Care After Death

- Care after death includes caring for the body with dignity and sensitivity and in a manner consistent with the client's religious or cultural beliefs.

- Explain how the nurse can support the family through the organ and tissue request process.

_____

_____

_____

_____

𝒩𝓅 Evaluation

Client Care

- Grieving is an individual process, and resolution of loss does not follow a set schedule.

- The care of the dying client requires the nurse to evaluate the client's level of comfort with illness and the client's quality of life.

Client Expectations

- The client expects individualized care, including relief of symptoms, preservation of dignity, and support of the family to maximize quality of life.

Review Questions

The student should select the appropriate answer and cite the rationale for choosing that particular answer.

1. Which statement about loss is accurate?
   a. Loss is only experienced when there is an actual absence of something valued.
   b. The more an individual has invested in what is lost, the less the feeling of loss.
   c. Loss may be maturational, situational, or both.
   d. The degree of stress experienced is unrelated to the type of loss.

   Answer: _____ Rationale: _____

   _____

   _____

2. The developmental stage at which the child is first able to understand logical explanations about death is:
   a. Toddlerhood
   b. Preschool-age
   c. School-age
   d. Adolescence

   Answer: _____ Rationale: _____

   _____

   _____

3. A hospice program emphasizes:
   a. Curative treatment and alleviation of symptoms
   b. Palliative treatment and control of symptoms
   c. Hospital-based care
   d. Prolongation of life

   Answer: _____ Rationale: _____

   _____

   _____

4. Trying questionable and experimental forms of therapy is a behaviour that is characteristic of which stage of dying?
   a. Anger
   b. Depression
   c. Bargaining
   d. Acceptance

Answer: _____ Rationale: _____
_____
_____

5. All of the following are crucial needs of the dying client *except:*
   a. Control of pain
   b. Preservation of dignity and self-worth
   c. Love and belonging
   d. Freedom from decision making

Answer: _____ Rationale: _____
_____
_____

Critical Thinking Model for Nursing Care Plan for Ineffective Coping

Imagine that you are the student nurse in the Care Plan on page 525 of your text. Complete the *evaluation phase* of the critical thinking model by writing your answers in the appropriate boxes of the model shown. Think about the following:

- In evaluating Mrs. Miller's plan of care, what knowledge did you apply?

- In what way might your previous experience influence your evaluation of Mrs. Miller's care?

- During evaluation, what intellectual and professional standards were applied to Mrs. Miller's care?

- In what way do critical thinking attitudes play a role in how you approach evaluation of Mrs. Miller's care?

- How might you adjust Mrs. Miller's care?

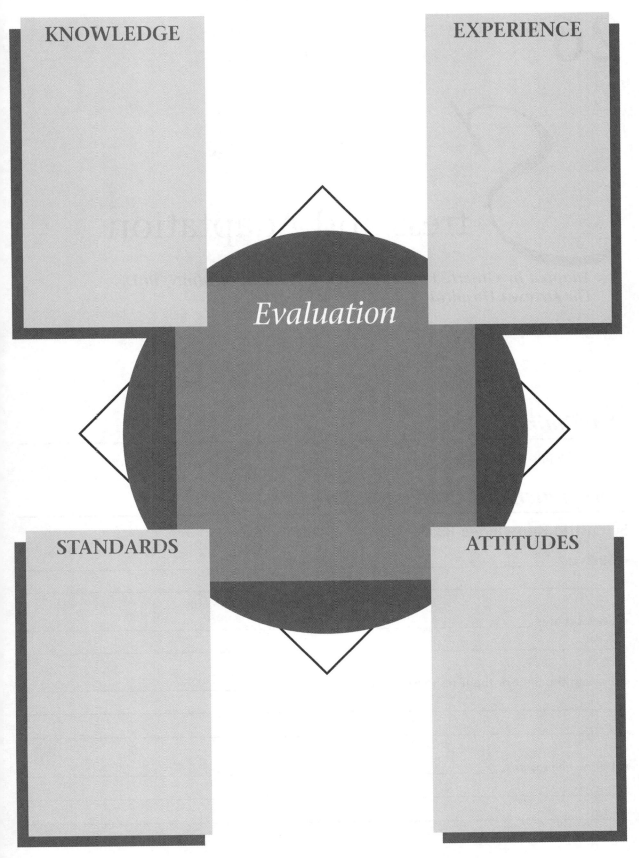

KNOWLEDGE

EXPERIENCE

Evaluation

STANDARDS

ATTITUDES

CHAPTER 25 Critical Thinking Model for Nursing Care Plan for *Ineffective Coping*

See answers on page 589.

26

$\mathcal{S}$tress and Adaptation

Adapted by Ginette Lemire Rodger, RN, BScN, MAdmN, PhD,
The Ottawa Hospital

$\mathcal{P}$reliminary Reading

Chapter 26, pp. 539-560

Comprehensive Understanding

Scientific Knowledge Base

- Stress is: _____
  _____

- Stressors are: _____
  _____

- Explain the fight-or-flight response to stress. _____
  _____
  _____

- Define *homeostasis*. _____
  _____
  _____

- Explain the following mechanisms of response to a stressor.

  a. Medulla oblongata: _____

  _____

  b. Reticular formation: _____

  _____

  c. Pituitary gland: _____

  _____

General Adaptation Syndrome

- List (in sequence) and briefly describe the three stages of the general adaptation syndrome (GAS).

  a. _____

  b. _____

  c. _____

Reaction to Psychological Stress

- Explain the following terms.

  a. Primary appraisal: _____

  b. Secondary appraisal: _____

  c. Coping: _____

  d. Ego-defense mechanisms: _____

Types of Stress

- Distinguish between the two different types of stress.

  a. Distress: _____

  _____

  b. Eustress: _____

  _____

- Explain *post-traumatic stress disorder.* _____

  _____

- Explain the two types of crisis.

  a. Developmental crisis: _____

  b. Situational crisis: _____

Nursing Knowledge Base

- Summarize the following models related to stress and coping.

  a. Neuman systems model: _____

  _____

  b. Pender's health promotion model: _____

  _____

- The following factors can potentially be stressors. Explain:

  a. Situational factors: _____

  _____

  b. Maturational factors: _____

  _____

  c. Socio-cultural factors: _____

  _____

Nursing Process

Assessment

- When assessing a client's stress level and coping resources, the nurse must ask the client to share personal and sensitive information. Therefore, the nurse must first establish a trusting nurse-client relationship.

- Give an example of each of the following factors to assess.

  a. Perception of stressor: _____

  b. Coping resources: _____

  c. Maladaptive coping used: _____

  d. Adherence to healthy practices: _____

- Identify six physical indicators of stress.

  a. _____

  b. _____

  c. _____

  d. _____

  e. _____

  f. _____

Chapter 26: Stress and Adaptation 135

𝒩𝒟 Nursing Diagnosis

- Stress can result in multiple diagnostic statements.

𝒩𝒟 Planning

- Desirable outcomes for persons experiencing stress are:

  a. _____

  b. _____

  c. _____

  d. _____

- Nursing interventions are designed within the framework of primary, secondary, and tertiary prevention.

𝒩𝒟 Implementation

Health Promotion

- Identify the primary modes of intervention for stress.

  a. _____

  b. _____

  c. _____

- Explain how the following methods reduce stressors.

  a. Time management: _____
  _____

  b. Regular exercise: _____
  _____

  c. Guided imagery and visualization: _____
  _____

  d. Support systems: _____
  _____

  e. Progressive muscle relaxation: _____
  _____

  f. Assertiveness training: _____
  _____

  g. Journal writing: _____
  _____

  h. Stress management in the nurse's workplace:
  _____

Acute Care

- Crisis intervention is: _____
  _____

- Crises occur: _____
  _____

Restorative and Continuing Care

- Briefly explain when recovery from stress occurs. _____
  _____

𝒩𝒟 Evaluation

- Briefly explain the client's care in relation to:
  a. Client's perceptions of stress: _____
  b. Client's expectations: _____

Review Questions

The student should select the appropriate answer and cite the rationale for choosing that particular answer.

1. Which definition does *not* characterize stress?
   a. Any situation in which a non-specific demand requires an individual to respond or take action
   b. A phenomenon affecting social, psychological, developmental, spiritual, and physiological dimensions
   c. A condition eliciting an intellectual, behavioural, or metabolic response
   d. Efforts to maintain relative constancy within the internal environment

Answer: _____   Rationale: _____

_____

_____

2. Which statement about homeostasis is inaccurate?
   a. Homeostatic mechanisms provide long-term and short-term control over the body's equilibrium.
   b. Homeostatic mechanisms are self-regulatory.
   c. Homeostatic mechanisms function through negative feedback.
   d. Illness may inhibit normal homeostatic mechanisms.

Answer: _____   Rationale: _____

_____

_____

3. Major homeostatic mechanisms are controlled by all of the following *except:*
   a. Thymus gland
   b. Medulla oblongata
   c. Reticular formation
   d. Pituitary gland

Answer: _____   Rationale: _____

_____

_____

4. Which of the following is a stage of the general adaptation syndrome?
   a. Alarm reaction
   b. Fight-or-flight response
   c. Ego-defense mechanisms
   d. Inflammatory response

Answer: _____   Rationale: _____

_____

_____

5. The general adaptation syndrome consists of three stages. During which stage does the body stabilize and hormone levels return to normal?
   a. Exhaustion
   b. Regeneration
   c. Adaptation
   d. Compensation

Answer: _____   Rationale: _____

_____

_____

6. Crisis intervention is a specific measure used for helping a client resolve a particular, immediate stress problem. This approach is based on:
   a. The ability of the nurse to solve the client's problems
   b. An in-depth analysis of a client's situation
   c. Teaching the client how to use ego-defense mechanisms
   d. Effective communication between the nurse and client

Answer: _____   Rationale: _____

_____

_____

Chapter 26: Stress and Adaptation   137

Critical Thinking Model for Nursing Care Plan for Caregiver Role Strain

Imagine that you are Maya, the nurse in the Care Plan on page 552 of your text. Complete the *evaluation phase* of the critical thinking model by writing your answers in the appropriate boxes of the model shown. Think about the following:

- In evaluating the care of Carl and Evelyn, what knowledge did Maya apply?

- In what way might Maya's previous experience influence the evaluation of Carl's care?

- During evaluation, what intellectual and professional standards were applied to Carl's care?

- In what way do critical thinking attitudes play a role in how Maya approaches the evaluation of Carl's care?

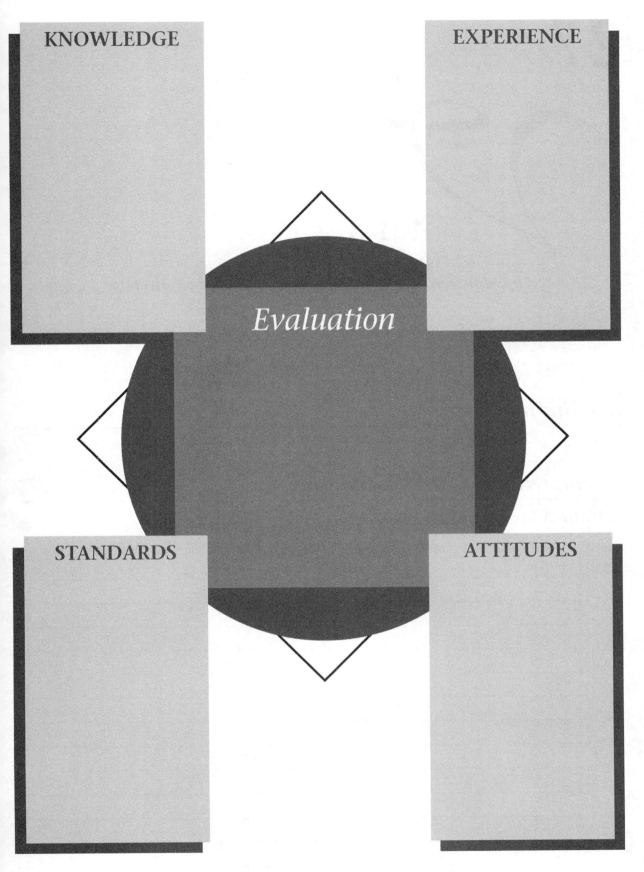

KNOWLEDGE

EXPERIENCE

Evaluation

STANDARDS

ATTITUDES

CHAPTER *26* Critical Thinking Model for Nursing Care Plan for *Caregiver Role Strain*

See answers on page 590.

27

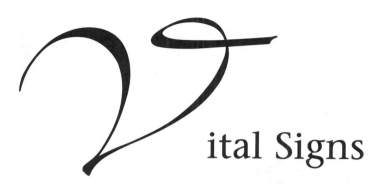

$\mathcal{V}$ital Signs

Adapted by Maureen McQueen, RN, MN, Athabasca University

$\mathcal{P}$reliminary Reading

Chapter 27, pp. 561-615

$\mathcal{C}$omprehensive Understanding

Guidelines for Measuring Vital Signs

- Identify the guidelines that assist the nurse to incorporate vital sign measurement into practice.

  a. _____

  b. _____

  c. _____

  d. _____

  e. _____

  f. _____

  g. _____

  h. _____

  i. _____

  j. _____

  k. _____

  l. _____

  m. _____

Body Temperature

Physiology

- The body temperature is the difference between the _____ and the amount _____.

- Define *core temperature*. _____
  _____

- Define *thermoregulation*. _____
  _____

- Briefly summarize how neural and vascular mechanisms control body temperature. _____
  _____
  _____

- List four sources, or mechanisms, for heat production.
  a. _____
  b. _____
  c. _____
  d. _____

- Explain the following mechanisms of body heat loss and give an example of each.
  a. Radiation: _____
  _____
  b. Conduction: _____
  _____
  c. Convection: _____
  _____
  d. Evaporation: _____
  _____
  e. Diaphoresis: _____
  _____

- Briefly explain the skin's role in temperature regulation.
  a. Insulation of the body: _____
  b. Vasoconstriction: _____
  c. Temperature sensation: _____

- Identify four factors that must be present for a person to control body temperature.
  a. _____
  b. _____
  c. _____
  d. _____

Factors Affecting Body Temperature

- Changes in body temperature within the normal range occur when the relationship between heat production and heat loss is altered by physiological or behavioural variables. Summarize the following variables.
  a. Age: _____
  _____
  b. Exercise: _____
  _____
  c. Circadian rhythm: _____
  _____
  d. Stress: _____
  _____
  e. Environment: _____
  _____

- Temperature alterations can be related to _____, _____, _____, _____, or any combination of these alterations.

- Pyrexia, or fever, occurs because _____
  _____

- Explain how a fever works as an important defense mechanism. _____
  _____

- Explain how a fever serves a diagnostic purpose. _____
  _____

- Explain how a fever affects metabolism. ____
  _____

- Define the following terms:
  a. Hyperthermia: _____
  b. Malignant hyperthermia: _____

- Define and explain the causes of heat stroke.
  _____
  _____
  _____

- Define and explain the causes of heat exhaustion. _____
  _____
  _____

- Define and explain the causes of hypothermia.
  _____
  _____
  _____

- Frostbite occurs when: _____
  _____
  _____

Nursing Process and Thermoregulation

- Independent measures can be implemented to increase or minimize heat loss, to promote heat conservation, and to increase comfort.

Assessment

- List the routine assessment sites for intermittent temperature measurement.
  a. _____
  b. _____
  c. _____
  d. _____

- State the formulas for the following conversions:
  a. Fahrenheit to centigrade: _____
  b. Centigrade to Fahrenheit: _____

- Identify three types of thermometers and list advantages and disadvantages of each.
  a. _____
  b. _____
  c. _____

Nursing Diagnosis

- Identify three nursing diagnoses related to thermoregulation.
  a. _____
  b. _____
  c. _____

Planning

- The plan of care depends on the nurse's assessment of the client's perception and acceptance of the body temperature alteration.

- Care also depends on the extent to which the client's internal compensatory mechanisms and behaviours have adjusted to the temperature alteration.

ℕℙ Implementation

Health Promotion

- Health promotion for clients at risk of altered temperature is directed to: _____

  _____

  _____

- Identify the risk factors for hypothermia.

  _____

  _____

  _____

Acute Care

- The procedures used to intervene and treat an elevated temperature depend on the fever's cause; its adverse effects; and its strength, intensity, and duration.

- Explain the differences related to febrile states in each of the following.

  a. Children: _____

  _____

  b. Hypersensitivity to drugs: _____

  _____

- Give three examples of each type of fever therapy.

  a. Pharmacological:

  1. _____

  2. _____

  3. _____

  b. Non-pharmacological:

  1. _____

  2. _____

  3. _____

- Identify an independent and a dependent nursing intervention to control shivering.

  _____

  _____

  _____

- First aid treatment for heatstroke is: _____

  _____

  _____

- Summarize the treatment for hypothermia.

  _____

  _____

  _____

Restorative and Continuing Care

- Summarize the client teaching in regard to the treatment of a fever. _____

  _____

  _____

ℕℙ Evaluation

- After any intervention, the nurse measures the client's temperature to evaluate it for any change.

- Other evaluative measures are _____ and _____.

Pulse

- Define *pulse*. _____

  _____

Physiology and Regulation

- Define the following terms.

  a. Stroke volume: _____

  b. Cardiac output: _____

- _____, _____, and _____ factors regulate the strength of the heart's contractions and its stroke volume.

Assessment of Pulse

- Identify the two most common peripheral pulse sites to assess.

  a. _____

  b. _____

- Identify the five major parts of the stethoscope.

  a. _____

  b. _____

  c. _____

  d. _____

  e. _____

Character of the Pulse

- List four characteristics to identify during peripheral pulse assessment. By using an asterisk, specify the two characteristics to identify when assessing an apical pulse.

  a. _____

  b. _____

  c. _____

  d. _____

- Define the following.

  a. Tachycardia:_____

  b. Bradycardia:_____

  c. Dysrhythmia: _____

  d. Pulse deficit: _____

Nursing Process and Pulse Determination

- Pulse assessment determines the general state of cardiovascular health and the response to other system imbalances.

- The nurse evaluates client outcomes by assessing the pulse _____, _____, _____, and _____ following each intervention.

Respiration

- Define the following.

  a. Ventilation:_____

  b. Diffusion: _____

  c. Perfusion: _____

Physiological Control

- Breathing is a passive process. The respiratory centre in the brainstem regulates the involuntary control of respirations.

- Ventilation is controlled by levels of _____, _____, and _____ in the arterial blood.

- The most important factor in the control of ventilation is the level of _____.

- *Hypoxemia* is: _____
  _____
  _____

Mechanics of Breathing

- Briefly summarize the process of inspiration.
  _____
  _____
  _____

- Define the following terms.

  a. Tidal volume: _____

  b. Eupnea:_____

Assessment of Ventilation

- Accurate measurement requires _____ and _____ of the chest wall movement.

- List three objective measurements used in respiratory status assessment.

  a. _____

  b. _____

  c. _____

- Define the following alterations in breathing patterns.

  a. Bradypnea: _____

  b. Tachypnea:_____

  c. Hyperpnea: _____

  d. Apnea:_____

e. Hypoventilation/hyperventilation: _____

f. Cheyne-Stokes respiration: _____

g. Kussmaul's respiration: _____

h. Biot's respiration: _____

Assessment of Diffusion and Perfusion

- The respiratory processes of diffusion and perfusion can be evaluated by measuring the oxygen saturation of the blood.

- The percent of saturation of arterial blood is _____, and venous blood is _____.

- Explain the purpose of a pulse oximeter. _____
_____
_____

Nursing Process and Respiratory Vital Signs

- Vital sign measurement of respiratory rate, pattern, and depth, along with SpO_2, allows the nurse to assess ventilation, diffusion, and perfusion.

- The nurse evaluates client outcomes by assessing the _____, _____, _____, and _____ following each intervention.

Blood Pressure

- Define the following terms.

  a. Blood pressure: _____

  b. Systolic: _____

  c. Diastolic: _____

- The difference between the systolic and diastolic pressure is the _____.

Physiology of Arterial Blood Pressure

- Blood pressure reflects the interrelationships of the following: _____
_____
_____

- Briefly explain each.

  a. Cardiac output: _____

  b. Peripheral resistance: _____

  c. Blood volume: _____

  d. Viscosity: _____

  e. Elasticity: _____

Factors Influencing Blood Pressure

- List six factors that influence blood pressure.

  a. _____

  b. _____

  c. _____

  d. _____

  e. _____

  f. _____

Hypertension

- Identify the criteria for the diagnosis of hypertension in an adult. _____
_____
_____

- Briefly summarize the physiology of hypertension. _____
_____
_____

- List five risk factors that are linked to hypertension.

  a. _____

  b. _____

  c. _____

  d. _____

  e. _____

Hypotension

- Identify the criteria for the diagnosis of hypotension in an adult. _____
_____
_____

- Explain the physiology of hypotension and its causes. _____
_____
_____

- Orthostatic hypotension occurs when: _____
_____
_____

- Explain how you would assess a client for orthostatic hypotension. _____
_____
_____

Measurement of Blood Pressure

- Identify two methods for measuring blood pressure.

  a. _____

  b. _____

- Identify the two types of sphygmomanometers, and list their advantages and disadvantages.

  a. _____

  b. _____

- The sounds heard over an artery distal to the blood pressure cuff are Korotkoff sounds. Describe each.

  a. First: _____

  b. Second: _____

  c. Third: _____

  d. Fourth: _____

  e. Fifth: _____

- During the initial assessment the nurse should obtain and record the blood pressure in both arms.

- Pressure differences between the arms greater than _____ mm Hg indicate vascular problems.

- Identify five common mistakes in blood pressure assessment.

  a. _____

  b. _____

  c. _____

  d. _____

  e. _____

- Identify four reasons why the measurement of blood pressure in infants and children is difficult.

  a. _____

  b. _____

  c. _____

  d. _____

- Explain the rationale for the use of an ultrasonic stethoscope. _____
_____
_____

- Identify the method the nurse may use to assess blood pressure when Korotkoff sounds are not audible with the standard stethoscope.
_____
_____
_____

- Define *auscultatory gap*. _____
_____
_____

- Give an example of when you would assess a client's blood pressure using the client's lower extremities. _____
_____
_____

- Identify the advantages and disadvantages of using automatic blood pressure devices. _____

_____

_____

- List the benefits of blood pressure self-measurement.

  a. _____

  b. _____

  c. _____

  d. _____

Nursing Process and Blood Pressure Determination

- The assessment of blood pressure and pulse is used to evaluate the general state of cardiovascular health and responses to other system imbalances.

- The nurse evaluates client outcomes by assessing the blood pressure following each intervention.

Health Promotion and Vital Signs

- When teaching clients and their families the importance of vital sign measurements, the client's age is an important factor.

- Identify some of the common variations in the older adult.

  a. Temperature: _____

  b. Pulse rate: _____

  c. Blood pressure: _____

  d. Respirations: _____

Recording Vital Signs

- In addition to the vital sign values, the nurse records in the nurses' notes any accompanying or precipitating symptoms.

- The nurse needs to document any intervention initiated as a result of a vital sign measurement.

Review Questions

The student should select the appropriate answer and cite the rationale for choosing that particular answer.

1. The skin plays a role in temperature regulation by:
   a. Insulating the body
   b. Constricting blood vessels
   c. Sensing external temperature variations
   d. All of the above

Answer: _____ Rationale: _____

_____

_____

2. The nurse bathes the client who has a fever with cool water. The nurse does this to increase heat loss by means of:
   a. Radiation
   b. Convection
   c. Condensation
   d. Conduction

Answer: _____ Rationale: _____

_____

_____

3. The nurse is assessing a client suspected of having the nursing diagnosis *hyperthermia related to vigourous exercise in hot weather*. In reviewing the data, the nurse knows that the most important sign of heatstroke is:
   a. Confusion
   b. Hot, dry skin
   c. Excess thirst
   d. Muscle cramps

Answer: _____ Rationale: _____
_____
_____

4. When taking a client's radial pulse, the nurse notes a dysrhythmia. The most appropriate action is to:
   a. Inform the physician immediately
   b. Wait 5 minutes and retake the radial pulse
   c. Take the pulse apically for 1 full minute
   d. Check the client's record for the presence of a previous dysrhythmia

Answer: _____ Rationale: _____
_____
_____

5. The nurse is auscultating Mrs. McKinnon's blood pressure. The nurse inflates the cuff to 180 mm Hg. At 156 mm Hg, the nurse hears the onset of a tapping sound. At 130 mm Hg the sound changes to a murmur or swishing. At 100 mm Hg the sound momentarily becomes sharper, and at 92 mm Hg it becomes muffled. At 88 mm Hg the sound disappears. Mrs. McKinnon's blood pressure is:
   a. 180/92
   b. 180/130
   c. 156/88
   d. 130/88

Answer: _____ Rationale: _____
_____
_____

148   Chapter 27: Vital Signs

28

$\mathscr{H}$ealth Assessment and Physical Examination

Adapted by D. Lynn Skillen, PhD, RN, University of Alberta
Rene A. Day, RN, PhD, University of Alberta
Marjorie C. Anderson, RN, PhD, University of Alberta
Tracey Stephen, RN, BScN, MN, University of Alberta
Julie A. Gilbert, RN, BScN, MN, University of Alberta

$\mathscr{P}$reliminary Reading

Chapter 28, pp. 616-782

$\mathscr{C}$omprehensive Understanding

Purposes of Physical Examination

- Physical assessment skills allow the nurse to _____ and _____.

- The nurse's success in providing care depends on his or her ability to recognize a change in the client's status and to modify therapies so that the client gains the most desirable outcome.

- Whether a complete or partial physical assessment is performed, an examination should be integrated into routine care.

- List the five nursing purposes for performing a physical assessment.

  a. _____

  b. _____

c. _____

d. _____

e. _____

Analyzing Signs and Symptoms

- The main objective of the nurse/client interaction is for the nurse to find out what is central to the client's concerns and to help the client find solutions.

- After collecting a history, the nurse conducts a physical examination to _____, _____, or _____ the existing database.

- A complete assessment is needed to form a definitive diagnosis.

- The nurse learns to group significant findings into patterns of data that reveal actual or high-risk nursing diagnoses.

- The baseline is: _____

_____

General Appearance and Behaviour

- Summarize the 14 specific observations of the client's general appearance and behaviour.

a. _____

b. _____

c. _____

d. _____

e. _____

f. _____

g. _____

h. _____

i. _____

j. _____

k. _____

l. _____

m. _____

n. _____

Physical Examination Modes

Inspection

- Define *inspection*. _____

_____

- List six principles to facilitate accurate inspection of body parts.

a. _____

b. _____

c. _____

d. _____

e. _____

f. _____

Palpation

- Define *palpation*. _____

_____

- Identify the parts of the hand used to assess each of the following.

a. Temperature: _____

b. Pulsations: _____

c. Vibrations: _____

d. Turgor: _____

- Briefly explain the following.

a. Light palpation: _____

b. Deep palpation: _____

c. Percussion: _____

- Identify the information obtained through percussion. _____

_____

_____

- Explain the two types of percussion.

a. Direct: _____

b. Indirect: _____

- Percussion produces five types of sounds. Identify them.

  a. _____

  b. _____

  c. _____

  d. _____

  e. _____

Auscultation

- Define *auscultation*. _____

  _____

- Briefly explain the following characteristics of sound.

  a. Frequency: _____

  b. Loudness: _____

  c. Quality: _____

  d. Duration: _____

Preparation for the Physical Examination

Client Preparation

- Briefly explain the following pre-examination preparations.

  a. Physical: _____

  b. Positioning: _____

  c. Psychological: _____

Assessment According to Age Groups

- List at least six variations in the nurse's individual style that are appropriate when examining children.

  a. _____

  b. _____

  c. _____

  d. _____

  e. _____

  f. _____

- List at least five variations in the nurse's individual style that are appropriate when examining older adults.

  a. _____

  b. _____

  c. _____

  d. _____

  e. _____

Environment Preparation

- List at least three environmental factors that the nurse should attempt to control before performing a physical examination.

  a. _____

  b. _____

  c. _____

Nurse Preparation

- Examination techniques cause the nurse to contact body fluids and discharge. Standard precautions should be used throughout the examination.

- Hand-washing is done before equipment preparation and before the examination.

- All equipment should be checked to see that it functions properly.

Organization of the Examination

- List eight principles to follow for a well-organized examination.

  a. _____

  b. _____

  c. _____

  d. _____

  e. _____

  f. _____

  g. _____

  h. _____

General Survey

- List three assessment components of the general survey.

  a. _____

  b. _____

  c. _____

Vital Signs

- Assessment of vital signs is the first part of the physical assessment.

Height, Weight, and Circumference

- A person's general level of health can be reflected in the ratio of height and weight.

- List three actions that should be taken to ensure accurate weight measurement of a hospitalized client.

  a. _____

  b. _____

  c. _____

- In the infant a chest circumference can be compared with the head circumference to rule out problems in head or chest size.

Assessing Mental and Emotional Status

- There are five areas that Folstein's Mini-Mental State tool assesses. Name them.

  a. _____

  b. _____

  c. _____

  d. _____

  e. _____

- An alteration in mental or emotional status may reflect a disturbance in cerebral functioning.

- List three factors that may change cerebral function.

  a. _____

  b. _____

  c. _____

- Define *delirium* and list the clinical criteria for it. _____

  _____

Level of Consciousness

- The level of consciousness exists along a continuum, from full awakening, alertness, and cooperation to unresponsiveness to any form of external stimuli.

- Identify the tool and the three factors to assess consciousness. _____

  _____

  _____

Behaviour and Appearance

- Behaviour, moods, hygiene, grooming, and choice of dress reveal pertinent information about mental status.

- Explain the function of the cerebral cortex in language. _____

  _____

Intellectual Function

- Intellectual function includes the following. Briefly explain how each is assessed.

  a. Abstract thinking: _____

  b. Judgment: _____

  c. Memory: _____

  d. Knowledge: _____

- There are two types of aphasia. Describe each one.

  a. _____

  b. _____

Assessing Sensory and Motor Function

Sensory Function

- The sensory pathways of the central nervous system conduct sensations of _____, _____, _____, _____, and _____.

- Summarize how a nurse would assess the client's sensory function. _____
  _____
  _____
  _____

Motor Function

- Identify the functions of the cerebellum. _____
  _____

- Describe the maneuvers used to assess balance and gross motor function.
  a. _____
  b. _____
  c. _____

Assessing the Integumentary System

Skin

- The skin provides the body's _____ and _____ and acts as a sensory organ for _____, _____, _____, and _____.

- The physical assessment skills of _____ and _____ are used to assess the integument's function and integrity.

- Assessment of the skin can reveal a variety of conditions including changes in _____, _____, _____, and _____.

- List at least four risks for skin lesions in the hospitalized client.
  a. _____
  b. _____
  c. _____
  d. _____

- Define the following terms:
  a. Melanoma: _____
  b. Basal cell carcinoma: _____

- For each skin colour variation, identify the mechanism that produces colour change, common causes of the variation, and the optimal sites for assessment. (See the following table.)

Skin Color	Mechanisms	Causes	Assessment Sites
Cyanosis			
Pallor			
Jaundice			
Erythema			

- Define *hyperpigmentation* and *hypopigmentation*. _____ _____

- Define *moisture*. _____ _____

- Excessive dryness can worsen skin conditions such as _____ and _____.

- The temperature of the skin depends on the amount of _____ circulating through the dermis.

- The character of the skin's surface and the feel of deeper portions are its _____.

- Define *skin turgor* and describe normal findings. _____ _____ _____

- Petechiae are: _____ _____

- Identify the two causes of edema.
  a. _____
  b. _____

- Explain the following terms related to lesions.
  a. Senile keratosis: _____
  b. Cherry angiomas: _____

- When a lesion is detected, it is inspected for _____, _____, _____, _____, _____, _____, and _____.

- Briefly describe the following primary skin lesions.
  a. Macule: _____
  b. Papule: _____
  c. Nodule: _____
  d. Tumour: _____
  e. Wheal: _____
  f. Vesicle: _____
  g. Pustule: _____
  h. Ulcer: _____
  i. Atrophy: _____

154   Chapter 28: Health Assessment and Physical Examination

Hair and Scalp

- When inspecting the hair, the nurse notes the

  _____, _____,

  _____, _____, and

  _____.

- Define.

  a. Alopecia: _____

  b. Hirsutism: _____

- Name the three types of lice.

  a. _____

  b. _____

  c. _____

Nails

- When inspecting the nail bed, the nurse notes

  the _____, _____,

  _____, _____,

  _____, and _____.

- The nurse palpates the nail base to determine:

  _____

  _____

- Briefly describe the following abnormalities of the nail bed.

  a. Clubbing: _____

  b. Beau's lines: _____

  c. Koilonychia: _____

  d. Splinter hemorrhages: _____

  e. Paronychia: _____

Assessing the Head and the Neck

Head

Inspection	Palpation	Percussion	Auscultation

- Define the following head abnormalities.

  a. Hydrocephalus: _____

  _____

  b. Acromegaly: _____

  _____

Eyes

Inspection	Palpation	Percussion	Auscultation
Visual Acuity			
Visual Fields			
Extraocular			
Movements			

Inspection and Internal Eye Structures

Inspection	Palpation	Percussion	Auscultation
Eyebrows			
Eyelids			
Lacrimal Apparatus			
Conjunctivae and Sclerae			
Corneas, Pupils, and Irises			

- Define the following common eye and visual abnormalities.

  a. Exophthalmos: _____

  b. Strabismus: _____

  c. Hyperopia: _____

  d. Myopia: _____

  e. Presbyopia: _____

  f. Astigmatism: _____

  g. Nystagmus: _____

- Identify the six structures you would assess in the internal eye.

  a. _____

  b. _____

  c. _____

  d. _____

  e. _____

  f. _____

Ears

Inspection	Palpation	Percussion	Auscultation
External Ear			
Middle Ear			
Inner Ear			

- Identify the mechanisms for sound transmission.

  a. _____

  b. _____

  c. _____

  d. _____

  e. _____

- Identify the types of problems that affect the ear.

  a. _____

  b. _____

  c. _____

  d. _____

- The three types of hearing loss are _____, _____, and _____.

- Define *ototoxicity*. _____ _____

- Briefly explain how a tuning fork works. ____ _____

- Define *Weber's test*. _____ _____

- Define *Rinné test*. _____ _____

Chapter 28: Health Assessment and Physical Examination   157

Nose and Paranasal Sinuses

Inspection	Palpation	Percussion	Auscultation
Nose			
Sinuses			

Mouth and Pharynx

Inspection	Palpation	Percussion	Auscultation
Lips			
Buccal Mucosa, Gums, and Teeth			
Tongue and Floor of Mouth			
Palate			
Pharynx			

- Define the following conditions of the mouth.

  a. Caries: _____

  b. Leukoplakia: _____

  c. Varicosities: _____

  d. Exostosis: _____

Neck

Inspection	Palpation	Percussion	Auscultation
Neck Muscles			
Lymph Nodes			
Thyroid Gland			
Carotid Artery and Jugular Vein			
Trachea			

Cranial Nerve Function

- Identify the 12 cranial nerves:

a. _____

b. _____

c. _____

d. _____

e. _____

f. _____

g. _____

h. _____

i. _____

j. _____

k. _____

l. _____

Assessing the Torso

Thorax and Lungs

Inspection	Palpation	Percussion	Auscultation
Posterior Thorax			
Lateral Thorax			
Anterior Thorax			

- Accurate physical assessment of the thorax and lungs requires review of the ventilatory and respiratory functions of the lung.

- Define *vocal* or *tactile fremitus*. _____
  _____
  _____

- Identify the normal breath sounds and where they are located.
  _____
  _____

- Complete the following table of adventitious breath sounds:

Sound	Auscultation Site	Cause	Character
Crackles			
Rhonchi			
Wheezes			
Pleural Friction Rub			

Assessing the Heart

- Assessment of heart function involves a review of signs and symptoms from the nursing history, pulse assessment, and direct examination of the heart.

- Answer the following questions regarding the PMI:

  a. What is the PMI? _____

  b. Where is the PMI normally located in the infant and young child? _____

  _____

  c. Where is the PMI located in the older child and adult? _____

  _____

  d. What techniques may be used to locate the PMI? _____

  _____

- Define what occurs during the two phases of the cardiac cycle.

  a. Systole: _____

  _____

  b. Diastole: _____

  _____

- Define the following heart sounds.

  S_1: _____

  S_2: _____

  S_3: _____

  S_4: _____

- Define *dysrhythmia*. _____

  _____

  _____

- Define *murmur*. _____

  _____

- List the six factors to assess when a murmur is detected.

  a. _____

  b. _____

  c. _____

  d. _____

  e. _____

  f. _____

- Define *thrill*. _____

  _____

  _____

Assessing the Breasts

- It is important to examine the breasts of female and male clients.

Inspection	Palpation	Percussion	Auscultation
Breasts			

- The American Cancer Society (1998) recommends the following guidelines for early detection of breast cancer.

  a. _____

  b. _____

  c. _____

  d. _____

  e. _____

- Briefly explain the proper technique for palpating breast tissue. _____

  _____

  _____

- List seven characteristics that should be included when describing an abnormal breast mass.

  a. _____

  b. _____

  c. _____

  d. _____

  e. _____

  f. _____

  g. _____

- Define the following terms.

  a. Metastasize: _____

  b. Fibrocystic breast disease: _____

Assessing the Abdomen

- The abdominal examination includes an assessment of the lower GI tract in addition to the liver, stomach, uterus, ovaries, kidneys, and bladder.

- Describe four techniques used to help the client relax during assessment of the abdomen.

  a. _____

  b. _____

  c. _____

  d. _____

Inspection	Palpation	Percussion	Auscultation
Abdomen

Liver | | | |

- Define the following.

  a. Hernias: _____

  b. Distention: _____

  c. Peristalsis: _____

  d. Paralytic ileus: _____

  e. Borborygmi: _____

  f. Rebound tenderness: _____

  g. Aneurysm: _____

Assessing the Female Genitalia and Reproductive Tract

- Briefly explain the preparation of a client for a complete examination of the genitalia and reproductive tract. _____

  _____

  _____

  _____

Inspection	Palpation	Percussion	Auscultation
External Genitalia			
Cervix			
Vagina			

- Define the following terms.

  a. Chancres: _____

  b. Cystocele: _____

  c. Rectocele: _____

- Speculum examination of the internal genitalia includes: _____

  _____

Assessing the Male Genitalia

- An examination of the male genitalia includes assessment of the external genitalia and the inguinal ring and canal.

Inspection	Palpation	Percussion	Auscultation
Penis			
Scrotum			
Inguinal Ring and Canal			
Rectum and Anus			

- Summarize how the nurse would assess sexual maturity. _____

_____

Assessing the Anus, Rectum, and Prostate

- The purpose of digital palpation is:

_____.

Assessing the Extremities

- The assessment of musculoskeletal function focuses on determining the range of joint motion, muscle strength and tone, and joint and muscle condition.

Joint Motion

Inspection	Palpation	Percussion	Auscultation
Joint Motion			

- Define:

  a. Hypertonicity: _____

  b. Hypotonicity: _____

  c. Kyphosis: _____

  d. Osteoporosis: _____

  e. Goniometer: _____

Neurological System

- The neurological system is responsible for many functions including _____

_____

Reflexes

- Eliciting reflex reactions allows the nurse to assess the integrity of sensory and motor pathways of the reflex arc and specific spinal cord segments.

- Briefly explain the two categories of normal reflexes. _____

_____

Vascular System

Inspection	Palpation	Percussion	Auscultation
Carotid Arteries			
Jugular Veins			
Peripheral Arteries			
Peripheral Veins			
Lymphatic System			

- Examination of the vascular system includes measurement of the blood pressure and a thorough assessment of the integrity of the peripheral vascular system.

- Explain the following conditions that are related to the vascular system.

   a. Syncope: _____

   b. Occlusion: _____

   c. Stenosis: _____

   d. Atherosclerosis: _____

   e. Bruit: _____

Chapter 28: Health Assessment and Physical Examination   165

- Explain the steps the nurse would use to assess venous pressure.

  a. _____

  b. _____

  c. _____

  d. _____

  e. _____

- The Allen's test is used to:

  _____

  _____

- The 3 Ps that characterize an occlusion are _____, _____, and _____.

- Phlebitis is:

  _____

  _____

$\mathcal{R}$eview Questions

The student should select the appropriate answer and cite the rationale for choosing that particular answer.

1. The component that should receive the highest priority before a physical examination is:
   a. Preparation of the environment
   b. Preparation of the equipment
   c. Physical preparation of the client
   d. Psychological preparation of the client

Answer: _____ Rationale: _____

_____

_____

2. The nurse assesses the skin turgor of the client by:
   a. Grasping a fold of skin on the back of the forearm and releasing
   b. Palpating the skin with the dorsum of the hand
   c. Pressing the skin for 5 seconds, releasing, and noting each centimeter of depth
   d. Inspecting the buccal mucosa with a penlight

Answer: _____ Rationale: _____

_____

_____

3. While examining Mr. Polanzsky, the nurse notes a circumscribed elevation of skin filled with serous fluid on his upper lip. The lesion is 0.4 cm in diameter. This type of lesion is called a:
   a. Macule
   b. Nodule
   c. Vesicle
   d. Pustule

Answer: _____ Rationale: _____

_____

_____

4. When assessing the client's thorax, the nurse should:
   a. Complete the left side and then the right side
   b. Change the position of the stethoscope between inspiration and expiration
   c. Compare symmetrical areas from side to side
   d. Begin with the posterior lobes on the right side

Answer: _____ Rationale: _____

_____

_____

5. In a client with pneumonia, the nurse hears high-pitched, continuous musical sounds over the bronchi on expiration. These sounds are called:
   a. Crackles
   b. Rhonchi
   c. Wheezes
   d. Friction rubs

Answer: _____ Rationale: _____

_____

_____

6. The second heart sound (S$_2$) occurs when:
   a. The mitral and tricuspid valves close
   b. There is rapid ventricular filling
   c. Systole begins
   d. The aortic and pulmonic valves close

Answer: _____ Rationale: _____

_____

_____

29

*I*nfection Control

Adapted by Jennifer Medves, RN, PhD, Queen's University

*P*reliminary Reading

Chapter 29, pp. 783-831

*C*omprehensive Understanding

Scientific Knowledge Base

- An infection is: _____

  _____

- Define *communicable*. _____

  _____

Chain of Infection

- Development of an infection occurs in a cycle that depends on the following elements:

  a. _____

  b. _____

  c. _____

  d. _____

  e. _____

  f. _____

- Micro-organisms include _____ and _____.

- Define: _____
  a. Virulence: _____
  b. Immuno-compromised: _____

- The potential for micro-organisms to cause disease depends on four factors. Name them.
  a. _____
  b. _____
  c. _____
  d. _____

- Define *reservoir*. _____
  _____

- Define *carriers*. _____
  _____

- To thrive, organisms require the following. Briefly explain each one.
  a. Food: _____
     _____
  b. Oxygen (or no oxygen): _____
     _____
  c. Water: _____
     _____
  d. Temperature: _____
     _____
  e. pH: _____
     _____
  f. Minimal light: _____
     _____

- What is a portal of exit? Give examples. _____
  _____

- List the major modes of transmission of micro-organisms from the reservoir to the host.
  _____

The Infectious Process

- The severity of the client's illness depends on the _____, the _____, and_____.

- Describe the two types of infections.
  a. Localized: _____
     _____
  b. Systemic: _____
     _____

Defences Against Infection

- The inflammatory response is: _____
  _____

- Explain the normal body defenses against infection.
  a. Normal flora: _____
     _____
  b. Body system defenses: _____
     _____
  c. Inflammation: _____
     _____

- For each body system or organ in the grid that follows, identify at least one defense mechanism and the primary action to prevent infection.

System/Organ	Defense Mechanism	Action
Skin		
Mouth		
Respiratory Tract		
Urinary Tract		
Gastrointestinal Tract		

- The inflammatory response includes the following. Explain each briefly.

   a. Vascular and cellular responses: _____

   _____

   b. Inflammatory exudate: _____

   _____

   c. Tissue repair: _____

   _____

- Briefly explain the following vascular and cellular responses.

   a. Edema: _____

   _____

   b. Phagocytosis: _____

   _____

Nosocomial Infections

- Define *nosocomial infection*. _____

   _____

- Define the following types of nosocomial infections.

   a. Iatrogenic: _____

   _____

   b. Exogenous: _____

   _____

   c. Endogenous: _____

   _____

- Identify at least three factors that increase a hospitalized client's risk of acquiring a nosocomial infection.

  a. _____

  b. _____

  c. _____

- Identify the major sites for nosocomial infection. _____

_____

The Nursing Process in Infection Control

Assessment

- The nurse assesses the client's _____, _____, and _____.

- Knowing the factors that increase the client's susceptibility or risk for infection, the nurse is better able to plan preventive therapy that includes aseptic technique.

- Any reduction in the body's primary or secondary defenses against infection places a client at risk. List at least four risk factors of each.

  a. Inadequate primary defenses:_____

  _____

  b. Inadequate secondary sources:_____

  _____

- The following factors influence client susceptibility to infection. Explain each one.

  a. Age: _____

  _____

  b. Nutritional status: _____

  _____

  c. Stress: _____

  _____

d. Disease process: _____

_____

e. Medical therapy:_____

_____

Clinical Appearance

- Describe the signs and symptoms of each type of infection.

  a. Local: _____

  _____

  b. Systemic: _____

  _____

- Describe how an infection is manifested in an older adult. _____

_____

Laboratory Data

- List at least five laboratory values that may indicate infection.

  a. _____

  b. _____

  c. _____

  d. _____

  e. _____

Clients With Infection

- The ways in which infection can affect the client's and family's needs may be _____, _____, _____, or _____,.

Nursing Diagnosis

- The nurse may diagnose a risk for infection or make diagnoses that result from the effects of infection on health status.

ℳℳ Planning

- List four common goals for the client with an actual or potential risk for infection.

  a. _____

  b. _____

  c. _____

  d. _____

ℳℳ Implementation

Health Promotion

- List five ways a nurse may prevent an infection from developing or spreading.

  a. _____

  b. _____

  c. _____

  d. _____

  e. _____

- List preventive interventions to protect a client from invasion by pathogens. _____

  _____

Acute Care Measures

- The nurse follows certain principles and procedures to prevent infection and to control its spread. Briefly explain what is meant by the concepts of *asepsis* and *medical asepsis*. _____

  _____

  _____

- Explain the following methods of controlling or eliminating infectious agents.

  a. Cleaning: _____

  _____

  b. Disinfection: _____

  _____

  c. Sterilization: _____

  _____

---

  d. Control or elimination of reservoirs: _____

  _____

  e. Control of portals of exit: _____

  _____

  f. Control of transmission: _____

  _____

  g. Hand hygiene: _____

  _____

- Describe the CDC guidelines on hand-washing and the use of alcohol-based waterless antiseptics:

  a. _____

  b. _____

  c. _____

  d. _____

  e. _____

  f. _____

  g. _____

  h. _____

  i. _____

- Many measures that control the exit of microorganisms also control the entrance of pathogens. Give at least five examples.

  a. _____

  b. _____

  c. _____

  d. _____

  e. _____

- A client's resistance to infection improves as the nurse protects the body's normal defenses against infection. Explain. _____

  _____

172   Chapter 29: Infection Control

- Standard precautions/routine practices call for the appropriate use of protective devices and clothing, including _____, _____, _____ and _____.

- Barrier protection is indicated for use with all clients because every client has the potential to _____.

- The CDC's isolation guidelines (1996) contain a two-tiered approach. Explain.

  a. Standard Precautions (Tier 1): _____ _____

  b. Transmission-Based (Isolation) Precautions (Tier 2): _____ _____

- List some basic principles common to all categories of isolation precautions. _____ _____

- Briefly summarize the psychological implications of isolation. _____ _____

- Explain the techniques for collecting specimens from the client with a suspected infection.

  a. Wound: _____ _____

  b. Blood: _____ _____

  c. Stool: _____ _____

  d. Urine: _____ _____

- Explain Health Canada's recommendations for bagging garbage or linen. _____ _____

- Describe how you would transport a client with an infection. _____ _____

Infection Prevention and Control for Hospital Personnel

- List eight responsibilities of the infection-control professional.

  a. _____

  b. _____

  c. _____

  d. _____

  e. _____

  f. _____

  g. _____

  h. _____

Client Education

- List six topics the nurse needs to discuss with the client in relation to infection-control practices.

  a. _____

  b. _____

  c. _____

  d. _____

  e. _____

  f. _____

Surgical Asepsis

- Explain when surgical asepsis must be used. _____ _____

- List three teaching points that reduce the risk of client-associated contamination during sterile procedures or treatments.

  a. _____

  b. _____

  c. _____

- List the seven principles of surgical asepsis.

  a. _____

  b. _____

  c. _____

  d. _____

  e. _____

  f. _____

  g. _____

- List and briefly explain the nine steps in performing a sterile procedure.

  a. _____

  b. _____

  c. _____

  d. _____

  e. _____

  f. _____

  g. _____

  h. _____

  i. _____

Evaluation

- The success of infection-control techniques is measured by determining whether the goals for reducing or preventing infection are achieved.

- Two important skills in evaluation are the ability to correctly assess wounds for healing and the ability to conduct a physical assessment of body systems.

- A clear description of any signs and symptoms of systemic or local infection is necessary to give all nurses a baseline for comparative evaluation.

- The client at risk for infection must understand the measures needed to reduce or prevent micro-organism growth and spread.

Review Questions

The student should select the appropriate answer and cite the rationale for choosing that particular answer.

1. Of the following, which is not an element in the chain of infection?
   a. Infectious agent or pathogen
   b. Reservoir for pathogen growth
   c. Mode of transmission
   d. Formation of immunoglobulin

   Answer: _____ Rationale: _____

   _____

   _____

2. Pathogenic organisms include all of the following *except:*
   a. Bacteria
   b. Leukocytes
   c. Viruses
   d. Fungi

   Answer: _____ Rationale: _____

   _____

   _____

3. The severity of a client's illness will depend on all of the following *except:*
   a. Extent of infection
   b. Pathogenicity of the microorganism
   c. Susceptibility of the host
   d. Incubation period

   Answer: _____ Rationale: _____

   _____

   _____

4. Which of the following best describes an iatrogenic infection?
   a. It results from a diagnostic or therapeutic procedure.
   b. It occurs when clients are infected with their own organisms as a result of immuno-deficiency.
   c. It involves an incubation period of 3 to 4 weeks before it can be detected.
   d. It results from an extended infection of the urinary tract.

Answer: _____ Rationale: _____

_____

_____

5. The nurse sets up a sterile field on the client's over-bed table. In which of the following instances is the field contaminated?
   a. The nurse keeps the top of the table above his or her waist.
   b. Sterile saline solution is spilled on the field.
   c. Sterile objects are kept within a 2.5-cm border of the field.
   d. The nurse, who has a cold, wears a double mask.

Answer: _____ Rationale: _____

_____

_____

6. When a client on airborne or droplet isolation precautions must be transported to another part of the hospital, which of the following is *not* required of the nurse?
   a. Place a mask on the client before leaving the room.
   b. Obtain a physician's order to prohibit the client from being transported.
   c. Advise personnel in diagnostic or procedural areas that the client is under isolation precautions.
   d. Provide the client with tissues and a bag for proper disposal of secretions.

Answer: _____ Rationale: _____

_____

_____

30

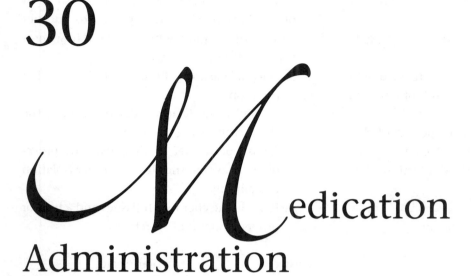

$\mathcal{M}$edication Administration

Adapted by Debbie Fraser Askin, RNC, MN, University of Manitoba

$\mathcal{P}$reliminary Reading

Chapter 30, pp. 832-919

$\mathcal{C}$omprehensive Understanding

Scientific Knowledge Base

- A medication is a substance used in the diagnosis, treatment, cure, relief, or prevention of health alterations.

Pharmacological Concepts

- A single medication may have three different names. Define each one.

  a. Chemical name: _____

  _____

  b. Generic name: _____

  _____

  c. Trade name: _____

  _____

- A medication classification indicates: _____

  _____

- The form of the medication determines its:

  _____

  _____

Medication Legislation and Standards

- Briefly summarize the role of the federal government in regulation. _____

  _____

- Explain the *Food and Drug Act*. _____

  _____

- The Health Protection Branch is responsible for: _____

  _____

- Summarize the role of the provincial government in drug regulation. _____

  _____

- Summarize the role of health care institutions.

  _____

  _____

Pharmacokinetics as the Basis of Medication Actions

- Pharmacokinetics is the study of: _____

  _____

Absorption

- Define *absorption*. _____

  _____

- Briefly explain the following factors that influence drug absorption.

  a. Route of administration: _____

  _____

  b. Ability of a medication to dissolve: _____

  _____

c. Blood flow to the area of absorption: _____

  _____

d. Body surface area: _____

e. Lipid solubility of a medication: _____

  _____

Distribution

- The rate and extent of distribution depend on the physical and chemical properties of the drug and on the physiological makeup of the person taking the drug.

- Explain how each of the following affect the rate and extent of medication distribution.

  a. Circulation: _____

  _____

  b. Membrane permeability: _____

  _____

  c. Protein binding: _____

  _____

Metabolism

- Define *biotransformation* and identify where it occurs. _____

  _____

Excretion

- After drugs are metabolized, they exit the body through the _____,

  _____, _____,

  _____, and _____.

- Identify the primary organ for drug excretion and explain what happens if this organ function declines. _____

  _____

Types of Medication Action

- Define the following predicted or unintended effects of drugs.

  a. Therapeutic effects: _____
  _____

  b. Side-effects: _____
  _____

  c. Adverse effects: _____
  _____

  d. Toxic effects: _____
  _____

  e. Idiosyncratic reactions: _____
  _____

  f. Allergic reactions: _____
  _____

  g. Anaphylactic reactions: _____
  _____

Medication Interactions

- A medication interaction is: _____
  _____

- A synergistic effect is: _____
  _____

Medication Dose Responses

- When a medication is prescribed, the goal is to achieve a constant blood level within a safe therapeutic range.

- Repeated doses are required to achieve a constant therapeutic concentration of a medication because a portion of a drug is always being excreted.

- Define the following.

  a. Serum concentration: _____
  _____

  b. Serum half-life: _____
  _____

- Explain the following time intervals of medication actions.

  a. Onset of drug action: _____
  _____

  b. Trough: _____
  _____

  d. Duration of action: _____
  _____

  e. Plateau: _____
  _____

Routes of Administration

- The route prescribed for a drug's administration depends on its properties, the desired effect, and the client's physical and mental condition.

Oral Routes

- The oral route is the easiest and the most commonly used route.

- Identify the types of oral routes, explain how the oral routes are used, and identify the effects of using these routes. _____
  _____

Parenteral Routes

- The parenteral route involves administering a drug through injection into body tissues.

- List the four major types of parenteral injections.

  a. _____

  b. _____

  c. _____

  d. _____

- Define the following advanced techniques of medication administration.

  a. Epidural: _____

  _____

  b. Intrathecal: _____

  _____

  c. Intraosseous: _____

  _____

  d. Intraperitoneal: _____

  _____

  e. Intrapleural: _____

  _____

  f. Intraarterial: _____

  _____

Topical Administration

- Medications that are applied to the skin and mucous membranes generally have local effects.

- Identify five methods for applying medications to mucous membranes.

  a. _____

  b. _____

  c. _____

  d. _____

  e. _____

Inhalation Route

- Describe the three passages through which inhalations can be administered.

  a. Nasal: _____

  _____

  b. Oral: _____

  _____

  c. Endotracheal or tracheal: _____

  _____

Intraocular Route

- Intraocular administration involves inserting a medication disk, similar to a contact lens, into the client's eye.

Systems of Medication Measurement

- The following are measurements used in drug therapy. Briefly explain their basic units.

  a. Metric system: _____

  _____

  b. Apothecary system: _____

  _____

  c. Household measurements: _____

  _____

- A solution is: _____

  _____

Clinical Calculations

Conversions Within One System

- Indicate which direction the decimal point is moved for the following mathematical calculations in the metric system.

  a. Division: _____

  b. Multiplication: _____

Conversion Between Systems

- To make actual drug calculations, it is necessary to work with units in the same measurement system.

- Before making a conversion, the nurse compares the measurement system available with that which has been ordered.

- Complete the following measurement equivalents:

Metric	Apothecary	Household
1 ml	_____ minims	_____ drops
_____ ml	_____ fluid drams	1 tablespoon
30 ml	_____ fluid ounce(s)	_____ tablespoon
_____ ml	_____ fluid ounce(s)	1 cup
_____ ml	1 pint	_____ pint
_____ ml	_____ quart	1 quart

- Complete the following conversions:

  a. 100 mg = _____ g

  b. 2.5 L = _____ mL

  c. 500 mL = _____ L

  d. 15 mg = _____ gr

  e. 30 gtt = _____ mL

  f. gr 1/6 = _____ mg

Dosage Calculations

- Write out the formula used to determine the correct dose when preparing solid or liquid forms of medications: _____

  _____

- Define the following.

  a. Dose ordered: _____

  b. Dose on hand: _____

  c. Amount on hand: _____

Pediatric Dosages

- Write out the formula applied to accurately calculate pediatric dosages. _____

  _____

- The nurse who is administering the medications is accountable for: _____

  _____

Nursing Knowledge Base

Prescriber's Role

- Identify the primary responsibilities of the prescriber in giving medications to clients.

  _____

Types of Orders

- Briefly explain the four common types of medication orders.

  a. Standing or routine: _____

  _____

  b. PRN: _____

  _____

  c. Single (one-time): _____

  _____

  d. STAT: _____

  _____

- List the six parts of a prescription.

  a. _____

  b. _____

  c. _____

  d. _____

  e. _____

  f. _____

- Identify the primary responsibility of the pharmacist in the administration of medications.

  _____

- List the three medication distribution systems and identify the advantages and disadvantages of each.

  a. _____

  b. _____

  c. _____

- Summarize the nurse's primary responsibilities when administering medications. _____

  _____

Critical Thinking

Knowledge

- Summarize the knowledge needed from other disciplines to safely administer medications.

  _____

- Psychomotor skills, the client's attitudes, knowledge, physical and mental status, and responses can make medication administration a complex experience.

- Demonstrating accountability and responsibility when administering medications means that the nurse: _____

  _____

- A medication error is: _____

  _____

Standards

- List the "six rights" of medication administration and briefly explain each one.

  a. _____

  b. _____

  c. _____

  d. _____

  e. _____

  f. _____

- Briefly summarize seven client rights related to medication administration. _____

  _____

Nursing Process and Medication Administration

Assessment

- Explain the following factors for assessment.

  a. History: _____

  _____

  b. History of allergies: _____

  _____

  c. Medication data: _____

  _____

  d. Diet history: _____

  _____

  e. Client's perceptual or coordination problems: _____

  _____

  f. Client's current condition: _____

  _____

  g. Client's attitude about medication use:

  _____

  _____

  h. Client's knowledge and understanding of medication therapy: _____

  _____

  i. Client's learning needs: _____

  _____

Nursing Diagnosis

- Assessment provides data on the client's condition, ability to self-administer medications, and medication use patterns. This information can be used to determine actual or potential problems with medication therapy.

Planning

- The nurse organizes care activities to ensure the safe administration of medications.

- Identify a goal and related outcomes that the nurse or client needs to meet before administration of medications.

  a. _____

  b. _____

  c. _____

  d. _____

Implementation

Health Promotion

- Identify factors that can influence the client's compliance with the medication regimen.

  _____

  _____

- Explain information that needs to be taught to the client and family in relation to medications.

  _____

  _____

Acute Care

- Explain why the following interventions are essential for safe and effective medication administration.

  a. Receiving medication orders: _____

  _____

  b. Correct transcription and communication of orders: _____

  _____

  c. Accurate dose calculation and measurement: _____

  _____

  d. Correct administration: _____

  _____

  e. Recording medication administration:

  _____

  _____

Restorative Care

- Regardless of the type of medication activity, the nurse is responsible for: _____

  _____

Special Considerations for Administering Medications to Specific Age Groups

Infants and Children

- Identify the appropriate nursing action used in administering medications to an infant or child.

  _____

Older Adults

- List the five behavioural patterns of medication use characteristic of the older adult and briefly explain each one.

  a. _____

  b. _____

  c. _____

  d. _____

  e. _____

Evaluation

- The nurse must know the therapeutic action and common side effects of each medication in order to monitor a client's response to that medication.

- Many different evaluation measures can be used in the context of medication administration. Name some of them. _____

  _____

- The most common type of measurement is:

  _____

  _____

Medication Administration

Oral Administration

- The easiest and most desirable way to administer medications is by mouth.

- The primary contraindication to giving oral medications is: _____

  _____

- To protect the client against possible aspiration, the nurse: _____

  _____

Topical Medication Applications

- Topical medications are applied locally, most often to intact skin. They can also be applied to mucous membranes.

Skin Applications

- Explain the procedure for administering the following skin applications.

  a. Ointment: _____

  _____

  b. Lotion: _____

  _____

  c. Powder: _____

  _____

Nasal Instillation

- Summarize the rationale for nasal instillations.

  _____

  _____

Eye Instillation

- List three principles for administering eye instillations.

  a. _____

  b. _____

  c. _____

Ear Instillation

- Explain the procedure for administering ear instillations.

  a. Adult: _____

  _____

  b. Children: _____

  _____

Vaginal Instillation

- Vaginal medications are available as

  _____, _____,

  _____, or _____.

Rectal Instillation

- Explain the differences between vaginal and rectal suppositories and the reason for these differences. _____

  _____

Administering Medications by Inhalation

- To maximize the effect of metered dose inhalers, the nurse advises the client to: _____

  _____

Administering Medications by Irrigations

- Identify the principles the nurse follows when performing irrigations. _____

  _____

Administering Parenteral Medications

- Each type of injection requires certain skills to ensure that the drug reaches the proper location.

- When medications are administered parenterally, it is an invasive procedure that must be performed using aseptic techniques.

Equipment

- Identify the three major types of syringes.

  a. _____

  b. _____

  c. _____

- Identify three factors that must be considered when selecting a needle for an injection.

  a. _____

  b. _____

  c. _____

- Identify the advantages of using the Tubex or Carpuject injection systems. _____

_____

Preparing an Injection From an Ampule

- An ampule is: _____

_____

- The procedure for withdrawing medications from ampules is outlined in Skill 30-7 on page 885 of your textbook.

Preparing an Injection From a Vial

- A vial is a: _____

_____

- The vial is a closed system, and air must be injected into it to permit easy withdrawal of the solution.

- The procedure for withdrawal of medications from vials is outlined in Skill 30-7 on page 885 of your textbook.

Mixing Medications

- It is possible to mix two drugs together into one injection if the total dosage is within accepted limits.

- List the three principles to follow when mixing medications from two vials:

  a. _____

  b. _____

  c. _____

- When mixing medications from an ampule and a vial, which medication should be prepared first?

_____

Insulin Preparation

- Insulin is: _____

_____

- Explain why insulin must be administered by injection. _____

_____

- Insulin is classified by: _____

- _____ is the only insulin used for sliding scales.

- Identify the simple guidelines for mixing two kinds of insulin in the same syringe.

_____

_____

Administering Injections

- The characteristics of the tissues injected influence the: _____

_____

- List the techniques used to minimize client discomfort that is associated with injections.

  a. _____

  b. _____

  c. _____

  d. _____

  e. _____

  f. _____

  g. _____

Subcutaneous Injections

- Subcutaneous injections involve placing the medications into the loose connective tissue under the dermis.

- Explain the differences in absorption between a subcutaneous and an intramuscular injection.

  _____

  _____

- The best sites for SQ injections include

  _____, _____, and

  _____.

- The site most frequently recommended for heparin injection is _____.

- The site chosen should be free of

  _____, _____, and

  _____.

- Identify the maximum amount of water-soluble medication given by the SQ route. ___

  _____

- State the rule that may be followed to determine if a SQ injection should be given at a 90- or 45-degree angle. _____

  _____

Intramuscular Injections

- Identify the major risk of using the IM route.

  _____

  _____

- The angle of insertion for an IM injection is _____ degrees.

- Indicate the maximum volume of medication for IM injection in each of the following groups.

  a. Well-developed adult: _____

  b. Older children, older adults, or thin adults:

  _____

  c. Older infants and small children: _____

Sites

- List the assessment criteria for selecting an IM site.

  a. _____

  b. _____

  c. _____

  d. _____

- Describe the advantages and disadvantages of the following injection sites.

  a. Vastus lateralis: _____

  _____

  b. Ventrogluteal: _____

  _____

  c. Dorsogluteal: _____

  _____

  d. Deltoid: _____

  _____

Special Techniques in IM Injections

- Explain the rationale for administering an intramuscular injection using the air-lock technique.

  _____

  _____

- Explain the rationale for using the Z-track method of injection. _____

  _____

  _____

Intradermal Injections

- Explain the rationale for administering an intradermal injection. _____

  _____

Safety in Administering Medications by Injection

- Explain the rationale for each of the following.

  a. Needleless device: _____

  _____

  b. One-handed needle recapping technique:

  _____

  _____

IV Administration

- The nurse administers medications intravenously by the following methods. _____

  _____

  _____

- Identify the advantage and disadvantage of the large-volume infusion method. _____

  _____

  _____

- Explain the advantage and disadvantage of the IV bolus route of administration. _____

  _____

  _____

- List the advantages of using volume-controlled infusions.

  a. _____

  b. _____

  c. _____

- Piggyback sets are: _____

  _____

- A tandem setup is: _____

  _____

- Volume-control administration sets are: _____

  _____

- A mini-infusor pump is: _____

  _____

- List the three advantages of using intermittent venous access devices.

  a. _____

  b. _____

  c. _____

Administration of Intravenous Therapy in the Home

- When receiving home intravenous therapy, client education should include: _____

  _____

Review Questions

The student should select the appropriate answer and cite the rationale for choosing that particular answer.

1. The study of how drugs enter the body, reach their sites of action, are metabolized, and exit from the body is called:
   a. Pharmacology
   b. Pharmacokinetics
   c. Pharmacopoeia
   d. Biopharmaceutica

Answer: _____ Rationale: _____

_____

_____

2. Which statement correctly characterizes drug absorption?

a. Many drugs must enter the systemic circulation to have a therapeutic effect.

b. Mucous membranes are relatively impermeable to chemicals, making absorption slow.

c. Oral medications are absorbed more quickly when administered with meals.

d. Drugs administered subcutaneously are absorbed more quickly than those injected intramuscularly.

Answer: _____ Rationale: _____

_____

_____

3. The onset of drug action is the time it takes for a drug to:

a. Produce a response

b. Accelerate the cellular process

c. Reach its highest effective concentration

d. Produce blood serum concentration and maintenance

Answer: _____ Rationale: _____

_____

_____

4. Which of the following is *not* a parenteral route of administration?

a. Buccal

b. Subcutaneous

c. Intramuscular

d. Intradermal

Answer: _____ Rationale: _____

_____

_____

5. Using the body surface area formula, what dose of drug X should a child who weighs 12 kg (body surface area = 0.54 m^2) receive if the normal adult dose of drug X is 300 mg?

a. 50 mg

b. 90 mg

c. 100 mg

d. 200 mg

Answer: _____ Rationale: _____

_____

_____

6. The nurse is preparing an insulin injection in which both short-acting (clear) and long-acting (cloudy) insulin will be mixed. Into which vial should the nurse inject air first?

a. The vial of long-acting insulin

b. The vial of short-acting insulin

c. Either vial, as long as long-acting insulin is drawn up first

d. Neither vial; it is not necessary to put air into vials before withdrawing medication

Answer: _____ Rationale: _____

_____

_____

31

Complementary and Alternative Therapies

Adapted by Jean McClennon-Leong, RN, MN, APNP, Northeast Wisconsin Technical College

Preliminary Reading

Chapter 31, pp. 920-939

Comprehensive Understanding

Complementary or Alternative Medicine Therapies in Health Care

• Describe the difference between the following terms.

a. Complementary therapies: _____

_____

b. Alternative therapies: _____

_____

• Explain the following alternative medical systems and give an example of each.

a. Acupuncture: _____

_____

b. Ayurveda: _____

_____

c. Homeopathic medicine: _____

_____

d. Latin American practices: _____

_____

e. Traditional Aboriginal medicine: _____

_____

f. Naturopathic medicine: _____

_____

g. Traditional Chinese medicine: _____

_____

- Describe integrative medical programs. _____

_____

Nursing-Accessible Therapies

Relaxation Therapy

- Define *stress response*. _____

_____

- Relaxation is: _____

_____

- Progressive relaxation training helps to: _____

_____

- Passive relaxation involves teaching: _____

_____

- Relaxation techniques lower _____,

  decrease _____, improve

  _____, and reduce _____.

- The type of relaxation intervention should be

  matched to: _____

_____

- Identify the limitations of relaxation therapy.

_____

_____

Meditation and Breathing

- Meditation is: _____

_____

- Identify the clinical applications of medita-

  tion. _____

_____

- Identify the limitations of meditation. _____

_____

Imagery

- Imagery is: _____

_____

- Creative visualization is: _____

_____

- Identify the clinical applications of imagery.

_____

_____

- Identify the limitations of imagery. _____

_____

Training-Specific Therapies

Biofeedback

- Biofeedback is: _____

_____

- Identify the clinical applications of biofeed-

  back. _____

_____

- Identify the limitations of biofeedback. _____

_____

Therapeutic Touch

- Therapeutic touch is: _____

_____

Chapter 31: Complementary and Alternative Therapies   189

- Therapeutic touch consists of five phases. Explain each one.

  a. Centring: _____

  _____

  b. Assessment: _____

  _____

  c. Unruffling: _____

  _____

  d. Treatment: _____

  _____

  e. Evaluation: _____

  _____

- Identify the physiological indicators of energy imbalance. _____

  _____

- Identify the clinical applications for therapeutic touch. _____

  _____

- Identify the limitations of therapeutic touch.

  _____

  _____

Chiropractic Therapy

- Chiropractic therapy is: _____

  _____

- Describe the clinical applications of chiropractic therapy. _____

  _____

- Identify the limitations of chiropractic therapy. _____

  _____

Traditional Chinese Medicine

- Traditional Chinese Medicine (TCM) comprises several healing modalities, including

  _____

- Explain the concept of yin and yang. _____

  _____

- *Qi* is: _____

  _____

- Traditional Chinese medicine classifies disease into three categories. State the influences of each.

  a. External causes: _____

  _____

  b. Internal causes: _____

  _____

  c. Non-external, non-internal causes: _____

  _____

- Define *meridians*. _____

  _____

Acupuncture

- Acupuncture is: _____

  _____

- Describe the clinical applications of acupuncture. _____

  _____

- Identify the limitations of acupuncture. _____

  _____

Herbal Therapies

- The goal of herbal therapy is: _____

  _____

- Describe the clinical applications of herbal therapy. _____

  _____

- Explain what a natural product number is.

  _____

  _____

- Identify the limitations of herbal therapy.

  _____

  _____

- Herbal products should be used cautiously with: _____

  _____

Nursing Role in Complementary and Alternative Therapies

- Summarize the role of the nurse regarding complementary and alternative medicine therapies.

  _____

  _____

*R*eview Questions

The student should select the appropriate answer and cite the rationale for choosing that particular answer.

1. Clients choose to use unconventional therapy because:
   a. They are willing to pay more to feel better.
   b. It is now widely accepted by Health Canada's Office of Natural Health Products.
   c. They are dissatisfied with conventional medicine.
   d. They want religious approval for the remedies they use.

   Answer: _____ Rationale: _____

   _____

   _____

2. An herb considered safe for the treatment of mild depression is:
   a. Milk thistle
   b. St. John's Wort
   c. Pokeroot
   d. Hawthorn

   Answer: _____ Rationale: _____

   _____

   _____

3. Nurses can best assess their client's use of alternative therapies by:
   a. Asking the client true/false questions about their health
   b. Asking for a thorough medical history
   c. Reviewing laboratory studies that assess levels of certain herbs
   d. Asking open-ended questions on alternative therapies

   Answer: _____ Rationale: _____

   _____

   _____

4. Which of the following steps should nurses take to be better informed about alternative therapies?
   a. Keep abreast of the current research on alternative therapies.
   b. Familiarize themselves with recent case studies on alternative therapies.
   c. Familiarize themselves with general principles of phytotherapy.
   d. Review herb manufacturer's literature on specific herbs.

   Answer: _____ Rationale: _____

   _____

   _____

32

*A*ctivity and Exercise

Adapted by Ann Brokenshire, RN, BScN, MEd, Ryerson University

*P*reliminary Reading

Chapter 32, pp. 940-969

*C*omprehensive Understanding

Scientific Knowledge Base

- *Body mechanics* include: _____
  _____
  _____

Overview of Body Mechanics, Exercise, and Activity

- The coordinated efforts of the musculoskeletal and nervous systems to maintain _____,
  _____, and _____ during lifting, bending, moving, and performing _____
  provide the foundation for body mechanics.

- Define *body alignment*. _____
  _____

- *Body balance* is achieved when: _____
  _____

- Proper body alignment and posture are maintained by using two simple techniques. Name them.

    a. _____

    b. _____

- Define *centre of gravity*. _____

    _____

- Coordinated body movement is the result of

    _____, _____, and

    _____.

- Define *friction*. _____

    _____

- List two techniques that minimize friction.

    a. _____

    b. _____

- *Activity tolerance* is: _____

    _____

- There are three categories of exercises. Briefly explain and give an example of each.

    a. Isotonic contraction: _____

    _____

    b. Isometric contraction: _____

    _____

    c. Resistive isometric: _____

    _____

Regulation of Movement

- List three systems responsible for coordinating body movements.

    a. _____

    b. _____

    c. _____

- List five functions of the skeletal system.

    a. _____

    b. _____

    c. _____

    d. _____

    e. _____

- Describe the following.

    a. Joints: _____

    b. Cartilaginous joint: _____

    c. Fibrous joint: _____

    d. Synovial joint: _____

    e. Ligaments: _____

    f. Cartilage: _____

    g. Tendons: _____

- Briefly describe how skeletal muscles affect movement. _____

    _____

- Briefly explain the work of muscles concerned with:

    a. Movement: _____

    _____

    b. Posture: _____

    _____

- The nervous system regulates and coordinates the following different muscle groups. Briefly explain each.

    a. Antagonistic muscles: _____

    _____

    b. Synergistic muscles: _____

    _____

    c. Antigravity muscles: _____

    _____

- Briefly describe how movement and posture are regulated by the nervous system. _____

    _____

- Define *proprioception*. _____

    _____

Chapter 32: Activity and Exercise   193

- The structures in the ear that assist in maintaining balance are the _____.

Principles of Body Mechanics

- List at least five principles of body mechanics.

    a. _____

    _____

    b. _____

    _____

    c. _____

    _____

    d. _____

    _____

    e. _____

    _____

Pathological Influences on Body Mechanics

- Briefly explain how the following pathological conditions may affect body alignment and mobility.

    a. Congenital abnormalities: _____

    _____

    b. Disorders of bones, joints, and muscles:

    _____

    _____

    c. Central nervous system damage: _____

    _____

    d. Musculoskeletal trauma: _____

    _____

Nursing Knowledge Base

- _____, _____,

    _____, _____, and

    _____ are important aspects of an individual that must be incorporated into the plan of care.

Developmental Changes

- The greatest change and impact on the maturational process is observed in _____ and _____.

- Identify the descriptive characteristics of body alignment and mobility related to the following developmental changes.

    a. Infants: _____

    _____

    b. Toddlers: _____

    _____

    c. Adolescents: _____

    _____

    d. Young to middle adults: _____

    _____

    e. Older adults: _____

    _____

Behavioural Aspects

- Clients are more likely to incorporate an exercise program into their daily life if they have _____ and _____.

Environmental Issues

- Explain the exercise and activity issues related to the following sites.

    a. Work: _____

    _____

    b. Schools: _____

    _____

    c. Community: _____

    _____

Cultural and Ethnic Influences

- The nurse must consider what motivates and what is deemed appropriate and enjoyable when developing a physical fitness program for culturally diverse populations. Design a comprehensive fitness program for two different ethno-cultural groups with which you interact.

_____

_____

_____

_____

Family and Social Support

- Briefly explain how a family may be a motivational tool in regard to physical fitness. _____

_____

Nursing Process

Assessment

- Throughout the assessment, the nurse will be able to determine _____,

_____, and _____.

- Briefly explain how assessment of body alignment and posture is carried out.

  a. Standing: _____

  _____

  b. Sitting: _____

  _____

  c. Recumbent: _____

  _____

- There are three components to assess in regard to mobility. Explain each.

  a. Range of motion: _____

  _____

  b. Gait: _____

  _____

  c. Exercise: _____

  _____

- Identify some factors that affect activity tolerance. _____

_____

Nursing Diagnosis

- Assessment of the _____,

_____, _____, and

_____ provides clusters of data or defining characteristics that lead the nurse to identify nursing diagnoses.

- Give five examples of nursing diagnoses related to exercise and activity.

  a. _____

  b. _____

  c. _____

  d. _____

  e. _____

Planning

- The plan should include consideration of:

  a. _____

  b. _____

  c. _____

  d. _____

  e. _____

Implementation

Health Promotion

- List the five recommendations for exercise.

  a. _____

  b. _____

  c. _____

  d. _____

  e. _____

- Explain how to calculate the client's maximum heart rate (MHR). _____
  _____

- An exercise program should include the following. Explain each one.
  a. Aerobic exercise: _____
     _____
  b. Stretching and flexibility exercises: _____
     _____
  c. Resistance training: _____
     _____

- Briefly explain proper lifting techniques. ____
  _____

Acute Care

- The musculoskeletal system can be maintained by encouraging the use of stretching and isometric-type exercises.

- Briefly explain the technique of stretching exercises. _____
  _____

- Explain how the nurse would maintain or improve joint mobility. _____
  _____

- Explain how walking affects joint mobility.
  _____
  _____

- Explain how the nurse would assist the client to walk. _____
  _____

Restorative and Continuing Care

- The nurse, in collaboration with others, promotes activity and exercise by teaching the use of assistive devices most appropriate for a client's condition. Briefly explain the appropriate use of the following.

  a. Canes: _____
  b. Crutches: _____
  c. Walkers: _____

- Explain the following crutch gaits.
  a. Four-point: _____
     _____
  b. Three-point: _____
     _____
  c. Two-point: _____
     _____
  d. Swing-through: _____
     _____

- Explain how the nurse would instruct the client in each of the following.
  a. Crutch walking on stairs: _____
     _____
  b. Sitting in the chair with crutches: _____
     _____

- Explain how the nurse would implement a plan of care to increase activity and exercise in the following specific disease conditions.
  a. Coronary heart disease: _____
     _____
  b. Hypertension: _____
     _____
  c. Chronic obstructive pulmonary disease:
     _____
     _____
  d. Diabetes mellitus: _____
     _____

Evaluation

Client Care

- This phase of the nursing process evaluates the actual care delivered by the health team based on the expected outcomes.

- Comparisons are made with baseline measures that include _____, _____, _____, _____, and _____.

Client Expectations

- The nurse needs to know the client's expectations concerning activity and exercise.

Review Questions

The student should select the appropriate answer and cite the rationale for choosing that particular answer.

1. Which of the following is true of body mechanics?
   a. The narrower the base of support, the greater the stability of the nurse.
   b. The higher the centre of gravity, the greater the stability of the nurse.
   c. When friction is reduced between the object to be moved and the surface on which it is moved, less force is required to move it.
   d. Rolling, turning, or pivoting requires more work than lifting.

Answer: _____ Rationale: _____

_____

_____

2. White, shiny, flexible bands of fibrous tissue binding joints together and connecting various bones and cartilage types are known as:
   a. Muscles
   b. Ligaments
   c. Joints
   d. Tendons

Answer: _____ Rationale: _____

_____

_____

3. The nurse would expect all of the following physiological effects of exercise on the body systems *except*:
   a. Decreased cardiac output
   b. Increased respiratory rate and depth
   c. Increased muscle tone, size, and strength
   d. Change in metabolic rate

Answer: _____ Rationale: _____

_____

_____

4. Which of the following is *not* true of the two-point gait with crutches?
   a. The client requires at least partial weight bearing on each foot.
   b. The client is required to bear all of the weight on one foot.
   c. The client moves one crutch at the same time as the opposing leg.
   d. Crutch movements are similar to arm motion during normal walking.

Answer: _____ Rationale: _____

_____

_____

5. Which of the following is a possible nursing diagnosis related to activity and exercise?
   a. Altered thought processes
   b. Altered oral mucous membrane
   c. Relocation stress syndrome
   d. Impaired gas exchange

Answer: _____ Rationale: _____

_____

_____

Critical Thinking for Nursing Care Plan for Activity Intolerance

Imagine that you are Erich, the nurse in the Care Plan on page 954 of your text. Complete the *planning phase* of the critical thinking model by writing your answers in the appropriate boxes of the model shown. Think about the following:

- In developing Mrs. Smith's plan of care, what knowledge did Erich apply?

- In what way might Erich's previous experience assist in developing a plan of care for Mrs. Smith?

- When developing a plan of care, what intellectual or professional standards were applied to Mrs. Smith?

- What critical thinking attitudes might have been applied in developing Mrs. Smith's plan?

- How will Erich accomplish his goals?

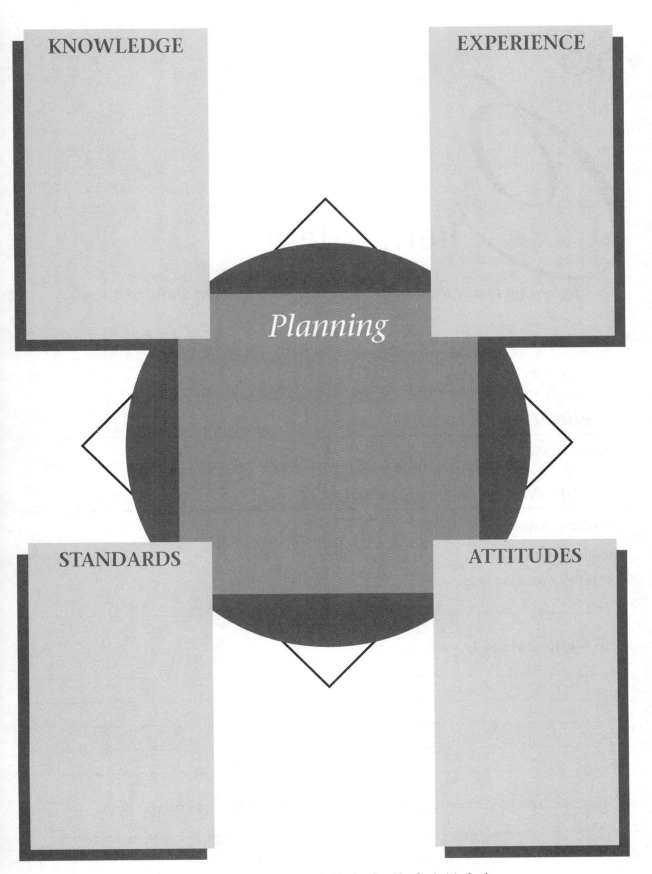

KNOWLEDGE

EXPERIENCE

Planning

STANDARDS

ATTITUDES

CHAPTER 32 Critical Thinking Model for Nursing Care Plan for *Activity Intolerance*

See answers on page 591.

33

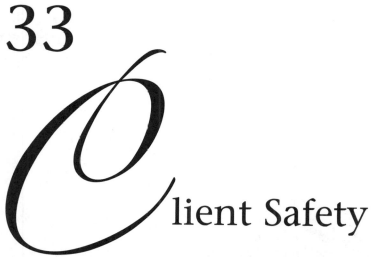

Client Safety

Adapted by Daria Romaniuk, RN, BN, MN, Ryerson University

Preliminary Reading

Chapter 33, pp. 970-1010

Comprehensive Understanding

Scientific Knowledge Base

Environmental Safety

- A client's environment includes: _____

  _____

- List five characteristics of a safe environment.

  a. _____

  b. _____

  c. _____

  d. _____

  e. _____

- Give an example of the four basic physiological needs that influence a person's safety.

  a. Oxygen: _____

  b. Nutrition: _____

  c. Temperature: _____

  d. Humidity: _____

- Physical hazards in the community and health care settings place clients at risk for accidental injury and death. List four physical hazards that contribute to falls.

  a. _____

  b. _____

  c. _____

  d. _____

- Define *pathogen*. _____
  _____

- Identify the most effective method for limiting the transmission of pathogens. _____
  _____

- Define *immunization*. _____
  _____

- Describe the two types of immunity.

  a. Active: _____

  b. Passive: _____

- Describe how the human immunodeficiency virus (HIV) is transmitted and who is at risk.
  _____
  _____

- A healthy environment is free from pollution. A pollutant is: _____
  _____

- Define the following types of pollution.

  a. Air: _____

  b. Land: _____

  c. Water: _____

  d. Noise: _____

Nursing Knowledge Base

- In addition to being knowledgeable about the environment, nurses must be familiar with:

  a. _____

  b. _____

  c. _____

  d. _____

  e. _____

Risks at Developmental Stages

- Identify at least three threats to safety in the following developmental stages.

  a. Infant, toddler, preschooler: _____

  b. School-age: _____

  c. Adolescents: _____

  d. Adult: _____

  e. Older adult: _____

Individual Risk Factors

- Explain how the following risk factors threaten safety.

  a. Lifestyle: _____
  _____

  b. Impaired mobility: _____
  _____
  _____

  c. Sensory or communication impairment:
  _____
  _____

  d. Lack of safety awareness: _____
  _____

Risks in the Health Care Agency

- List the four major risks to client safety in the health care environment.

  a. _____

  b. _____

  c. _____

  d. _____

Safety and the Nursing Process

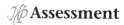Assessment

- In order to conduct a thorough client assessment, the nurse will consider possible threats to the client's safety, including the client's immediate environment and any individual risk factors.

- Identify the specific assessments a nurse needs to make in the following settings.

  a. The client's home: _____

  b. A health care facility: _____

- Explain the following health care environment risks.

  a. Risk for falls: _____

  _____

  b. Risk for medical errors: _____

  _____

Nursing Diagnosis

- Identify four actual or potential nursing diagnoses for safety risks.

  a. _____

  b. _____

  c. _____

  d. _____

Planning

- Identify common goals that focus on the client's need for safety.

  a. _____

  b. _____

  c. _____

Implementation

Health Promotion

- In order to promote an individual's health it is necessary for the individual to be in a safe environment and to practice a lifestyle that minimizes risk of injury.

- Identify at least four interventions for each of the following developmental age groups.

  a. Infant, toddler, preschooler: _____

  b. School-age: _____

  c. Adolescent: _____

  d. Adult: _____

  e. Older adult: _____

- Nurses can contribute to a safer environment by helping the client _____.

Acute Care

- List eight measures to prevent falls in the health care setting.

  a. _____

  b. _____

  c. _____

  d. _____

  e. _____

  f. _____

  g. _____

  h. _____

- A physical restraint is _____.

- The immobility imposed by restraining a client can lead to the following complications.

  a. Physical: _____

  _____

  b. Psychological: _____

  _____

- Use of restraints must meet the following objectives.

  a. _____

  b. _____

  c. _____

  d. _____

- Explain why an Ambularm is used. _____

  _____

- Explain the use of side rails. _____

  _____

- Describe four fire-containment guidelines.

  a. _____

  b. _____

  c. _____

  d. _____

- A poison is: _____

  _____

- List five teaching strategies for prevention of electrical hazards.

  a. _____

  b. _____

  c. _____

  d. _____

  e. _____

- A seizure is: _____

  _____

- Identify the measures with which the nurse must be familiar to reduce exposure to radiation. _____

  _____

Evaluation

Client Care

- The nurse continually assesses the client and family's need for additional support services such as _____, _____, and _____.

Client Expectations

The expected outcomes include a _____ and _____ environment.

Review Questions

The student should select the appropriate answer and cite the rationale for choosing that particular answer.

1. Which of the following would most threaten an individual's safety?
   a. 70% humidity
   b. Carbon dioxide
   c. Unrefrigerated fresh vegetables
   d. Lack of water supply

   Answer: _____ Rationale: _____

   _____

   _____

2. The developmental stage that carries the highest risk of an injury from a fall is:
   a. Preschool
   b. School-age
   c. Adulthood
   d. Older adulthood

   Answer: _____ Rationale: _____

   _____

   _____

3. Mrs. Gupta falls asleep while smoking in bed and drops the burning cigarette on her blanket. When she awakens, her bed is on fire, and she quickly calls the nurse. On observing the fire, the nurse should immediately:
   a. Report the fire
   b. Attempt to extinguish the fire
   c. Assist Mrs. Gupta to a safe place
   d. Close all windows and doors to contain the fire

   Answer: _____ Rationale: _____
   _____
   _____

4. Sixteen-year-old Simon is admitted to an adolescent unit with a diagnosis of substance abuse. The nurse examines Simon and finds that he has bloodshot eyes, slurred speech, and an unstable gait. He smells of alcohol and is unable to answer questions appropriately. The appropriate nursing diagnosis would be:
   a. Self-care deficit related to alcohol abuse
   b. Altered thought processes related to sensory overload
   c. Knowledge deficit related to alcohol abuse
   d. High risk for injury related to impaired sensory perception

   Answer: _____ Rationale: _____
   _____
   _____

5. If a client receives an electric shock, the nurse's first action should be to:
   a. Assess the client's pulse
   b. Assess the client for thermal injury
   c. Notify the physician
   d. Notify the maintenance department

   Answer: _____ Rationale: _____
   _____
   _____

Critical Thinking for Nursing Care Plan for Risk for Injury

Imagine that you are Mr. Key, the nurse in the Care Plan on page 984 of your text. Complete the *assessment phase* of the critical thinking model by writing your answers in the appropriate boxes of the model shown. Think about the following:

- In developing Ms. Cohen's plan of care, what knowledge did Mr. Key apply?

- In what way might Mr. Key's previous experience assist in this case?

- What intellectual or professional standards were applied to Ms. Cohen's case?

- What critical thinking attitudes might have been applied in this case?

- As you review your assessment, what key areas did you cover?

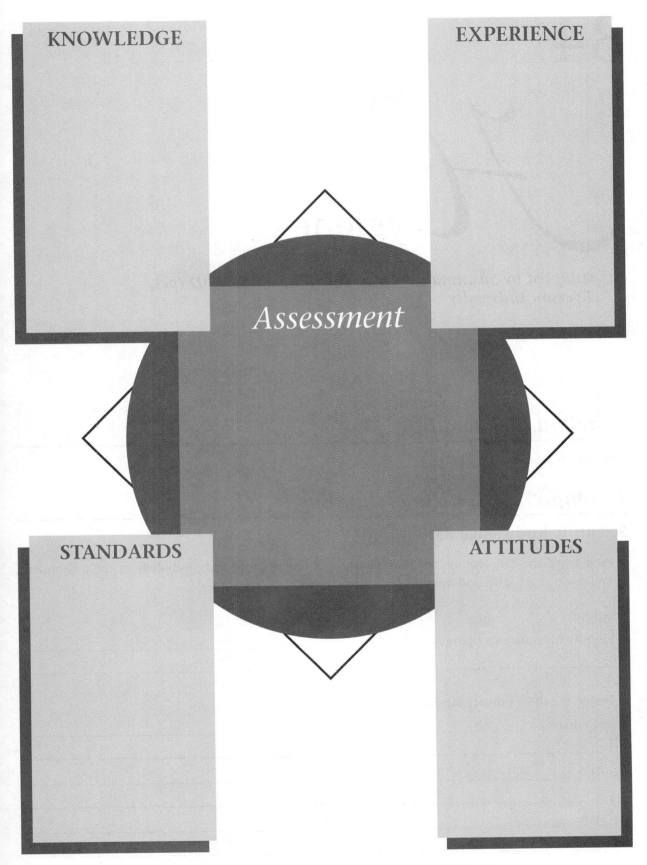

KNOWLEDGE

EXPERIENCE

Assessment

STANDARDS

ATTITUDES

CHAPTER *33* Critical Thinking Model for Nursing Care Plan for *Risk for Injury*

See answers on page 592.

34

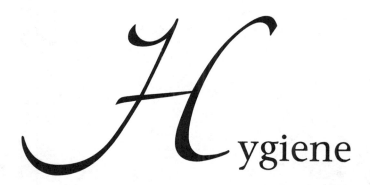

Hygiene

*Adapted by Susanna Edwards, RN, BScN, MSc, PhD (pc),
Ryerson University*

Preliminary Reading

Chapter 34, pp. 1011-1076

Comprehensive Understanding

Scientific Knowledge Base

- Proper hygiene care requires an understanding of the anatomy and physiology of the integument, oral cavity, eyes, ears, and nose.

The Skin

- Identify the functions of the skin. _____
  _____

- Define the three primary layers.

  a. Epidermis: _____
  _____

  b. Dermis: _____
  _____

  c. Subcutaneous: _____
  _____

The Feet, Hands, and Nails

- Define the following terms.

  a. Cuticle: _____

  _____

  b. Lunula: _____

  _____

The Oral Cavity

- There are three pairs of salivary glands that secrete about 1 litre of saliva a day.

- The buccal glands are: _____

  _____

- Teeth are organs of chewing, or _____, and are designed to _____.

- Regular oral hygiene is necessary to maintain the integrity of tooth surfaces and to prevent:

  _____

The Hair

- Identify the factors that can affect the hair's characteristics. _____

  _____

The Eyes, Ears, and Nose

- Cleansing of the sensitive sensory tissues should be done to prevent injury and client discomfort.

Nursing Knowledge Base

- Briefly explain each of the following factors influencing hygiene habits.

  a. Social practices: _____

  _____

  b. Personal preferences:_____

  _____

  c. Body image:_____

  _____

d. Socio-economic status: _____

_____

e. Health beliefs and motivation: _____

_____

f. Cultural variables: _____

_____

g. Physical condition: _____

_____

The Nursing Process

Assessment

Skin

- When inspecting the skin, the nurse thoroughly examines:

  a. _____

  b. _____

  c. _____

  d. _____

  e. _____

  f. _____

- Common skin problems can affect how hygiene is administered. Describe the hygiene provided for the following.

  a. Dry skin: _____

  b. Acne: _____

  c. Skin rashes: _____

  d. Contact dermatitis: _____

  e. Abrasion: _____

- Briefly explain the six conditions that place clients at risk for impaired skin integrity.

  a. Immobilization: _____

  _____

  b. Reduced sensation: _____

  _____

c. Nutrition and hydration alterations: _____

_____

d. Secretions and excretions on the skin: ____

_____

e. Vascular insufficiency: _____

_____

f. External devices:_____

_____

Feet and Nails

- Assessment of the feet involves a thorough examination of all skin surfaces, including the soles of the feet and the areas between the toes.

- Inspection of the feet for lesions includes noting areas of:

    a. _____

    b. _____

    c. _____

- Define neuropathy. _____

_____

- Describe a nursing assessment for neuropathy.

_____

_____

- Identify the characteristics of the following foot and nail problems.

    a. Calluses: _____

    b. Corns: _____

    c. Plantar warts: _____

    d. Athlete's foot: _____

    e. Ingrown nails: _____

    f. Ram's horn nails: _____

    g. Paronychia: _____

    h. Foot odours: _____

Oral Cavity

- The nurse inspects all areas of the oral cavity for:

    a. _____

    b. _____

    c. _____

    d. _____

Hair

- Describe the characteristics of the following hair and scalp conditions.

    a. Dandruff: _____

    b. Ticks: _____

    c. Pediculosis: _____

    d. Pediculosis capitis: _____

    e. Pediculosis corporis: _____

    f. Pediculosis pubis: _____

    g. Alopecia: _____

Eyes, Ears, and Nose

- Identify the normal assessment findings for the following.

    a. Eyes: _____

    b. Nose: _____

    c. Ears: _____

Developmental Changes

Skin

- For each developmental stage, briefly describe normal conditions that create a high risk for impaired skin integrity.

    a. Neonate: _____

    b. Toddler: _____

    c. Adolescent: _____

    d. Older adult: _____

Feet and Nails

- Identify the common foot problems of the older adult._____

_____

The Mouth

- Identify the factors associated with aging that can result in poor oral care. _____

_____

Hair

- Throughout life, changes in the growth, distribution, and condition of hair influence hygiene. Explain. _____

_____

Self-Care Ability

- Identify the factors that are assessed to determine a client's ability to perform routine hygiene.

_____

Cultural Factors

- Explain how culture affects a client's hygiene needs. _____

_____

Clients at Risk for Hygiene Problems

- Provide examples of clients at risk for the following.
  - a. Oral problems: _____
  - b. Skin problems: _____
  - c. Foot problems: _____
  - d. Eye care problems: _____

Special Considerations in Hygiene Assessment

- Explain how footwear may predispose a client to foot and nail problems. _____

_____

Nursing Diagnosis

- List four possible nursing diagnoses that apply to clients in need of hygiene care.
  - a. _____
  - b. _____
  - c. _____
  - d. _____

Planning

- List factors to consider when planning hygiene care. _____

_____

Implementation

Health Promotion

- List four guidelines for educating clients about hygiene care.
  - a. _____
  - b. _____
  - c. _____
  - d. _____

Bathing and Skin Care

- A complete bed bath is: _____

_____

- A partial bed bath involves: _____

_____

- Identify guidelines the nurse should follow when assisting or providing a client with any type of bath. _____

_____

- Explain bag baths and identify the advantages of this method. _____

_____

Chapter 34: Hygiene   209

- Define *perineal care* and identify the clients at risk for skin breakdown in the perineal area.

  _____

- A back rub promotes:

  a. _____

  b. _____

  c. _____

  d. _____

  e. _____

- Routine morning care involves:

  a. _____

  b. _____

  c. _____

  d. _____

  e. _____

  f. _____

  g. _____

  h. _____

Foot and Nail Care

- List at least eight guidelines to include when advising clients with peripheral neuropathy or vascular insufficiency about foot care.

  a. _____

  b. _____

  c. _____

  d. _____

  e. _____

  f. _____

  g. _____

  h. _____

Oral Hygiene

- Oral hygiene helps maintain: _____

  _____

- Briefly explain the following interventions in relation to oral hygiene.

  a. Diet:_____

  b. Brushing and flossing: _____

  c. Oral care for the unconscious client: _____

  d. Denture care:_____

Hair and Scalp Care

- Briefly describe the rationale for the following.

  a. Brushing and combing: _____

  b. Shampooing: _____

  c. Shaving: _____

  d. Mustache and beard care: _____

Care of the Eyes, Ears, and Nose

- Care focuses on preventing infection and maintaining normal sensory function.

- Describe basic eye care for a client. _____

  _____

- Describe the correct procedure for cleaning eyeglasses. _____

  _____

- Briefly describe proper contact lens care technique._____

  _____

- Describe each of the following techniques necessary in caring for an artificial eye.

  a. Removal: _____

  _____

  b. Cleansing: _____

  _____

  c. Reinsertion: _____

  _____

  d. Storage: _____

  _____

Ear Care

- Describe the procedure for removing cerumen from the ear. _____ _____

- Describe the following types of hearing aids.
  a. In-the-canal (ITC): _____
  b. In-the-ear (ITE): _____
  c. Behind-the-ear (BTE): _____

Nasal Care

- Describe three interventions used to remove secretions from the nose.
  a. _____
  b. _____
  c. _____

Client's Room Environment

Maintaining Comfort

- Identify four factors the nurse can control to create a more comfortable environment:
  a. _____
  b. _____
  c. _____
  d. _____

Room Equipment

- A typical hospital room contains the following basic pieces of furniture.
  a. _____
  b. _____
  c. _____
  d. _____
  e. _____

- A client's bed must be frequently inspected to ensure the linens are _____, _____, and _____.

- Identify the factors a nurse considers when making a client's bed. _____ _____

Evaluation

Client Care

- Evaluation of hygiene measures occurs both during and after each particular skill.

- The standards for evaluation are the expected outcomes established in the planning stage of the client's care.

Client Expectations

- The client's expectations are important guidelines in determining client satisfaction.

Review Questions

The student should select the appropriate answer and cite the rationale for choosing that particular answer.

1. Mr. Ng is a 19-year-old client in the rehabilitation unit. He is completely paralyzed below the neck. The most appropriate bath for Mr. Ng is a:
   a. Partial bed bath
   b. Complete bed bath
   c. Sitz bath
   d. Tepid bath

   Answer: _____ Rationale: _____ _____ _____

2. All of the following will help maintain skin integrity in the older adult *except:*
   a. Environmental air that is cold and dry
   b. Use of warm water and mild cleansing agents for bathing
   c. Bathing every other day
   d. Drinking 8 to 10 glasses of water a day

   Answer: _____ Rationale: _____

   _____

   _____

3. When preparing to give complete AM care to a client, what would the nurse do first?
   a. Gather the necessary equipment and supplies.
   b. Remove the client's gown or pajamas while maintaining privacy.
   c. Assess the client's preferences for bathing practices.
   d. Lower the side rails and assist the client to assume a comfortable position.

   Answer: _____ Rationale: _____

   _____

   _____

4. Mrs. Veech has diabetes. Which intervention should be included in her teaching plan regarding foot care?
   a. Use a pumice stone to smooth corns and calluses.
   b. File toenails straight across and square.
   c. Apply powder to dry areas along the feet and between the toes.
   d. Wear elastic stockings to improve circulation.

   Answer: _____ Rationale: _____

   _____

   _____

5. Assessment of the hair and scalp reveals that a client has head lice. An appropriate intervention would be:
   a. Shave hair off the affected area
   b. Place oil on the hair and scalp until all of the lice are dead
   c. Use a pediculosis shampoo and repeat 7 to 10 days later
   d. Shampoo with regular shampoo and dry with hair-dryer set at the hottest setting

   Answer: _____ Rationale: _____

   _____

   _____

Critical Thinking for Nursing Care Plan for Hygiene

Imagine that you are Jeannette, the nurse in the Care Plan on page 1031 of your text. Complete the *planning phase* of the critical thinking model by writing your answers in the appropriate boxes of the model shown. Think about the following:

- In developing Mrs. Wyatt's plan of care, what knowledge did Jeannette apply?

- In what way might Jeannette's previous experience assist in developing a plan of care for Mrs. Wyatt?

- When developing a plan of care, what intellectual and professional standards were applied?

- What critical thinking attitudes might have been applied in developing Mrs. Wyatt's plan of care?

- How will Jeannette accomplish the goals?

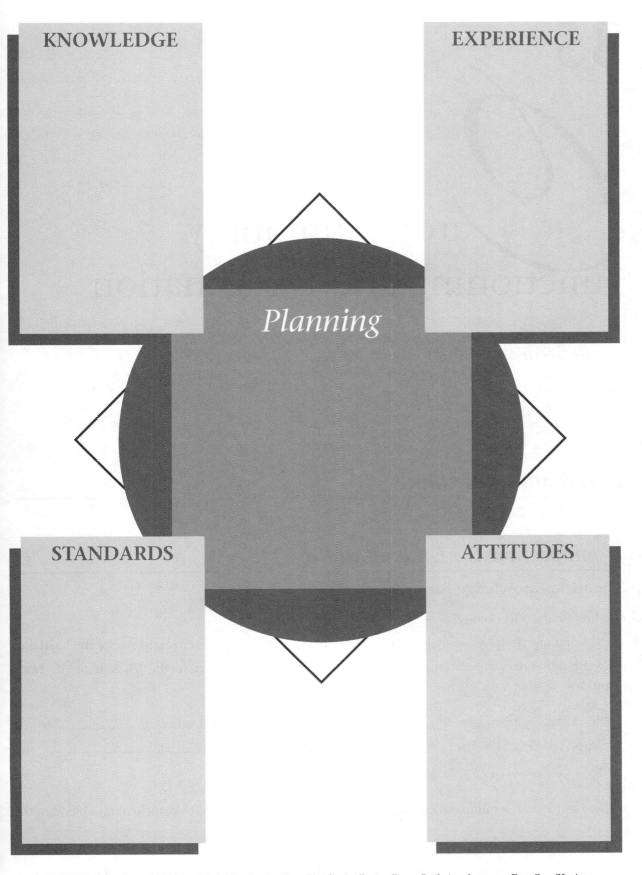

KNOWLEDGE

EXPERIENCE

Planning

STANDARDS

ATTITUDES

CHAPTER *34* Critical Thinking Model for Nursing Care Plan for *Ineffective Tissue Perfusion, Improper Foot Care/Hygiene*

See answers on page 593.

35

Cardiopulmonary Functioning and Oxygenation

Adapted by Zoraida DeCastro Beekhoo, RN, MA,
University of Toronto

Preliminary Reading

Chapter 35, pp. 1077-1143

Comprehensive Understanding

Scientific Knowledge Base

Cardiovascular Physiology

* Cardiopulmonary physiology involves delivery of _____ to the right side of the heart and to the pulmonary circulation, and _____ from the lungs to the left side of the heart and the tissues.

* The cardiac system delivers _____, _____, and other _____ to the tissues and removes the _____ through the _____, _____ and the _____.

* The right ventricle pumps blood through the _____. The left ventricle pumps blood to the _____.

* The four chambers of the heart fill with blood during _____ and empty during _____.

- Describe the Frank-Starling law of the heart.

  _____

  _____

  _____

- Briefly describe the flow of blood through the

  heart. _____

  _____

  _____

- Describe the following types of circulation.

  a. Coronary artery:_____

  b. Systemic: _____

- Describe the following terms related to blood flow regulation.

  a. Cardiac output: _____

b. Cardiac index: _____

c. Stroke volume: _____

d. Preload: _____

e. Afterload: _____

f. Myocardial contractility: _____

- Describe how the following affect the conduction system of the heart.

  a. Sympathetic nerve fibres:_____

  _____

  b. Parasympathetic nerve fibres: _____

  _____

- Diagram and label the electrical conduction system of the heart in the box below.

- Diagram and label the components of the ECG waveform for normal sinus rhythm (NSR) in the box below.

```



```

Respiratory Physiology

- The three steps in the process of oxygenation are _____, _____ and _____.

- The _____, _____, _____, and _____ are essential for ventilation, perfusion, and exchange of respiratory gases.

- Define *ventilation*. _____ _____

- Define the following terms related to the work of breathing.

  a. Surfactant: _____ _____

  b. Accessory Muscles: _____ _____

  c. Compliance: _____ _____

  d. Airway Resistance: _____ _____

- Spirometry is used to: _____ _____

216   Chapter 35: Cardiopulmonary Functioning and Oxygenation

- Variations in lung volumes may be associated with health states such as _____, _____, _____, or _____ and _____ conditions of the lungs.

- The amount of _____, _____, and _____ can affect pressures and volumes within the lungs.

- Briefly describe the pulmonary circulation.

  _____

  _____

- Identify the normal distribution of pressures within the pulmonary circulation._____

  _____

- Respiratory gases are exchanged in the _____ and the _____ of the body tissue.

- Define *diffusion*. _____

  _____

- The rate of diffusion can be affected by: _____

  _____

- List four factors required for oxygen transport and delivery.

  a. _____

  b. _____

  c. _____

  d. _____

- Describe the breakdown of carbon dioxide as it is diffused into the red blood cells. _____

  _____

- Explain the two regulators that control the process of respiration.

  a. Neural: _____

  _____

  b. Chemical: _____

  _____

Factors Affecting Oxygenation

- List the four factors that influence oxygenation.

  a. _____

  b. _____

  c. _____

  d. _____

- Explain the following factors that affect the body's ability to meet oxygen demands. Give examples of each.

  a. Decreased carrying capacity:_____

  _____

  b. Decreased inspired oxygen concentration:

  _____

  c. Hypovolemia: _____

  _____

  d. Increased metabolic rate: _____

  _____

- Explain how the following conditions affect chest wall movement.

  a. Pregnancy: _____

  _____

  b. Obesity:_____

  _____

  c. Musculoskeletal abnormalities: _____

  _____

  d. Trauma:_____

  _____

  e. Neuromuscular diseases: _____

  _____

f. Central nervous system alterations: _____

_____

g. Influences of chronic disease: _____

_____

Alterations in Cardiac Functioning

- Illnesses and conditions that affect _____, _____, _____, and _____ cause alterations in cardiac functioning.

- Define *dysrhythmias*. _____

_____

- Briefly describe the following dysrhythmias.

  a. Sinus tachycardia: _____

  _____

b. Sinus bradycardia: _____

_____

c. Sinus dysrhythmia: _____

_____

d. PSVT: _____

_____

e. A-Fib: _____

_____

f. PVCs: _____

_____

g. Ventricular tachycardia: _____

_____

e. Ventricular fibrillation: _____

_____

- Failure of the myocardium to eject sufficient volume to the systemic and pulmonary circulations can result in left-sided and right-sided heart failure. Complete the grid below.

Type of Failure	Clinical Findings
Left-sided	
Right-sided	

- Define each of the following.

  a. Valvular heart disease: _____

  _____

  b. Stenosis: _____

  _____

  c. Regurgitation: _____

  _____

  d. Myocardial ischemia: _____

  _____

e. Angina pectoris: _____

_____

f. Myocardial infarction: _____

_____

- Describe the chest pain associated with myocardial infarction. _____

_____

- Briefly explain acute coronary syndrome (ACS). _____
_____

Alterations in Respiratory Functioning

- The three primary alterations in respiratory function are _____,
_____, and _____.

- Complete the grid below.

Alterations	Causes	Signs and Symptoms
Hyperventilation		
Hypoventilation		
Hypoxia		

- Define the following terms.
   a. Atelectasis: _____
   b. Cyanosis: _____

Nursing Knowledge Base

Developmental Factors

- Identify at least one physiological factor influencing tissue oxygenation for each developmental level listed.
   a. Infants and toddlers: _____
   _____
   b. School-age children and adolescents:
   _____
   _____
   c. Young and middle-age adults: _____
   _____
   d. Older adults: _____
   _____

Lifestyle Risk Factors

- Briefly describe how the following lifestyle factors influence respiratory function.
   a. Poor nutrition: _____
   _____
   b. Inadequate exercise: _____
   _____
   c. Smoking: _____
   _____
   d. Substance abuse: _____
   _____
   e. Stress: _____
   _____

Environmental Factors

- List four occupational pollutants.

  a. _____

  b. _____

  c. _____

  d. _____

Nursing Process

Assessment

- The nursing assessment of a client's cardiopulmonary functioning should include data from the following areas. Briefly explain each.

  a. Health history: _____

  _____

  b. Physical examination:_____

  _____

  c. Diagnostic tests: _____

  _____

- Define the following terms.

  a. Fatigue: _____

  _____

  b. Dyspnea:_____

  _____

  c. Orthopnea: _____

  _____

  d. Cough: _____

  _____

  e. Productive cough: _____

  _____

  f. Hemoptysis: _____

  _____

  g. Wheezing: _____

  _____

- Briefly explain the following techniques used during the physical examination to assess tissue oxygenation.

  a. Inspection: _____

  _____

  b. Palpation: _____

  _____

  c. Percussion: _____

  _____

  d. Auscultation: _____

  _____

- Describe the following tests that determine myocardial contraction and blood flow.

  a. Echocardiography: _____

  _____

  b. Scintigraphy: _____

  _____

  c. Cardiac catheterization and angiography:

  _____

  _____

- Describe the following diagnostic tests used to determine the adequacy of the cardiac conduction system.

  a. Electrocardiogram: _____

  _____

  b. Holter monitor: _____

  _____

  d. ECG exercise stress test: _____

  _____

  e. Electrophysiological studies: _____

  _____

- Describe the following tests used to measure the adequacy of ventilation and oxygenation.

  a. Pulmonary function tests:_____

  _____

  b. CT scan: _____

  _____

c. Arterial blood gases: _____

_____

d. Pulse oximetry: _____

_____

e. Chest X-Ray exam: _____

_____

f. Lung Scan: _____

_____

- Describe the following tests used to determine abnormal cells or infection in the respiratory tract.

    a. Bronchoscopy: _____

    _____

    b. Sputum specimens: _____

    _____

    c. Thoracentesis: _____

    _____

Nursing Diagnosis

- Clients with an altered level of oxygenation can have nursing diagnoses that are primarily from a cardiovascular or pulmonary origin.

Planning

- List four goals appropriate for a client with actual or potential oxygenation needs.

    a. _____

    b. _____

    c. _____

    d. _____

Implementation

Health Promotion

- Describe the purpose of the influenza and pneumococcal vaccines and explain for whom the vaccines are recommended. _____

_____

- Identify some healthy lifestyle behaviours that decrease the risk of cardiopulmonary disease.

_____

Acute Care

- Nursing interventions for the client with acute pulmonary illnesses are directed toward _____, _____, and _____.

- List four treatment modalities appropriate for a client with dyspnea.

    a. _____

    b. _____

    c. _____

    d. _____

- Describe selected nursing interventions used to promote and maintain adequate oxygenation by completing the grid that follows. Include the purpose of the intervention.

Chapter 35: Cardiopulmonary Functioning and Oxygenation   221

Nursing Interventions	Purpose
Cascade cough	
Huff cough	
Quad cough	
Oropharyngeal and nasopharyngeal suctioning	
Tracheal suctioning	
Oral airway	
Tracheal airway	

Mobilization of Pulmonary Secretions

- Nursing interventions that promote mobilization of pulmonary secretions include the following. Briefly explain each one.

  a. Hydration: _____

  _____

  b. Humidfication: _____

  _____

  c. Nebulization: _____

  _____

  d. Chest Physiotherapy (CPT): _____

  _____

- Briefly describe the three activities involved in CPT.

  a. Postural drainage: _____

  _____

  b. Chest percussion: _____

  _____

  c. Vibration: _____

  _____

- Briefly explain the following types of suctioning techniques.

  a. Oropharyngeal and nasophryngeal:

  _____

  _____

b. Orotracheal and nasotracheal: _____

_____

c. Tracheal: _____

_____

- Nursing interventions that maintain or promote lung expansion include the following noninvasive techniques. Briefly explain each one.

    a. Positioning: _____

    _____

    b. Incentive spirometry: _____

    _____

- Identify the three reasons for inserting chest tubes.

    a. _____

    b. _____

    c. _____

- Define the following.

    a. *Pneumothorax:* _____

    _____

    b. *Hemothorax:* _____

    _____

- List the two types of drainage systems used with chest tubes.

    a. _____

    b. _____

- Identify five special considerations the nurse needs to address when dealing with chest tubes.

    a. _____

    b. _____

    c. _____

    d. _____

    e. _____

- Promotion of lung expansion, mobilization of secretions, and maintenance of a patent airway assist the client in meeting oxygenation needs.

- Identify the goal of oxygen therapy. _____

    _____

- List five safety measures to institute when a client receives oxygen administration.

    a. _____

    b. _____

    c. _____

    d. _____

    e. _____

- Describe the following methods of oxygen delivery and identify the usual flow rates.

    a. Nasal cannula: _____

    _____

    b. Transtracheal oxygen: _____

    _____

    c. Face mask: _____

    _____

    d. Venturi mask: _____

    _____

- Identify the indications for a client to receive home oxygen therapy. _____

    _____

- Identify the teaching required by the client for use of home oxygen therapy. _____

    _____

- List the three goals of cardiopulmonary resuscitation (CPR).

    a. _____

    b. _____

    c. _____

Restorative Care and Continuing Care

- Cardiopulmonary rehabilitation is: _____

  _____

- Briefly explain the following breathing exercises used to improve ventilation and oxygenation.

  a. Pursed-lip breathing: _____

  _____

  b. Diaphragmatic breathing: _____

  _____

NP Evaluation

Client Care

- The nurse evaluates the actual care provided to the client by the health care team based on the expected outcomes.

- The client is the only person who can evaluate his or her degree of breathlessness.

- Evaluation   of   _____,

  _____, _____,

  _____, and _____ provide the nurse with objective measurements of the success of therapies and treatments.

Client Expectations

- Evaluate the care from the client's perspective.

- Working closely with the client will enable the nurse to redefine those client expectations that can be realistically met within the limitations of the client's condition and treatment.

*R*eview Questions

The student should select the appropriate answer and cite the rationale for choosing that particular answer.

1. Ventilation, perfusion, and exchange of gases are the major purposes of:
   a. Respiration
   b. Circulation
   c. Aerobic metabolism
   d. Anaerobic metabolism

   Answer: _____ Rationale: _____

   _____

   _____

2. *Afterload* refers to:
   a. The amount of blood ejected from the left ventricle each minute
   b. The amount of blood ejected from the left ventricle with each contraction
   c. The resistance to left ventricle ejection
   d. The amount of blood in the left ventricle at the end of diastole

   Answer: _____ Rationale: _____

   _____

   _____

3. The movement of gases into and out of the lungs depends on the:
   a. 50% oxygen content in the atmospheric air
   b. Pressure gradient between the atmosphere and the alveoli
   c. Use of accessory muscles of respiration during expiration
   d. Amount of carbon dioxide dissolved in the fluid of the alveoli

   Answer: _____ Rationale: _____

   _____

   _____

4. The client's ECG shows an abnormal rhythm that slows during inspiration and increases with expiration. The rate is 70 to 80 beats per minute. The P-wave, PR interval, and QRS complex are normal. This is referred to as:
   a. Sinus tachycardia
   b. Sinus dysrhythmia
   c. Supraventricular tachycardia
   d. Premature ventricular contractions

Answer: _____ Rationale: _____

_____

_____

5. Mr. Isaac comes to the ER complaining of difficulty breathing. An objective finding associated with his dyspnea might include:
   a. Statements about a sense of impending doom
   b. Complaints of shortness of breath
   c. Feelings of heaviness in the chest
   d. Use of accessory muscles of respiration

Answer: _____ Rationale: _____

_____

_____

6. The use of chest physiotherapy to mobilize pulmonary secretions involves the use of:
   a. Hydration
   b. Percussion
   c. Nebulization
   d. Humidification

Answer: _____ Rationale: _____

_____

_____

Critical Thinking for Nursing Care Plan for Respiratory Alterations

Imagine that you are the student nurse in the Care Plan on page 1104 of your text. Complete the *assessment phase* of the critical thinking model by writing your answers in the appropriate boxes of the model shown. Think about the following:

- What knowledge base was applied to Mr. Edwards?

- In what way might your previous experience apply in this case?

- What intellectual or professional standards were applied to Mr. Edwards?

- What critical thinking attitudes did you use in assessing Mr. Edwards?

- As you review your assessment, what key areas did you cover?

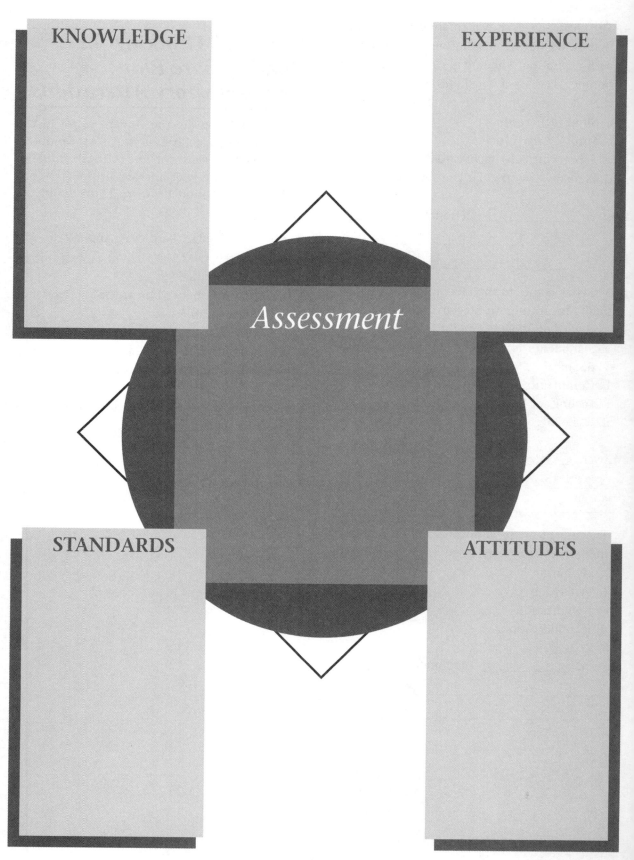

KNOWLEDGE

EXPERIENCE

Assessment

STANDARDS

ATTITUDES

CHAPTER *35* Critical Thinking Model for Nursing Care Plan for *Ineffective Airway Clearance/Retained Secretions*
See answers on page 594.

36

*F*luid, Electrolyte, and Acid-Base Balances

Adapted by Anita Molzahn, RN, BScN, MN, PhD,
University of Victoria

*P*reliminary Reading

Chapter 36, pp. 1144-1208

*C*omprehensive Understanding

Scientific Knowledge Base

- _____ is the largest single component of the body; 60% of the average adult's weight

  is _____.

Distribution of Body Fluids

- Body fluids are distributed in two distinct compartments. Briefly explain each one.

  a. Extracellular: _____

  _____

  b. Intracellular: _____

  _____

- Extracellular fluids (ECF) are divided into two smaller compartments. Explain each one.

  a. Interstitial: _____

  _____

  b. Intravascular: _____

  _____

Composition of Body Fluids

- Define *electrolyte*. _____

  _____

- Define the following terms related to the composition of body fluids.

  a. Cations: _____

  b. Anions: _____

  c. mmol/L: _____

  d. Solute: _____

  e. Solvent: _____

  f. Minerals: _____

Movement of Body Fluids

- Fluids and electrolytes constantly shift between compartments to facilitate body processes.

- List and briefly describe the four factors responsible for movement of body fluids.

  a. _____

  _____

  b. _____

  _____

  c. _____

  _____

  d. _____

  _____

- Define the following terms related to osmosis.

  a. Osmotic pressure: _____

  _____

  b. Isotonic: _____

  _____

  c. Hypotonic: _____

  _____

  d. Hypertonic: _____

  _____

- Define *hydrostatic pressure*. _____

  _____

Regulation of Body Fluids

- Body fluids are regulated by _____,

  _____, and _____. This

  balance is termed _____.

- Briefly describe the physiological stimuli triggering the thirst mechanism. _____

  _____

- For each hormone, identify the stimuli for its release and its influence on fluid and electrolyte balance in the grid below.

Hormone	Stimuli	Action
ADH		
Aldosterone		
Glucocorticoids		

228　Chapter 36: Fluid, Electrolyte, and Acid-Base Balances

- Fluid output occurs through four organs. List and explain each one.

  a. _____

  b. _____

  c. _____

  d. _____

- Define the following.

  a. Insensible water loss: _____

  _____

  b. Sensible water loss: _____

  _____

Regulation of Electrolytes

- The major cations within the body fluids include _____, _____, _____, and _____.

- The major anions are _____, _____, and _____.

- Give the normal values, function, and regulatory mechanisms for the major body electrolytes in the grid below.

Electrolyte	Values	Function	Regulatory Mechanism
Sodium			
Potassium			
Calcium			
Magnesium			
Chloride			
Bicarbonate			
Phosphate			

Regulation of Acid-Base Balance

- Identify and describe the acid-base regulatory mechanisms for each of the following buffering systems.

    a. Chemical regulation: _____

    _____

    b. Biological regulation: _____

    _____

    c. Physiological regulation: _____

    _____

- Describe the physiological mechanism through which the lungs regulate hydrogen ion concentration. _____

Disturbances in Electrolyte, Fluid, and Acid-Base Balances

- For each electrolyte disturbance, identify the diagnostic laboratory finding, and list at least four characteristic signs and symptoms in the grid below.

Imbalance	Lab Finding	Signs and Symptoms
Hyponatremia		
Hypernatremia		
Hypokalemia		
Hyperkalemia		
Hypocalcemia		
Hypercalcemia		
Hypomagnesemia		
Hypermagnesemia		

- The basic types of fluid imbalances are _____ and _____.

- Isotonic deficit and excess exist when _____.

- Osmolar imbalances are: _____
_____

- Arterial blood gas (ABG) analysis is the best way to evaluate acid-base balance. Give the normal value for each.

  a. pH: _____

  b. $PaCO_2$: _____

c. PaO_2: _____

d. SaO_2: _____

e. Base excess: _____

f. HCO_3: _____

- Complete the grid below giving the causes and signs and symptoms of the listed fluid disturbances.

Fluid Disturbances	Causes	Signs and Symptoms
Fluid volume deficit (FVD)		
Fluid volume deficit (FVE)		
Hyperosmolar imbalance		
Hypo-osmolar imbalance		

- Briefly explain the following components of the acid-base balance.

  a. pH: _____

  b. $PaCO_2$: _____

  c. PaO_2: _____

  d. Oxygen saturation: _____

e. Base excess: _____

f. Bicarbonate: _____

- The four primary types of acid-base imbalances are listed in the following grid. For each acid-base imbalance, identify the diagnostic laboratory finding and list the characteristic signs and symptoms.

Chapter 36: Fluid, Electrolyte, and Acid-Base Balances   231

Acid-Base Imbalance	Lab Findings	Signs and Symptoms
Respiratory acidosis		
Respiratory alkalosis		
Metabolic acidosis		
Metabolic alkalosis		

Nursing Knowledge Base

- List the five major risk factors that can affect fluid and electrolyte imbalances. Give two examples of each.

  a. _____

  _____

  b. _____

  _____

  c. _____

  _____

  d. _____

  _____

  e. _____

  _____

Nursing Process

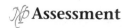 **Assessment**

- Briefly describe the fluid changes that are associated with aging and development.

  a. Infants: _____

  _____

  b. Children: _____

  _____

  c. Adolescents: _____

  _____

  d. Older adults: _____

  _____

- Explain how the following acute illnesses affect fluid, electrolyte, and acid-base balances.

  a. Surgery: _____

  _____

  b. Burns: _____

  _____

c. Respiratory disorders: _____

_____

d. Head injury: _____

_____

- Describe how the following chronic illnesses affect fluid, electrolyte, and acid-base imbalances.

  a. Cancer: _____

  _____

  b. Cardiovascular disease: _____

  _____

  c. Renal disorders: _____

  _____

  d. Gastrointestinal disturbances: _____

  _____

  e. HIV/AIDS: _____

  _____

- Briefly explain how the following affect fluid, electrolyte, and acid-base imbalances.

  a. Diet: _____

  _____

  b. Lifestyle factors: _____

  _____

  c. Medication: _____

  _____

- Indicate the possible fluid, electrolyte, or acid-base imbalances associated with each physical finding.

  a. Weight loss of 5% to 10%: _____

  b. Irritability: _____

  c. Lethargy: _____

  d. Periorbital edema: _____

  e. Sticky, dry mucous membranes: _____

  f. Distended neck veins: _____

  g. Dysrhythmias: _____

  h. Weak pulse: _____

i. Low blood pressure: _____

j. Third heart sound: _____

k. Increased respiratory rate: _____

l. Crackles: _____

m. Anorexia: _____

n. Abdominal cramps: _____

o. Poor skin turgor: _____

p. Oliguria or anuria: _____

q. Increased specific gravity: _____

r. Muscle cramps, tetany: _____

s. Hypertonicity of muscles on palpation:

_____

t. Decreased or absent deep tendon reflexes:

_____

u. Increased temperature: _____

v. Distended abdomen: _____

w. Cold, clammy skin: _____

x. Edema (dependant body parts): _____

- Recording intake and output (I&O) is essential for obtaining an accurate database. Accurate I&O measurements can identify both clients at risk for and clients who are experiencing fluid, electrolyte, and acid-base disturbances.

- Intake includes _____,

  _____, _____, and

  _____.

- Output includes _____,

  _____, _____,

  _____, and _____.

Nursing Diagnosis

- List five potential or actual nursing diagnoses for a client with fluid, electrolyte, or acid-base imbalances.

  a. _____

  b. _____

  c. _____

  d. _____

  e. _____

Planning

- List three goals that are appropriate for a client with altered fluid, electrolyte, or acid-base imbalances.

  a. _____

  b. _____

  c. _____

Implementation

Health Promotion

- Identify some common risk factors for imbalances for which the caregiver may implement appropriate preventive measures. _____

Acute Care

- When implementing specific measures to increase or decrease fluid, two interventions are necessary. Explain each one.

  a. Daily weights: _____

  _____

  b. I&O: _____

  _____

- List and briefly describe the enteral replacement of fluids.

  a. _____

  _____

  b. _____

  _____

- Briefly explain the need for a restricted fluid intake and how the nurse would implement the restriction. _____

  _____

- List the three methods of parenteral replacement.

  a. _____

  b. _____

  c. _____

- Vascular assist devices are: _____

  _____

- Total parenteral nutrition (TPN) is: _____

  _____

- Identify the primary goal of IV fluid administration. _____

  _____

- Define the following types of electrolyte solutions.

  a. Isotonic: _____

  _____

  b. Hypotonic: _____

  _____

  c. Hypertonic: _____

  _____

- List two major purposes of infusion pumps.

  a. _____

  b. _____

- List three groups of clients for whom venipunctures may be difficult.

  a. _____

  b. _____

  c. _____

- List four factors that may affect IV flow rates.

  a. _____

  b. _____

  c. _____

  d. _____

- List four interventions that can reduce the risk of infusion-related infections.

  a. _____

  b. _____

c. _____

d. _____

- Indicate the sequence to be followed when changing the gown of a client with an IV line.

  a. _____

  b. _____

  c. _____

  d. _____

  e. _____

  f. _____

- Complete the grid below describing complications of IV therapy.

Complication	Assessment Finding	Nursing Action
Infiltration		
Phlebitis		
Fluid overload		
Bleeding		

- Briefly summarize the procedure for discontinuing intravenous infusions. _____

  _____

- List three objectives for blood transfusion.

  a. _____

  b. _____

  c. _____

- Complete the grid below describing the major blood groups.

	A	B	O	AB
Antigens present				
Antibodies present				

- Define *autotransfusion*. _____
  _____

- Identify the five nursing interventions associated with blood transfusions and give the rationale for each.

  a. _____
  _____

  b. _____
  _____

  c. _____
  _____

  d. _____
  _____

  e. _____
  _____

- Define *transfusion reaction* and identify its cause. _____
  _____

- Identify types of transfusion reactions, their causes, and how they are managed.

  a. _____
  _____

  b. _____
  _____

  c. _____
  _____

  d. _____
  _____

  e. _____
  _____

  f. _____
  _____

- List the steps the nurse should follow if a transfusion reaction is suspected.

  a. _____
  b. _____
  c. _____
  d. _____
  e. _____
  f. _____
  g. _____
  h. _____

Restorative Care

- Older adults and clients with chronically illness require special considerations to prevent complications from developing. Briefly summarize the following.

    a. Home intravenous therapy: _____

    _____

    b. Nutritional support: _____

    _____

    c. Medication safety: _____

    _____

ℵℰ Evaluation

Client Care

- The nurse evaluates the actual care delivered by the health care team based on the expected outcomes.

- The nurse will perform evaluative measures and determine if changes have occurred from the last client assessment. The client's level of progress determines whether the nurse needs to continue or revise the care plan.

Client Expectations

- Nurses routinely review with their client their success in meeting expectations of care.

- Often the client's level of satisfaction with care also depends on the nurse's success in involving friends and family.

Review Questions

The student should select the appropriate answer and cite the rationale for choosing that particular answer.

1. The body fluids comprising the interstitial fluid and blood plasma are:
    a. Intracellular
    b. Extracellular
    c. Hypotonic
    d. Hypertonic

    Answer: _____ Rationale: _____

    _____

    _____

2. Which of the following statements is true with regard to the lungs' regulation of acid-base balance?
    a. The lungs serve a minor role in the physiological buffering of H ions.
    b. It takes several days for the lungs to restore pH to a normal level.
    c. The lungs correct imbalances by altering the rate and depth of respiration.
    d. The lungs maintain normal pH by either retaining or excreting bicarbonate.

    Answer: _____ Rationale: _____

    _____

    _____

3. Mrs. Singh's arterial blood gas results are as follows: pH, 7.32; $PaCO_2$, 52; PaO_2, 78; HCO_3, 24. Mrs. Singh has:
    a. Respiratory acidosis
    b. Respiratory alkalosis
    c. Metabolic acidosis
    d. Metabolic alkalosis

    Answer: _____ Rationale: _____

    _____

    _____

4. Mr. Frank is an 82-year-old client who has had a 3-day history of vomiting and diarrhea. Which symptom would you expect to find on a physical examination?
   a. Neck vein distention
   b. Crackles in the lungs
   c. Tachycardia
   d. Hypertension

Answer: _____ Rationale: _____

_____

_____

5. Which of the following is most likely to result in respiratory alkalosis?
   a. Fad dieting
   b. Hyperventilation
   c. Chronic alcoholism
   d. Steroid use

Answer: _____ Rationale: _____

_____

_____

Critical Thinking for Fluid and Electrolyte Alterations

Imagine that you are the student nurse in the Care Plan on page 1166 of your text. Complete the *planning phase* of the critical thinking model by writing your answers in the appropriate boxes of the model shown. Think about the following:

- When developing a plan of care, what intellectual and professional standards were applied?

- In developing Mrs. Bottomley's plan of care, what knowledge did you apply?

- In what way might your previous experience assist you in developing a plan of care for Mrs. Bottomley?

- What critical thinking attitudes might have been applied to developing Mrs. Bottomley's care?

- How will you accomplish your goals?

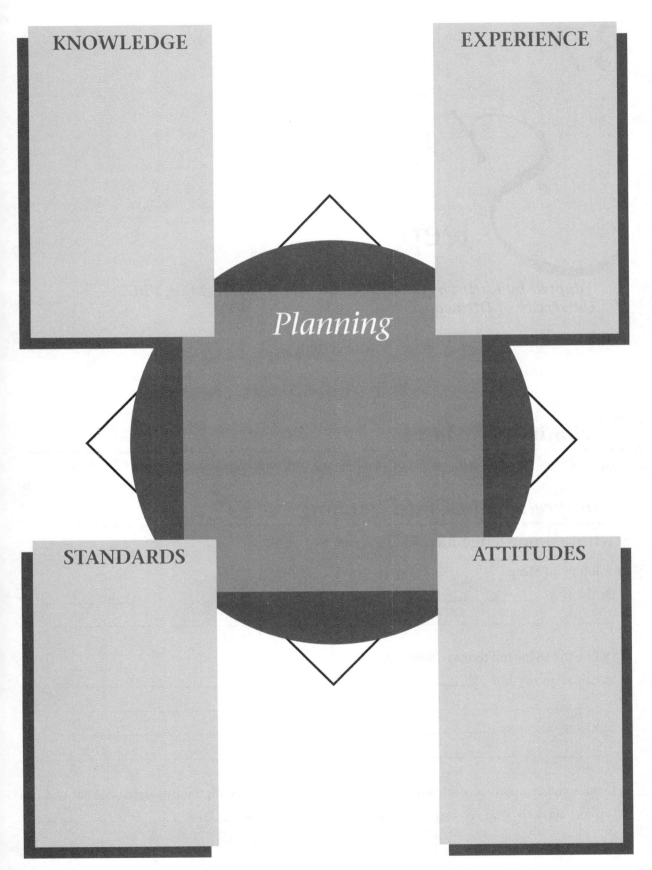

KNOWLEDGE

EXPERIENCE

Planning

STANDARDS

ATTITUDES

CHAPTER *36* Critical Thinking Model for Nursing Care Plan for *Fluid and Electrolyte Alterations*

See answers on page 595.

37

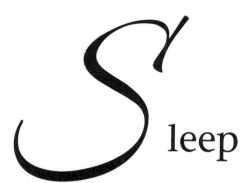

leep

*Adapted by Kathryn A. Smith Higuchi, RN, BScN, MEd, PhD,
University of Ottawa*

Preliminary Reading

Chapter 37, pp. 1209-1234

Comprehensive Understanding

Scientific Knowledge Base

Physiology of Sleep

• Define *sleep*. _____

_____

• Define the following terms related to sleep.

  a. Circadian rhythm: _____

  _____

  b. Biological clocks: _____

  _____

• Sleep involves a sequence of physiological states maintained by highly integrated central nervous system activity that is associated with changes in the _____, _____, _____, _____, and _____ systems.

- The control and regulation of sleep may depend on the interrelationship between two cerebral mechanisms that intermittently activate and suppress the brain's higher centres to control sleep and wakefulness.

- Summarize the function of the reticular activating system (RAS). _____ _____

- The area of the brain called the *bulbar synchronizing region* (BSR) is responsible for: _____ _____ _____

- Explain the two stages of sleep.
    a. NREM: _____
    b. REM: _____

- Describe the characteristics of the following cycles of sleep.
    a. Stage 1: _____
    b. Stage 2: _____
    c. Stage 3: _____
    d. Stage 4: _____
    e. REM: _____

Functions of Sleep

- Explain briefly the functions of sleep. _____ _____

Physical Illness

- Explain how the following conditions affect sleep.
    a. Discomfort: _____
    b. Respiratory disease: _____
    c. Hypertension: _____
    d. Hypothyroidism: _____
    e. Hyperthyroidism: _____
    f. Nocturia: _____
    g. Restless legs syndrome: _____

Sleep Disorders

- Briefly describe the following categories of sleep disorders.
    a. Dyssomnias: _____
    b. Parasomnias: _____
       _____

- Define *insomnia*. _____ _____

- List two conditions that are associated with insomnia.
    a. _____
    b. _____

- Define *sleep apnea*. _____ _____

- Define the following types of apnea.
    a. Central sleep apnea: _____
       _____
    b. Obstructive sleep apnea: _____
       _____

- Briefly explain excessive daytime sleepiness (EDS). _____ _____

- Define *narcolepsy*. _____ _____

- Define the following terms related to narcolepsy.
    a. Cataplexy: _____
       _____
    b. Hypnagogic hallucinations: _____
       _____

- Identify the developmental stage in which narcolepsy symptoms first develop. _____ _____

- Identify the treatment modalities for a client with narcolepsy. _____
  _____

- Sleep deprivation is: _____
  _____

- List the physiological and psychological manifestations of sleep deprivation in the grid below.

- Explain the following parasomnias.
  a. Somnambulism: _____
     _____
  b. Nocturnal enuresis: _____
     _____
  c. Bruxism: _____
     _____

Physiological Symptoms	Psychological Symptoms

Nursing Knowledge Base

Sleep and Rest

- Define *rest*. _____
  _____

Normal Sleep Requirements and Patterns

- Complete the grid that follows listing the normal sleep patterns and rituals for the various developmental stages.

Factors Affecting Sleep

- A number of factors affect the quantity and quality of sleep.

- Sleepiness and sleep deprivation are common side effects of medications. Describe how each of the following affects sleep and give an example of each.

  a. Drugs and substances: _____
     _____

  b. Lifestyle: _____
     _____

Developmental Stage	Sleep Patterns	Usual Rituals
Neonates		
Infants		
Toddlers		
Preschoolers		
School-age children		
Adolescents		
Young adults		
Middle adults		
Older adults		

- List three alterations in routine that can disrupt sleep patterns.

  a. _____

  b. _____

  c. _____

- Explain how emotional stress affects sleep. _____

  _____

- List and briefly describe three environmental factors that affect sleep.

  a. _____

  _____

  b. _____

  _____

  c. _____

  _____

- Explain how exercise promotes sleep. _____
  _____

- List and briefly describe five foods that affect sleep and why.

  a. _____
     _____

  b. _____
     _____

  c. _____
     _____

  d. _____
     _____

  e. _____

Nursing Process

Assessment

- Sleep and restfulness are subjective experiences.

- Assessment is aimed at understanding the characteristics of a sleep problem and the client's sleep habits.

- Identify three sources for sleep assessment.

  a. _____
  b. _____
  c. _____

- List seven components of a sleep history.

  a. _____
  b. _____
  c. _____
  d. _____
  e. _____
  f. _____
  g. _____

- List and briefly describe the six areas to assess with a client when asking about the nature of a sleeping problem.

  a. _____
     _____

  b. _____
     _____

  c. _____
     _____

  d. _____
     _____

  e. _____
     _____

  f. _____
     _____

- Identify the information recorded in a sleep–wake log. _____
  _____

- Briefly explain how the following factors interfere with sleep.

  a. Physical and psychological illness: _____

  _____

  b. Current life events: _____

  _____

  c. Bedtime routines: _____

  _____

  d. Bedtime environment: _____

  _____

- List four behaviours a client may manifest with sleep deprivation.

  a. _____

  b. _____

  c. _____

  d. _____

Nursing Diagnosis

- If a sleep pattern disturbance is identified, the nurse specifies the condition.

- Assessment should also identify the related factor or probable cause of the sleep disturbance.

Planning

- It is important for the plan of care to include strategies that are appropriate for the client's environment and lifestyle.

- List four goals appropriate for a client needing rest or sleep.

  a. _____

  b. _____

  c. _____

  d. _____

Implementation

- Nursing interventions designed to improve the quality of a person's sleep are largely focused on health promotion.

Health Promotion

- Many factors affect the ability to gain adequate rest and sleep. Briefly give examples of each of the following.

  a. Environmental control: _____

  b. Promoting bedtime routines: _____

  c. Comfort: _____

  d. Periods of rest and sleep: _____

  e. Stress reduction: _____

  f. Bedtime snacks: _____

  g. Pharmacological approaches: _____

Acute Care

- For each of the following situations, give two examples of nursing measures that will promote sleep.

  a. Environmental control:

  1. _____

  2. _____

  b. Promoting comfort:

  1. _____

  2. _____

  c. Establishing periods of rest and sleep:

  1. _____

  2. _____

  d. Stress reduction:

  1. _____

  2. _____

Restorative or Continuing Care

- Give an example of the following interventions that are implemented in the restorative environment.

  a. Promoting comfort: _____

  b. Controlling physiological disturbances:

  _____

  c. Pharmacological approaches: _____

- Briefly describe the effect of benzodiazepines in promoting sleep. _____
  _____

- Identify three types of clients who should not use benzodiazepines and explain why.

  a. _____

  b. _____

  c. _____

- The regular use of sleeping medication can lead to: _____
  _____

ℳ Evaluation

Client Care

- The client is the only person who knows if sleep problems are improved and which interventions or therapies are successful.

Client Expectations

- Identify some subtle behaviours a client may exhibit that indicate satisfaction. _____
  _____

Review Questions

The student should select the appropriate answer and cite the rationale for choosing that particular answer.

1. The 24-hour day-night cycle is known as:
   a. Circadian rhythm
   b. Infradium rhythm
   c. Ultradian rhythm
   d. Non-REM rhythm

Answer: _____ Rationale: _____
_____
_____

2. Which of the following substances will promote normal sleep patterns?
   a. L-tryptophan
   b. Beta-blockers
   c. Alcohol
   d. Narcotics

Answer: _____ Rationale: _____
_____
_____

3. All of the following are symptoms of sleep deprivation *except:*
   a. Hyperactivity
   b. Irritability
   c. Rise in body temperature
   d. Decreased motivation

Answer: _____ Rationale: _____
_____
_____

4. Mrs. Phan complains of difficulty falling asleep, awakening earlier than desired, and not feeling rested. She attributes these problems to leg pain that is secondary to her arthritis. What would be the appropriate nursing diagnosis for her?
   a. *Sleep pattern disturbances related to arthritis*
   b. *Fatigue related to leg pain*
   c. *Knowledge deficit related to sleep hygiene measures*
   d. *Sleep pattern disturbances related to chronic leg pain*

Answer: _____ Rationale: _____
_____
_____

5. A nursing care plan for a client with sleep problems has been implemented. All of the following would be expected outcomes *except:*
   a. Client reports no episodes of awakening during the night.
   b. Client falls asleep within 1 hour of going to bed.
   c. Client reports satisfaction with amount of sleep.
   d. Client rates sleep as an 8 or above on the visual analogue scale.

Answer: _____ Rationale: _____

_____

_____

Critical Thinking for Nursing Care Plan for Disturbed Sleep Pattern

Imagine that you are the nurse in the Care Plan on page 1225 of your text. Complete the *evaluation phase* of the critical thinking model by writing your answers in the appropriate boxes of the model shown. Think about the following:

- What knowledge did you apply in evaluating Julie's care?

- In what way might your previous experience influence your evaluation of Julie's care?

- During evaluation, what intellectual and professional standards were applied to Julie's care?

- In what way do critical thinking attitudes play a role in how you approach the evaluation of Julie's care plan?

- How might you evaluate Julie's care plan?

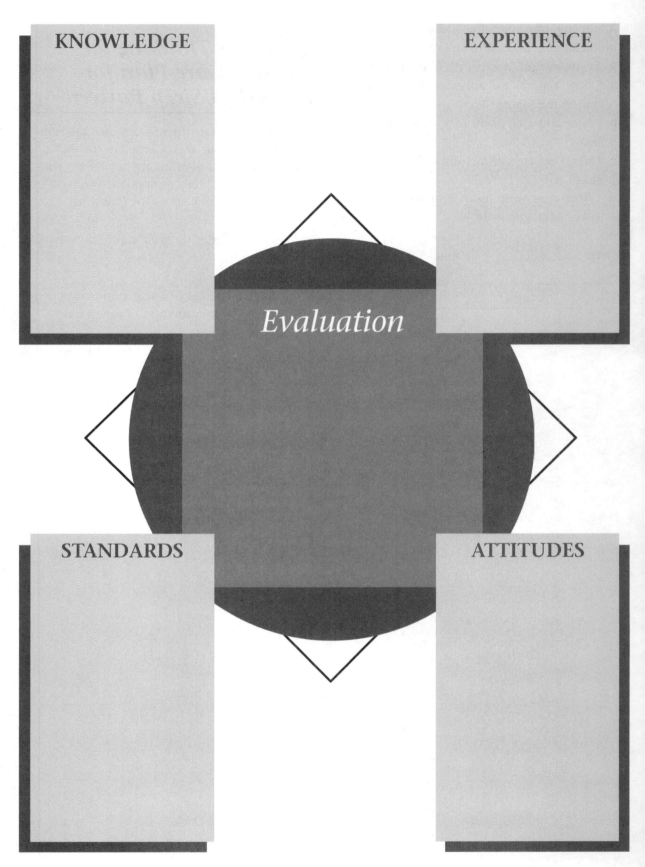

KNOWLEDGE

EXPERIENCE

Evaluation

STANDARDS

ATTITUDES

CHAPTER 37   Critical Thinking Model for Nursing Care Plan for *Disturbed Sleep Pattern*

See answers on page 596.

38

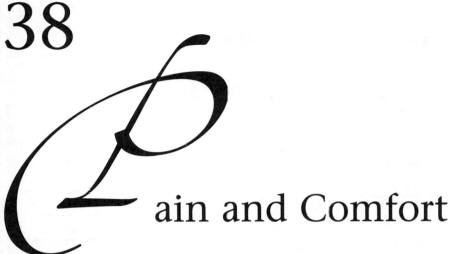

Pain and Comfort

Adapted by Fay F. Warnock, RN, PhD, University of British Columbia

Preliminary Reading

Chapter 38, pp. 1235-1277

Comprehensive Understanding

- Pain is subjective; no two people experience pain in the same way, and no two painful events create identical responses or feelings in a person.

- Pain and pain management options are viewed within the context of comfort; providing comfort is central to nursing.

- The relief from pain is considered a basic human right and is incorporated into the Canadian Pain Society's *Patient Pain Manifesto*.

Scientific Knowledge Base

Nature of Pain

- Define *pain*. _____

_____

Physiology of Pain

- Explain the four processes of nociceptive pain.

  a. Transduction: _____

  _____

b. Transmission: _____

_____

c. Perception: _____

_____

d. Modulation: _____

_____

- Explain the two types of neuroregulators.

a. Neurotransmitters: _____

_____

b. Neuromodulators: _____

_____

- Identify the neurophysiological function of the following neuroregulators:

a. Substance P: _____

b. Prostaglandins: _____

c. Serotonin: _____

d. Endorphins: _____

e. Bradykinin: _____

- Explain the gate-control theory of pain. _____

_____

- List some physiological reactions to pain.

a. Sympathetic stimulation:

1. _____

2. _____

3. _____

4. _____

5. _____

b. Parasympathetic stimulation:

1. _____

2. _____

3. _____

4. _____

5. _____

- Identify four behavioural changes that characterize a client experiencing pain.

a. _____

b. _____

c. _____

d. _____

- List four characteristics of acute pain.

a. _____

b. _____

c. _____

d. _____

- Define *chronic pain*. _____

_____

Nursing Knowledge Base

Knowledge, Attitudes, and Beliefs

- The medical model of illness describes pain as:

_____

_____

- Identify common biases and misconceptions about pain. _____

_____

Factors Influencing Pain

- Explain the developmental differences of client's reaction to pain.

a. Young children: _____

_____

b. Toddlers and preschoolers: _____

_____

c. Older adults: _____

_____

250 Chapter 38: Pain and Comfort

Copyright © 2006 Elsevier Canada, Inc. All rights reserved.

- Identify five misconceptions about pain in older clients.

  a. _____

  b. _____

  c. _____

  d. _____

  e. _____

- Fatigue heightens the perception of pain. Explain. _____

  _____

- Explain how a client's neurological function can influence pain. _____

  _____

- Give an example how the following influence pain.

  a. Attention: _____

  b. Previous experience: _____

  c. Family and social support: _____

  d. Spiritual factors: _____

- Explain how the following psychological factors affect pain.

  a. Anxiety: _____

  _____

  b. Coping style: _____

  _____

  c. Meaning of pain: _____

  _____

- Explain how cultural factors affect pain. _____

  _____

Nursing Process and Pain

- Pain management extends beyond pain relief, encompassing the client's _____ and ability to _____, _____, and _____.

Assessment

- For clients with an acute episode of pain, the nurse assesses and responds to the _____, _____, and _____ of the pain.

- Assessment of chronic pain should focus on _____, _____, and _____ dimensions of the pain and on its history and context.

- Explain what is meant by pain assessment and management "ABCDE."

  A: _____

  B: _____

  C: _____

  D: _____

  E: _____

- Identify examples of non-verbal expressions of pain. _____

  _____

- Cognitively impaired clients might require simple assessment approaches involving close observation of behaviour changes, especially movement.

- Briefly explain the common characteristics of pain.

  a. Onset and duration: _____

  _____

  b. Location: _____

  _____

  c. Intensity: _____

  _____

- Describe the following descriptive scales for measuring the severity of pain.

  a. Numerical rating scale (NRS): _____

  _____

Chapter 38: Pain and Comfort 251

b. Verbal descriptor scale (VDS): _____

_____

c. Visual analogue scale (VAS): _____

_____

d. FACES scale: _____

_____

- Identify some terms a client can use to describe the quality of pain. _____

_____

- Identify some measures a client may use to relieve pain. _____

_____

- Identify some contributing symptoms that may make pain worsen. _____

_____

- Summarize how pain affects the psychological well-being of the client. _____

_____

- Give examples of the following behavioural indicators of pain.
  a. Vocalizations: _____
  b. Facial expressions: _____
  c. Body movement: _____
  d. Social interaction: _____

- Explain how pain can influence activities of daily living in regard to the following.
  a. Sleep: _____

  _____

  b. Hygiene: _____

  _____

  c. Sexual relations: _____

  _____

  d. Employment: _____

  _____

e. Social activities: _____

_____

ℕ𝒟 Nursing Diagnosis

- The nursing diagnosis focuses on the nature of the pain so that the nurse can identify the best interventions for relieving pain and minimizing its effect on the client's lifestyle and function.

- List five potential or actual nursing diagnoses related to a client in pain.
  a. _____
  b. _____
  c. _____
  d. _____
  e. _____

ℕ𝒟 Planning

- An intervention that works for one client will not work for all clients.

- When developing a plan of care, the nurse selects priorities based on the client's level of pain and its effect on the client's condition.

- List the client outcomes appropriate for the client experiencing pain.
  a. _____
  b. _____
  c. _____
  d. _____
  e. _____

ℕ𝒟 Implementation

Health Promotion

- Teaching clients about the pain experience reduces anxiety and helps clients achieve a sense of control.

- Describe how you would teach a child about a painful procedure. _____
_____

- The Agency for Healthcare Research and Quality (AHRQ) guidelines for acute pain management cite non-pharmacological interventions appropriate for clients who meet certain criteria. List those criteria.

    a. _____

    b. _____

    c. _____

    d. _____

    e. _____

- Briefly explain how relaxation lessens pain.
_____
_____

- Briefly explain how the nurse would lead a client through guided imagery. _____
_____

- Briefly explain how the nurse would guide a client through progressive relaxation exercises. _____
_____

- Define *distraction*, and list one disadvantage and advantage of using distraction. _____
_____

- Describe the effects of using music as a distraction to control pain. _____
_____

- Define the following pain-relief measures and the rationale for their use.

    a. Biofeedback: _____
_____

- b. Cutaneous stimulation: _____
_____

- c. Herbals: _____
_____

- d. Reducing pain perception: _____
_____

- What is TENS, and how is it believed to reduce pain? _____
_____

Acute Care

Pharmacological Pain-Relief Interventions

- Analgesics are the most common method of pain relief.

- Identify the three types of analgesics and explain the conditions for which they are generally prescribed.

    a. _____
_____

    b. _____
_____

    c. _____
_____

- One way to maximize pain relief while minimizing drug toxicity is to administer the medication on a(n) _____ basis rather than on a(n) _____ basis.

- Describe four major principles for analgesic administration.

    a. _____

    b. _____

    c. _____

    d. _____

- Explain the benefits of patient-controlled analgesia (PCA). _____
_____

Chapter 38: Pain and Comfort   253

- Describe what a local anaesthetic is, how it may be applied, and possible side effects. _____
  _____

- Describe what a regional anaesthetic is and list 3 types. _____
  a. _____
  b. _____
  c. _____

- Explain an advantage of an epidural analgesia and how it is administered. _____
  _____

- Describe goals of nursing care for a client with epidural infusions. Explain one intervention for each goal.
  a. _____
  _____
  b. _____
  _____
  c. _____
  _____
  d. _____
  _____
  e. _____
  _____
  f. _____
  _____

- Explain the following surgical interventions for pain.
  a. Dorsal rhizotomy: _____
  _____
  b. Chordotomy: _____
  _____

- Identify the three-step approach to cancer pain management recommended by the World Health Organization (1990).
  a. _____
  _____
  b. _____
  _____
  c. _____
  _____

- Identify clients who are candidates for continuous infusions.
  a. _____
  b. _____
  c. _____
  d. _____

- List four guidelines for safe administration of morphine sulfate via ambulatory infusion pumps.
  a. _____
  b. _____
  c. _____
  d. _____

Restorative Care and Continuing Care

Explain hospice programs. _____
_____

Evaluation

Client Care

- If a client continues to have discomfort after an intervention, a different approach may be needed. For example, if an analgesic provides only partial relief, the nurse may add relaxation exercises or guided-imagery exercises.

- Pain assessment and responses to intervention should be accurately and thoroughly documented so that they can be communicated to others caring for the client.

Client Expectations

- The client, if able, is the best judge of whether pain-relief measures work.

- The family often is another valuable resource, particularly in the case of the client with cancer who may not be able to express discomfort during the latter stages of terminal illness.

*R*eview Questions

The student should select the appropriate answer and cite the rationale for choosing that particular answer.

1. Pain is a protective mechanism warning of tissue injury and is largely a(n):
   a. Symptom of a severe illness or disease
   b. Subjective experience
   c. Objective experience
   d. Acute symptom of short duration

Answer: _____ Rationale: _____

_____

_____

2. A substance that can cause analgesia when it attaches to opiate receptors in the brain is:
   a. Substance P
   b. Serotonin
   c. Prostaglandin
   d. Endorphin

Answer: _____ Rationale: _____

_____

_____

3. To adequately assess the quality of a client's pain, which question would be appropriate?
   a. "Tell me what your pain feels like."
   b. "Is your pain a crushing sensation?"
   c. "How long have you had this pain?"
   d. "Is it a sharp pain or a dull pain?"

Answer: _____ Rationale: _____

_____

_____

4. The use of client distraction in pain control is based on the principle that:
   a. Small C fibres transmit impulses via the spinothalamic tract.
   b. The reticular formation can send inhibitory signals to gating mechanisms.
   c. Large A fibres compete with pain impulses to close gates to painful stimuli.
   d. Transmission of pain impulses from the spinal cord to the cerebral cortex can be inhibited.

Answer: _____ Rationale: _____

_____

_____

5. Teaching a child about painful procedures is best achieved by:
   a. Early warnings of the anticipated pain
   b. Storytelling about the upcoming procedure
   c. Relevant play directed toward procedure activities
   d. Avoiding explanations until the pain is experienced

Answer: _____ Rationale: _____

_____

_____

Critical Thinking for Nursing Care Plan for Acute Pain

Imagine that you are the student nurse in the Care Plan on page 1256 of your text. Complete the *assessment phase* of the critical thinking model by writing your answers in the appropriate boxes of the model shown. Think about the following:

- What knowledge base was applied to Mrs. Mays?

- In what way might previous experience assist you in this case?

- What intellectual or professional standards were applied to the care of Mrs. Mays?

- What critical thinking attitudes did you use in assessing Mrs. Mays?

- As you review your assessment, what key areas did you cover?

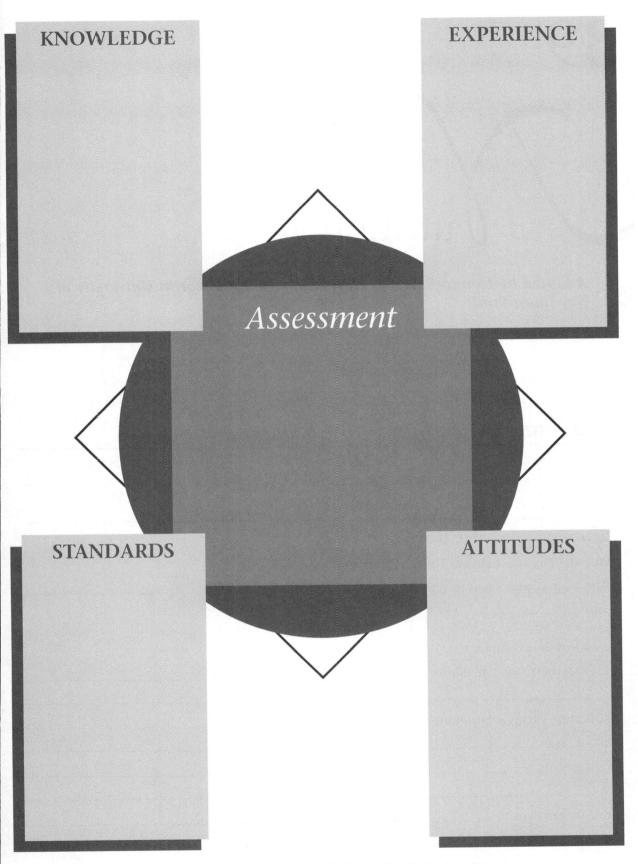

KNOWLEDGE

EXPERIENCE

Assessment

STANDARDS

ATTITUDES

CHAPTER 38   Critical Thinking Model for Nursing Care Plan for *Acute Pain*

See answers on page 597.

39

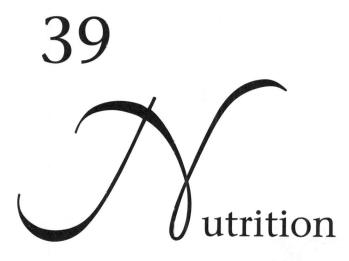

Nutrition

Adapted by Donna Best, RN, BN, MN, ACNP, Memorial University of Newfoundland

Preliminary Reading

Chapter 39, pp. 1278-1328

Comprehensive Understanding

Scientific Knowledge Base

Nutrients: The Biochemical Units of Nutrition

- The body requires fuel to provide energy for _____, _____, _____, and _____.

- Define the following terms.

  a. Basal metabolic rate (BMR): _____
  _____

  b. Resting energy expenditure (REE):_____
  _____

  c. Nutrients: _____
  _____

  d. Nutrient density: _____
  _____

- List the six categories of nutrients.

  a. _____

  b. _____

  c. _____

  d. _____

  e. _____

  f. _____

Carbohydrates

- Each gram of carbohydrate produces _____ kilocalories (kcal).

- Identify the three classifications of carbohydrates.

  a. _____

  b. _____

  c. _____

Proteins

- Proteins are essential for _____ in _____, _____, and _____.

- The simplest form of protein is the _____.

- Explain the two forms of protein.

  a. Essential amino acids: _____

  _____

  b. Non-essential amino acids: _____

  _____

- Define the following terms.

  a. Complete protein: _____

  _____

  b. Incomplete protein: _____

  _____

  c. Complementary proteins: _____

  _____

- Protein is the only major nutrient that contains _____ and is the only source of _____ for the body.

- *Nitrogen balance* is _____.

Fats

- Lipids (fats) are the most calorically dense nutrient, providing _____ kcal per gram.

- Describe the following composition of fats.

  a. Triglycerides: _____

  _____

  b. Fatty acids: _____

  _____

- Define the following types of fatty acids and give an example of each.

  a. Saturated: _____

  _____

  b. Unsaturated: _____

  _____

  c. Monounsaturated: _____

  _____

  d. Polyunsaturated: _____

  _____

  e. Trans: _____

  _____

Water

- Water composes _____ of total body weight.

- _____ have the greatest percentage of total body weight as water, and _____ people have the least.

- Fluid needs are met by _____ and by water produced during _____.

Chapter 39: Nutrition 259

Vitamins

- Vitamins are _____
  _____
  _____ .

- Identify the fat-soluble vitamins. _____
  _____

- Identify the water-soluble vitamins. _____
  _____

Minerals

- Minerals are _____
  _____ .

- Minerals are classified as _____ when the daily requirement is 100 mg or more, and _____ when less than 100 mg is needed daily.

Anatomy and Physiology of the Digestive System

- Digestion of food consists of the mechanical breakdown and chemical reactions by which food is reduced to its simplest form.

- Enzymes are _____
  _____ .

- The following activities of digestion are interdependent. Explain each one.
  a. Mechanical: _____
     _____
  b. Chemical: _____
     _____
  c. Hormonal: _____
     _____

- The major portion of digestion occurs in the _____
  _____ .

- Define the following terms.
  a. Peristalsis: _____
     _____
  b. Dysphagia: _____
     _____
  c. Chyme: _____
     _____

- The primary absorption site of nutrients is the _____
  _____ .

- The main source of water absorption is via the _____
  _____ .

- In addition to water, electrolytes and minerals are absorbed, and bacteria in the colon synthesize _____ vitamins.

- *Metabolism* refers to _____
  _____ .

- Describe the two types of metabolism.
  a. Anabolism: _____
     _____
  b. Catabolism: _____
     _____

- The body's major form of reserved energy is _____, which is stored as _____ .

- Glycogen is synthesized from _____ and provides _____ .

- Nutrient metabolism consists of three main processes. Explain each one.
  a. Glycogenolysis: _____
     _____

b. Glycogenesis:_____

_____

c. Gluconeogenesis: _____

_____

- Feces contain:_____

_____

Dietary Guidelines

- Explain the Dietary Reference Intakes (DRIs) format. _____

_____

- Using the space below, diagram and label *Canada's Food Guide to Healthy Living.*

- List the five dietary guidelines for Canadians identified in *Canada's Guidelines for Healthy Eating.*

  a. _____

  b. _____

  c. _____

  d. _____

  e. _____

- List the nutritional recommendations for Canadians identified in *Canada's Guidelines for Healthy Eating.*

  a. _____

  b. _____

  c. _____

d. _____

e. _____

f. _____

g. _____

h. _____

- List the parts of a food label. _____

_____

Nursing Knowledge Base

Nutrition During Human Growth and Development

Infants Through School-Age Children

- An energy intake of approximately _____ kcal/kg is needed in the first half of infancy, and an intake of _____ kcal/kg is needed in the second half.

- A full-term newborn is able to digest and absorb _____.

- Infants need _____ mL/kg/day of fluid.

- List at least four benefits for breast-feeding an infant.

    a. _____

    b. _____

    c. _____

    d. _____

- Explain why the following should not be used in infant formula.

    a. Cow's milk: _____

    _____

    b. Honey and corn syrup: _____

    _____

- The addition of solid foods to an infant's diet should be governed by the infant's _____, _____, and _____.

- The toddler needs _____ calories but an increased amount of _____ in relation to body weight.

- School-age children's diets should be assessed for: _____

_____

- Explain some reasons for the increase in childhood obesity. _____

_____

Adolescents

- Identify the common deficiencies in the following adolescent population groups.

    a. Girls: _____

    b. Boys: _____

    c. Those who eat fast food: _____

    d. Pregnant: _____

- Identify the diagnostic criteria for the following eating disorders.

    a. Anorexia nervosa: _____

    _____

    _____

    b. Bulimia nervosa: _____

    _____

    _____

Young and Middle Adults

- Obesity may become a problem because of:

_____

_____

- Adult women who use oral contraceptives need extra _____.

- The energy requirements of pregnancy are related to _____

  _____

- Supplementation is usually recommended along with dietary modification to increase intake of _____, _____,

  _____, _____, and

  _____.

- During lactation, there is an increased need for vitamins _____ and _____.

Older Adults

- List four factors that influence the nutritional status of the older adult.

  a. _____

  b. _____

  c. _____

  d. _____

Alternative Food Patterns

- Briefly describe the vegetarian diet. _____

  _____

  _____

Nursing Process and Nutrition

- Close daily contact with clients and their families enables nurses to make observations about their physical status, food intake, weight changes, and responses to therapy.

Assessment

- Define the following terms.

  a. Body mass index (BMI): _____

  _____

  b. Ideal body weight (IBW): _____

  _____

  c. Anthropometry: _____

  _____

- Identify the common laboratory tests used to study the nutritional status of a client. _____

  _____

- List the eight components of a dietary history and provide a sample question for each.

  a. _____

  b. _____

  c. _____

  d. _____

  e. _____

  f. _____

  g. _____

  h. _____

- For each assessment area, list at least two signs of good and poor nutrition.

  a. General appearance

  1. _____

  2. _____

  b. General vitality

  1. _____

  2. _____

  c. Weight

  1. _____

  2. _____

  d. Hair

  1. _____

  2. _____

  e. Skin

  1. _____

  2. _____

  f. Mouth, oral membranes

  1. _____

  2. _____

  g. Gastrointestinal function

  1. _____

  2. _____

h. Cardiovascular function

    1. _____

    2. _____

i. Nervous system function

    1. _____

    2. _____

j. Muscles

    1. _____

    2. _____

Nursing Diagnosis

- List three potential or actual nursing diagnoses for altered nutritional status.

    a. _____

    b. _____

    c. _____

Planning

- Nurses frequently collaborate with dietitians to ensure nutrition plans are appropriate and to learn how to obtain accurate data, for example, how to conduct calorie counts. A good care plan requires accurate exchange of information between disciplines.

- Provide an example of a goal and associated outcomes appropriate for a client with nutritional problems.

    a. _____

    b. _____

    c. _____

    d. _____

Implementation

Health Promotion

- Clients can prevent the development of many diseases by incorporating knowledge of nutrition into their lifestyle.

- Summarize meal planning and identify the factors that should be considered. _____

_____

Acute Care

- List three factors that can cause anorexia (loss of appetite) in acute care settings.

    a. _____

    b. _____

    c. _____

- Clients who are NPO and only receive standard IV fluids for more than seven days are at nutritional risk.

- List five ways that a nurse can promote appetite.

    a. _____

    b. _____

    c. _____

    d. _____

    e. _____

- List three complications of dysphagia.

    a. _____

    b. _____

    c. _____

- List eight nursing interventions to assist dysphagic clients with feeding.

    a. _____

    b. _____

    c. _____

    d. _____

    e. _____

    f. _____

    g. _____

    h. _____

- Define *enteral nutrition (EN)*. _____

_____

- Describe the following types of feeding tubes. Identify the tube(s) that can be inserted by a nurse.

  a. Nasogastric: _____

  _____

  b. Nasointestinal: _____

  _____

  c. Gastrostomy: _____

  _____

  d. Jejunostomy: _____

  _____

  e. PEG: _____

  _____

- If EN therapy is to be administered for less than 4 weeks, _____ tubes may be used. _____ tubes are preferred for long-term feeding (more than 4 weeks).

- Differentiate between the following types of formula.

  a. Polymeric: _____

  _____

  b. Modular: _____

  _____

  c. Elemental: _____

  _____

  d. Specialty: _____

  _____

- Explain the physiological changes and further complications caused by aspiration of enteral formula into the lungs. _____

  _____

- List five common conditions that increase the risk of aspiration during tube feedings.

  a. _____

  b. _____

  c. _____

  d. _____

  e. _____

- The most reliable method for testing the placement of a small bore feeding tube is ____

  _____

- Describe an alternative method that the nurse may use to test the placement of a small-bore feeding tube. _____

  _____

- List six major complications of enteral feedings and an intervention for each.

  a. _____

  b. _____

  c. _____

  d. _____

  e. _____

  f. _____

- Define *parenteral nutrition (PN).*_____

  _____

- List the three factors on which safe administration of PN depends.

  a. _____

  b. _____

  c. _____

- Lipid emulsions are: _____

  _____

- The need for continued PN is consistently re-evaluated with the goal of moving toward using the GI tract because disuse of the GI tract has been associated with _____.

- Briefly describe the rationale for each action associated with the initiation and maintenance of total parenteral nutrition.
  - a. Chest x-ray: _____
    _____
  - b. Beginning an infusion: _____
    _____
  - c. Infusion flow rate: _____
    _____

- List six potential complications of parenteral nutrition and identify the symptoms of each.
  - a. _____
  - b. _____
  - c. _____
  - d. _____
  - e. _____
  - f. _____

- Explain the goal of transition from PN to EN and/or oral feeding. _____
  _____

Restorative and Continuing Care

- Medical nutrition therapy (MNT) is: _____
  _____

- Identify the nutritional interventions for the following common disease states.
  - a. Gastrointestinal diseases
    1. Peptic ulcers: _____
    2. Inflammatory bowel disease: _____
    3. Malabsorption syndromes: _____
    4. Diverticulitis: _____
  - b. Diabetes mellitus (DM)
    1. Type 1: _____
    2. Type 2: _____
  - c. Cardiovascular disease: _____
  - d. Cancer: _____
  - e. HIV: _____

Np **Evaluation**

Multidisciplinary collaboration remains essential in the provision of nutritional support.

Client Care

- The effectiveness of nutritional interventions delivered by the health care team is based on the expected outcomes.

- The client's ability to incorporate dietary changes into his or her lifestyle with the least amount of stress or disruption will ensure that outcome measures are successfully met.

Client Expectations

- Clients expect competent and accurate care. The plan of care must be altered if the outcomes are not being met.

Review Questions

The student should select the appropriate answer and cite the rationale for choosing that particular answer.

1. Which nutrient is the body's most preferred energy source?
   a. Protein
   b. Fat
   c. Carbohydrate
   d. Vitamin

Answer: _____ Rationale: _____
_____
_____

2. Positive nitrogen balance would occur in which condition?
   a. Infection
   b. Starvation
   c. Burn injury
   d. Wound healing

Answer: _____ Rationale: _____
_____
_____

3. Mrs. Schultz is talking with the nurse about the dietary needs of her 23-month-old daughter, Anita. Which of the following responses by the nurse would be appropriate?
   a. "Use skim milk to cut down on the fat in Anita's diet."
   b. "Anita should be drinking at least 720 mL of milk per day."
   c. "Anita needs fewer calories in relation to her body weight now than she did as an infant."
   d. "Anita needs less protein in her diet now because she isn't growing as fast."

   Answer: _____ Rationale: _____
   _____
   _____

4. All of the following clients are at risk for alteration in nutrition *except:*
   a. Client J, who is 86 years old, lives alone, and has poorly fitting dentures
   b. Client K, who has been NPO for seven days following bowel surgery and is receiving 3000 ml of 10% dextrose per day
   c. Client L, whose weight is 10% above his ideal body weight
   d. Client M, a 17-year-old girl who weighs 40 kg and frequently complains about her baby fat

   Answer: _____ Rationale: _____
   _____
   _____

5. Which of the following is the most accurate method of bedside confirmation of placement of a small-bore nasogastric tube?
   a. Auscultate the epigastrium for gurgling or bubbling
   b. Test the pH of withdrawn gastric contents
   c. Assess the client's ability to speak
   d. Assess the length of the tube that is outside the client's nose

   Answer: _____ Rationale: _____
   _____
   _____

6. Dietary recommendations for people with high cholesterol include:
   a. Saturated fat: < 7% of total calories
   b. Total fat: 40% to 50% of total calories
   c. Carbohydrates: 25% to 35% of total calories
   d. Cholesterol: > 200 mg/day

   Answer: _____ Rationale: _____
   _____
   _____

Critical Thinking for Nursing Care Plan for Imbalanced Nutrition: Less Than Body Requirements

Imagine that you are Belinda, the nurse in the Care Plan on page 1299 of your text. Complete the *Planning phase* of the critical thinking model by writing your answers in the appropriate boxes of the model shown. Think about the following:

- In developing Mrs. Cooper's plan of care, what knowledge did Belinda apply?

- In what ways might Belinda's previous experience assist in developing Mrs. Cooper's plan of care?

- When developing a plan of care for Mrs. Cooper, what intellectual and professional standards were applied?

- What critical thinking attitudes might have been applied in developing Mrs. Cooper's plan of care?

- How will Belinda accomplish these goals?

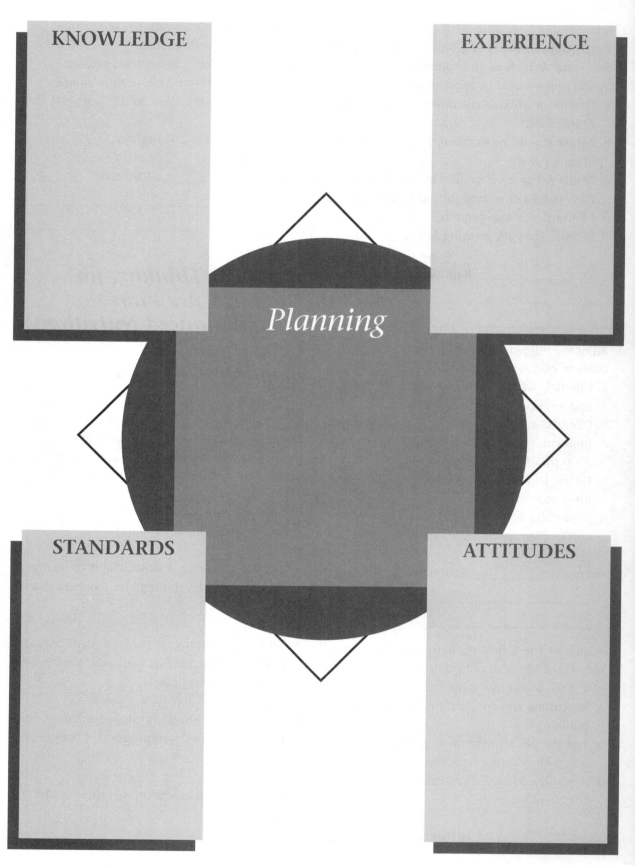

KNOWLEDGE

EXPERIENCE

Planning

STANDARDS

ATTITUDES

CHAPTER *39* Critical Thinking Model for Nursing Care Plan for *Imbalanced Nutrition: Less Than Body Requirements*

See answers on page 598.

40

$\mathscr{U}$rinary Elimination

Adapted by Jill Milne, RN, MN, PhD, University of Alberta

$\mathscr{P}$reliminary Reading

Chapter 40, pp. 1329-1383

$\mathscr{C}$omprehensive Understanding

Scientific Knowledge Base

- Summarize the function of each of the following organs in the urinary system.

  a. Kidneys: _____

  _____

  b. Ureters: _____

  _____

  c. Bladder: _____

  _____

  d. Urethra: _____

  _____

- Define the following terms related to urine elimination.

  a. Nephron: _____

  _____

  b. Proteinuria: _____

  _____

c. Erythropoietin: _____

_____

d. Renin: _____

_____

e. Micturition: _____

_____

f. Urethral meatus: _____

_____

- The ability of the urethra to maintain adequate closure is critical to continence.

- Briefly describe how the following contribute to urethral closure.

  a. Smooth muscle: _____

  _____

  b. Striated muscle: _____

  _____

  c. Rhabdosphincter (urethral sphinter, external sphincter): _____

  _____

Act of Urination

- Number the steps describing the normal act of micturition in sequential order.

  _____ The detrusor muscle contracts.

  _____ Urine volume stretches the bladder walls, sending impulses to the micturition centre in the spinal cord.

  _____ The urethral sphincter relaxes.

  _____ Impulses travel from the micturition centre, to the pontine centre, and then back to the micturition centre.

  _____ The bladder empties.

Factors Influencing Urination

- Problems related to the act of urination may be the result of cognitive, functional, or physical means resulting in incontinence, retention, or infection.

- Disease processes that primarily affect renal function (changes in urine volume or quality) are generally categorized as the following. Briefly explain:

  a. Prerenal: _____

  _____

  b. Renal: _____

  _____

  c. Postrenal: _____

  _____

- Define *oliguria*. _____

_____

- Define *anuria*. _____

_____

- List the characteristic signs of the uremic syndrome. _____

_____

- Briefly describe the two methods of dialysis.

  a. Peritoneal: _____

  _____

  b. Hemodialysis: _____

  _____

- Identify some indications for dialysis. _____

_____

- Discuss how each of the following can impact urinary elimination.

  a. Calculi (stones): _____

  _____

  b. Enlargement of prostate gland: _____

  _____

c. Parkinson's disease: _____

_____

d. Alzheimer's disease: _____

_____

e. Rheumatoid arthritis: _____

_____

- Explain how the following affect the balance of urine excreted.

  a. Alcohol: _____

  _____

  b. Caffeine drinks: _____

  _____

  c. Peripheral edema: _____

  _____

  d. Febrile conditions: _____

  _____

- List four types of medications that affect urination, and describe their major effect.

  a. _____

  _____

  b. _____

  _____

  c. _____

  _____

  d. _____

  _____

- Explain how pelvic floor muscle tone affects urinary elimination. _____

  _____

- Explain what a cystoscopy is and how it may affect urination. _____

  _____

- Briefly explain how the stress of surgery affects urine output. _____

  _____

- Briefly explain how anaesthetics and narcotic analgesics affect urine output. _____

  _____

Common Alterations in Urinary Elimination

- Most clients with urinary problems have disturbances in the act of micturition that involve a failure to store urine, a failure to empty urine, or both. List the three most common alterations in urinary elimination.

  a. _____

  b. _____

  c. _____

- Although many micro-organisms may cause urinary tract infections (UTIs), the most frequent causative pathogen is _____.

- Describe two host defense mechanisms specific to each of the following.

  a. Females: _____

  _____

  b. Males: _____

  _____

  c. Both females and males: _____

  _____

- List six signs or symptoms of UTIs.

  a. _____

  b. _____

  c. _____

  d. _____

  e. _____

  f. _____

- Identify the most common cause of UTIs.

  _____

- List four risk factors for UTI in women.

    a. _____

    b. _____

    c. _____

    d. _____

- Define the following terms related to UTIs.

    a. Bacteriuria: _____

    _____

    b. Dysuria: _____

    _____

    c. Hematuria: _____

    _____

    d. Pyelonephritis: _____

    _____

    e. Cystitis: _____

    _____

- Explain why residual urine is a risk factor for UTIs. _____

- Define *urinary incontinence*. _____

    _____

- Briefly describe the major types of urinary incontinence.

    a. Transient: _____

    _____

    b. Urge: _____

    _____

    c. Stress: _____

    _____

    d. Mixed: _____

    _____

    e. Functional: _____

    _____

    f. Overflow: _____

    _____

    g. Reflex: _____

    _____

- Explain the term *overactive bladder*. _____

    _____

- Define *urinary retention*. _____

    _____

- List five signs of urinary retention.

    a. _____

    b. _____

    c. _____

    d. _____

    e. _____

- Identify three indications for urinary diversions.

    a. _____

    b. _____

    c. _____

- Briefly describe the following urinary diversions.

    a. Ileal loop or conduit: _____

    _____

    b. Ureterostomy: _____

    _____

    c. Nephrostomy: _____

    _____

Nursing Knowledge Base

- The nurse needs to know concepts other than anatomy and physiology, such as infection control, hygiene measures, growth and development, and psychosocial influences.

- Hospital-acquired UTIs are often related to _____, _____, or _____.

- Briefly summarize the developmental changes that may influence urination. _____

    _____

272   Chapter 40: Urinary Elimination

- Identify the psychosocial and cultural factors that may influence urination. _____

Nursing Process and Alterations in Urinary Function

𝒩𝓅 Assessment

- List three factors to be explored when completing a health history related to urinary elimination.

  a. _____

  b. _____

  c. _____

- List five topics that should be included in a urinary diary.

  a. _____

  b. _____

  c. _____

  d. _____

  e. _____

- Describe the following symptoms of urinary alterations.

  a. Incontinence: _____

  b. Urgency: _____

  c. Dysuria: _____

  d. Frequency: _____

  e. Hesitancy: _____

  f. Polyuria: _____

  g. Oliguria: _____

  h. Nocturia: _____

  i. Dribbling: _____

  j. Hematuria: _____

  k. Retention: _____

  l. Residual urine: _____

- Briefly explain the four structures/organs that the nurse would assess to determine the presence and severity of urinary problems.

  a. _____
  _____

  b. _____
  _____

  c. _____
  _____

  d. _____
  _____

- Assessment of urine involves _____ and _____.

- Describe the following characteristics of urine.

  a. Colour: _____

  b. Clarity: _____

  c. Odour: _____

- Describe the following types of urine specimens collected for testing.

  a. Random: _____
  _____

  b. Clean-voided or midstream: _____
  _____

  c. Sterile: _____
  _____

  d. Timed urine: _____
  _____

- Common urine tests include the following. Briefly explain each.

  a. Urinalysis: _____
  _____

  b. Specific gravity: _____
  _____

  c. Urine culture: _____
  _____

Chapter 40: Urinary Elimination   273

- Briefly explain the following types of diagnostic examinations and give the nursing implications for each.

    a. Abdominal roentgenogram: _____

    _____

    b. Intravenous pyelogram (IVP): _____

    _____

    c. Renal scan: _____

    _____

    d. Computerized axial tomography (CT) scan:

    _____

    _____

    e. Ultrasound: _____

    _____

- List the three types of invasive diagnostic examinations and the nursing implications.

    a. _____

    b. _____

    c. _____

Nursing Diagnosis

- List six potential or actual nursing diagnoses related to urinary elimination.

    a. _____

    b. _____

    c. _____

    d. _____

    e. _____

    f. _____

Planning

- List two examples of goals appropriate for a client with a urinary elimination problem.

    _____

    _____

Implementation

Health Promotion

- Maintaining regular patterns of urinary elimination can help prevent many urination problems. The nurse should reinforce the importance of voiding regularly every _____ to _____ hours during the day.

- List three techniques that may be used to stimulate the micturition reflex.

    a. _____

    b. _____

    c. _____

- List several food substances that can be irritating to the bladder mucosa. _____

    _____

- Urine is normally acidic and tends to inhibit the growth of microorganisms. List four types of foods that increase urine acidity.

    a. _____

    b. _____

    c. _____

    d. _____

Acute Care

- Briefly explain how the nurse could help the hospitalized client maintain normal elimination habits. _____

    _____

- List and explain three types of medications that can be used to treat incontinence or retention.

    a. _____

    _____

    b. _____

    _____

    c. _____

    _____

- Briefly describe the following types of catheters.

  a. Straight: _____

  _____

  b. Foley: _____

  _____

  c. Coudé: _____

  _____

- List three indications for each of the following.

  a. Short-term catheterization: _____

  b. Long-term catheterization: _____

  c. Intermittent catheterization: _____

- Explain the following nursing measures taken to maintain client comfort, prevent infection, and maintain an unobstructed flow of urine in catheterized clients.

  a. Fluid intake: _____

  b. Perineal hygiene: _____

  c. Catheter care: _____

- Briefly describe catheter irrigations and instillations. _____

  _____

- Name two principles to follow when removing an in-dwelling catheter.

  a. _____

  b. _____

- Briefly explain the two alternatives for urinary catheterization and give the nursing implications for each.

  a. Suprapubic catheter: _____

  _____

  b. Condom catheter: _____

  _____

- Name two precautions that should be taken to ensure client safety and comfort when using a condom catheter.

  a. _____

  b. _____

- List the nursing measures used to maintain skin integrity when urine comes in contact with the skin.

  a. _____

  b. _____

  c. _____

  d. _____

- List comfort measures for a client with the following sources of discomfort.

  a. Inflamed tissues near urethral meatus: _____

  _____

  b. Painful distension: _____

Restorative Care

- List measures the nurse can teach the incontinent client to gain control over elimination.

  a. _____

  b. _____

  c. _____

  d. _____

  e. _____

  f. _____

  g. _____

  h. _____

  i. _____

  j. _____

  k. _____

- Behavioural therapies should be the first line of treatment because they are _____ and _____.

- Describe three lifestyle modifications that can improve symptoms of UI.

  a. _____

  b. _____

  c. _____

- Define *pelvic floor muscle exercises* (*PFMEs/Kegel exercises*) and list the types of incontinence for which they are generally indicated._____

  _____

- Describe a regimen of bladder training and the clients most likely to benefit. _____

  _____

- Describe the behavioural therapies most appropriate for clients with cognitive and/or physical impairment.

  a. _____

  b. _____

ℕ𝒫 Evaluation

Client Care

- The client is the best source of evaluation of outcomes and responses to nursing care; however, the nurse also evaluates interventions through comparisons with baseline data.

- The nurse evaluates for change in the _____, _____, and _____.

Client Expectations

- The nurse needs to confirm whether the client's expectations have been met to full satisfaction.

- The nurse can also assist the client in redefining unrealistic goals when an impairment is not likely to be altered as completely as the client might like.

ℛeview Questions

The student should select the appropriate answer and cite the rationale for choosing that particular answer.

1. All of the following factors will influence the production of urine *except:*
   a. Poor pelvic floor muscle tone
   b. Acute renal disease
   c. Febrile conditions
   d. Diuretic medications

   Answer: _____   Rationale: _____

   _____

   _____

2. Mrs. Rantz complains of a small amount of leaking urine when she coughs or laughs. This is known as:
   a. Transient incontinence
   b. Stress incontinence
   c. Urge incontinence
   d. Reflex incontinence

   Answer: _____   Rationale: _____

   _____

   _____

3. Ms. Worobetz has a urinary tract infection. Which of the following symptoms would you expect her to exhibit?
   a. Proteinuria
   b. Dysuria
   c. Oliguria
   d. Polyuria

   Answer: _____   Rationale: _____

   _____

   _____

4. The nurse is working with a client who is having an intravenous pyelogram. Which of the following complaints by the client is an abnormal response?
   a. Shortness of breath and audible wheezing
   b. Feeling dizzy and warm with obvious facial flushing
   c. Thirst and feeling "worn out"
   d. Frequent, loose stools

Answer: _____ Rationale: _____

_____

_____

5. A post-surgical client who has recently had her in-dwelling catheter removed complains of feeling the urge to void every 20 to 30 minutes, but is only voiding small amounts. Which of the following behavioural therapies would be most appropriate?
   a. Habit retraining
   b. Prompted voiding
   c. Pelvic floor muscle exercise
   d. Bladder training

Answer: _____ Rationale: _____

_____

_____

Critical Thinking for Nursing Care Plan for Functional Urinary Incontinence

Imagine that you are Kay, the home care nurse in the Care Plan on page 1354 of your text. Complete the *assessment phase* of the critical thinking model by writing your answers in the appropriate boxes of the model shown. Think about the following:

- What knowledge base was applied to the care of Mrs. Grayson?

- In what way might Kay's previous experience assist in this case?

- What intellectual or professional standards were applied to Mrs. Grayson?

- What critical thinking attitudes did you utilize in assessing Mrs. Grayson?

- As you review the assessment, what key areas did Kay cover?

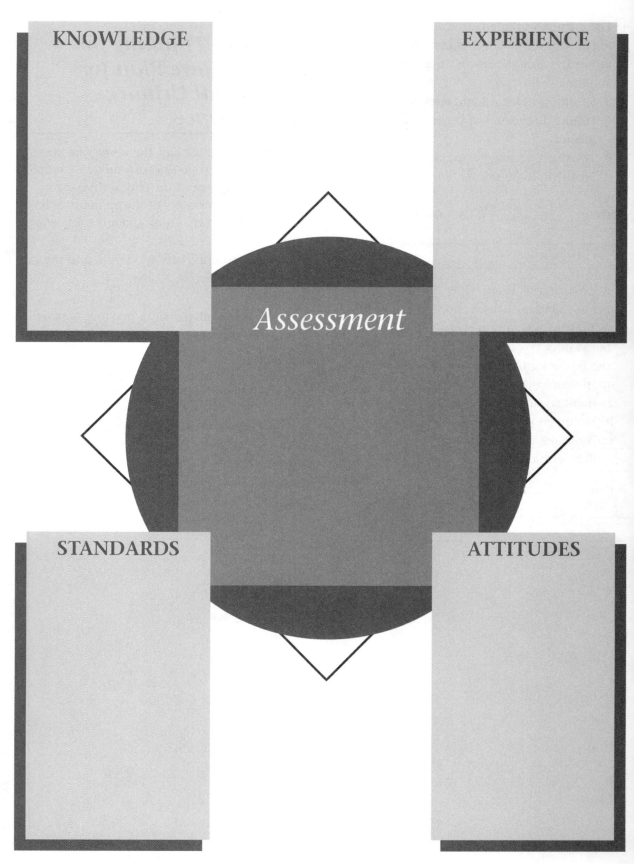

KNOWLEDGE

EXPERIENCE

Assessment

STANDARDS

ATTITUDES

CHAPTER 40 Critical Thinking Model for Nursing Care Plan for *Functional Urinary Incontinence*

See answers on page 599.

41

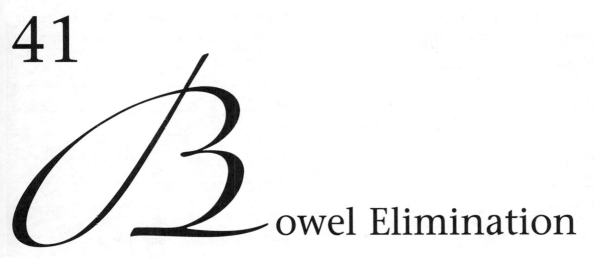

Bowel Elimination

Adapted by Jo-Ann E.T. Fox-Threlkeld, RN, BN, MSc, PhD,
McMaster University

Preliminary Reading

Chapter 41, pp. 1384-1433

Comprehensive Understanding

Scientific Knowledge Base

- The volume of fluids absorbed by the GI tract is high, making fluid and electrolyte balance a key function of the GI system.

- Summarize the functions of the following.

a. Mouth: _____

_____

b. Esophagus: _____

_____

c. Stomach: _____

_____

d. Small intestine: _____

_____

e. Large intestine: _____

_____

- Define the following terms and identify the portion of the GI tract to which they relate.

  a. Masticate: _____

  _____

  b. Bolus: _____

  _____

  c. Peristalsis: _____

  _____

  d. Chyme: _____

  _____

  e. Flatus: _____

  _____

  f. Feces: _____

  _____

- Indicate the correct sequence of mechanisms involved in normal defecation.

  _____ Abdominal muscles contract, increasing intra-rectal pressure.

  _____ The external sphincter relaxes.

  _____ The internal sphincter relaxes and awareness of the need to defecate occurs.

  _____ Movement in left colon, occurs moving stool toward anus.

- Describe the Valsalva manoeuvre and the risk it poses to certain clients. _____

  _____

Nursing Knowledge Base

Factors Affecting Bowel Elimination

- Briefly describe the normal elimination pattern of an infant. _____

  _____

- List six changes that occur in the GI system of the older adult that impair normal digestion and elimination.

  a. _____

  b. _____

  c. _____

  d. _____

  e. _____

  f. _____

- Identify the mechanisms that cause high-fibre diets to promote elimination. _____

  _____

- List five types of foods that are considered high in fibre (bulk).

  a. _____

  b. _____

  c. _____

  d. _____

  e. _____

- Define *lactose intolerance*. _____

  _____

- Summarize how an inadequate intake of fluids can affect the character of feces. _____

  _____

- Physical activity _____ peristalsis; immobilization _____ peristalsis.

- Weakened abdominal and pelvic floor muscles impair the ability to _____ and to _____.

- List two diseases of the GI tract that may be associated with stress.

  a. _____

  b. _____

- List four personal elimination habits that influence bowel function.

  a. _____

  b. _____

  c. _____

  d. _____

- Describe how the position of squatting facilitates defecation. _____

  _____

- List conditions that may result in painful defecation.

  a. _____

  b. _____

  c. _____

  d. _____

- Identify the common problems related to defecation that occur during pregnancy and explain why they occur. _____

  _____

- Summarize the effects of anaesthetic agents and peristalsis on defecation. _____

  _____

- Describe the effect of each medication on elimination.

  a. Mineral oil: _____

  _____

  b. Dicyclomine HCl (Bentyl): _____

  _____

  c. Narcotics: _____

  _____

  d. Anticholinergics: _____

  _____

  e. Antibiotics: _____

  _____

f. Histamines: _____

  _____

g. Non-steroidal anti-inflammatory drugs:

  _____

  _____

- List three types of diagnostic tests for visualization of GI structures.

  a. _____

  b. _____

  c. _____

Common Bowel Elimination Problems

- List five factors that place a client at risk for elimination problems.

  a. _____

  b. _____

  c. _____

  d. _____

  e. _____

- Define *constipation*. _____

  _____

- List and briefly describe four causes of constipation.

  a. _____

  _____

  b. _____

  _____

  c. _____

  _____

  d. _____

  _____

- List three groups of clients in whom constipation could pose a significant health hazard.

  a. _____

  b. _____

  c. _____

Chapter 41: Bowel Elimination   281

- Define *fecal impaction*. _____
  _____

- List four signs and symptoms of fecal impaction.
  a. _____
  b. _____
  c. _____
  d. _____

- Define *diarrhea*. _____
  _____

- Name the two major complications associated with diarrhea.
  a. _____
  b. _____

- List five conditions and the physiological effects that cause diarrhea.
  a. _____
  b. _____
  c. _____
  d. _____
  e. _____

- Define *fecal incontinence*. _____
  _____

- Flatulence is _____. It is a common cause of _____, _____, and _____.

- Define *hemorrhoids*: _____
  _____

- List four conditions that cause hemorrhoids.
  a. _____
  b. _____
  c. _____
  d. _____

Bowel Diversions
- Define the following.
  a. Stoma: _____
  _____
  b. Ileostomy: _____
  _____
  c. Colostomy: _____
  _____

- The location of the ostomy determines the consistency of the stool.

- Briefly explain each of the following types of colostomy construction.
  a. Loop colostomy: _____
  _____
  b. End colostomy: _____
  _____
  c. Double-barrel colostomy: _____
  _____

- Briefly describe the following surgical procedures that provide continence for selected colectomy clients.
  a. Ileoanal pouch anastomosis: _____
  _____
  b. Kock continent ileostomy: _____
  _____

- Identify a major physiological concern of a client with an ostomy. _____
  _____

Nursing Process and Bowel Elimination

Assessment

- List 16 factors that affect elimination that need to be included in a health history for clients with altered elimination status.

  a. _____

  b. _____

  c. _____

  d. _____

  e. _____

  f. _____

  g. _____

  h. _____

  i. _____

  j. _____

  k. _____

  l. _____

  m. _____

  n. _____

  o. _____

  p. _____

- Summarize the following steps for assessing the abdomen.

  a. Inspection: _____

  _____

  b. Auscultation: _____

  _____

  c. Palpation: _____

  _____

  d. Percussion: _____

  _____

- Summarize the assessment of the rectum.

  _____

  _____

- Briefly describe the appropriate technique for collecting a fecal specimen. _____

  _____

- Define *guaiac test*. _____

  _____

- Describe the normal fecal characteristics.

  a. Colour: _____

  _____

  b. Odour: _____

  _____

  c. Consistency: _____

  _____

  d. Frequency: _____

  _____

  e. Amount: _____

  _____

  f. Shape: _____

  _____

  g. Constituents: _____

  _____

- Indicate the possible cause for each of the following fecal characteristics.

  a. White or clay colour: _____

  b. Black or tarry: _____

  c. Melena: _____

  d. Liquid consistency: _____

  e. Narrow, pencil-shaped: _____

Nursing Diagnosis

- List five potential or actual nursing diagnoses for a client with alteration in bowel elimination.

  a. _____

  b. _____

  c. _____

  d. _____

  e. _____

𝒩𝓅 Planning

- List an example of a goal and five associated outcomes appropriate for clients with elimination problems.

  a. _____

  b. _____

  c. _____

  d. _____

  e. _____

𝒩𝓅 Implementation

Health Promotion

- Explain how the following can assist the client to evacuate his or her bowels.

  a. Sitting position: _____

  _____

  b. Positioning on the bedpan: _____

  _____

- Explain the proper technique for positioning a client on a bedpan._____

  _____

Acute Care

- Identify the primary action of the following.

  a. Cathartics: _____

  _____

  b. Laxatives: _____

  _____

  c. Anti-diarrheals: _____

  _____

- The primary reason for an enema is:_____

  _____

- Briefly describe the following types of enemas.

  a. Tap water:_____

  _____

b. Normal saline:_____

_____

c. Soapsuds: _____

_____

d. Hypertonic solution:_____

_____

e. Oil-retention: _____

_____

f. Carminative: _____

_____

- Explain the physician's order, "Give enemas till clear."_____

  _____

- List three complications of digital removal of stool.

  a. _____

  b. _____

  c. _____

- List four reasons to insert a nasogastric (NG) tube for decompression.

  a. _____

  b. _____

  c. _____

  d. _____

- Explain how the Salem sump tube works.

  _____

  _____

- Explain how the nurse would provide comfort to a client with a NG tube. _____

  _____

- Explain how an NG tube can cause distention and how it can be prevented. _____

  _____

Continuing and Restorative Care

Care of Ostomies

- List eight factors to consider when selecting a pouching system for an ostomate.

  a. _____

  b. _____

  c. _____

  d. _____

  e. _____

  f. _____

  g. _____

  h. _____

- Summarize the nutritional considerations for clients with ostomies. _____ _____

- Summarize the goals of a bowel-training program. _____ _____

- Briefly explain bowel training. _____ _____

- Describe two nursing interventions that promote comfort for clients who experience the following.

  a. Hemorrhoids:

     1. _____

     2. _____

  b. Risk to skin integrity:

     1. _____

     2. _____

Evaluation

Client Care

- The effectiveness of care depends on success in meeting the goals and expected outcomes of care.

- The client is the only one who is able to determine if the bowel elimination problems have been relieved and which therapies were the most effective.

Client Expectations

- The client will relate a feeling of comfort and freedom from pain as elimination needs are met within the limits of the client's condition and treatment.

Review Questions

The student should select the appropriate answer and cite the rationale for choosing that particular answer.

1. Most nutrients and electrolytes are absorbed in the:
   a. Esophagus
   b. Small intestine
   c. Colon
   d. Stomach

   Answer: _____ Rationale: _____

   _____

   _____

2. Regarding diagnostic examinations involving visualization of the lower GI structures, all of the following are true *except:*
   a. The client must drink fluids immediately before the test.
   b. The client will likely receive a prescribed bowel preparation before the test.
   c. The client is not allowed to eat or drink before the test.
   d. Changes in elimination may occur following the procedure until normal eating patterns resume.

   Answer: _____ Rationale: _____

   _____

   _____

3. Mrs. Ahmed is concerned about her breast-fed infant's stool, stating that it is yellow instead of brown. The nurse explains that:
   a. A change to formula may be necessary.
   b. Her infant is dehydrated and she should increase his fluid intake.
   c. The stool is normal for an infant.
   d. It will be necessary to send a stool specimen to the lab.

Answer: _____ Rationale: _____

_____

_____

4. After positioning a client on the bedpan, the nurse should:
   a. Leave the head of the bed flat.
   b. Raise the head of the bed 30 degrees.
   c. Raise the head of the bed to a 90-degree angle.
   d. Raise the bed to the highest working level.

Answer: _____ Rationale: _____

_____

_____

5. The physician has ordered a cleansing enema for 7-year-old Michael. The nurse realizes the maximum volume to be given would be:
   a. 100 to 150 mL
   b. 150 to 250 mL
   c. 300 to 500 mL
   d. 600 to 700 mL

Answer: _____ Rationale: _____

_____

_____

Critical Thinking for Nursing Care Plan for Constipation

Imagine that you are Javier, the nurse in the Care Plan on page 1406 of your text. Complete the *planning phase* of the critical thinking model by writing your answers in the appropriate boxes of the model shown. Think about the following:

- In developing Larry's plan of care, what knowledge did Javier apply?

- In what way might Javier's previous experience assist in developing a plan of care for Larry?

- When developing a plan of care, what intellectual and professional standards were applied?

- What critical thinking attitudes might have been applied in developing a plan for Larry?

- How will Javier accomplish the goals?

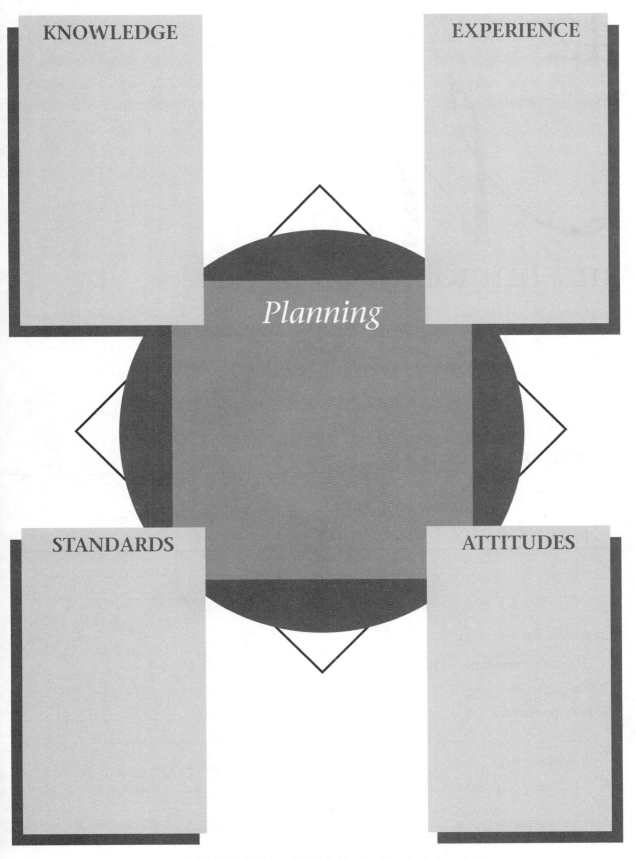

KNOWLEDGE

EXPERIENCE

Planning

STANDARDS

ATTITUDES

CHAPTER 41   Critical Thinking Model for Nursing Care Plan for *Constipation*

See answers on page 600.

42

$\mathcal{M}$obility and Immobility

Adapted by Jan Park Dorsay, RN, MN, ACPN(D), McMaster University

$\mathcal{P}$reliminary Reading

Chapter 42, pp. 1434-1496

$\mathcal{C}$omprehensive Understanding

- *Mobility* refers to: _____
  _____

Scientific Knowledge Base

Physiology and Principles of Body Mechanics

- Define the following.

  a. Body mechanics: _____
     _____

  b. Body alignment: _____
     _____

- Balance is required for _____, _____, and _____.

- The ability to balance can be compromised by _____, _____, _____,
  _____, _____, _____, and _____.

288 Chapter 42: Mobility and Immobility

Copyright © 2006 Elsevier Canada, Inc. All rights reserved.

Gravity and Friction

- Define *friction*. _____

  _____

- List two techniques that minimize friction.

  a. _____

  b. _____

Regulation of Movement

- List three systems responsible for coordinating body movements.

  a. _____

  b. _____

  c. _____

Skeletal System

- List four functions of the skeletal system.

  a. _____

  b. _____

  c. _____

  d. _____

- Describe what *pathological fractures* are. _____

  _____

- Describe the following types of joints and give an example of each.

  a. Synarthrotic joint: _____

  _____

  b. Cartilaginous joint: _____

  _____

  c. Fibrous joint: _____

  _____

  d. Synovial joint: _____

  _____

- Ligaments are: _____

  _____

- Tendons are: _____

  _____

- Cartilage is: _____

  _____

Skeletal Muscle

- Briefly describe how skeletal muscles cause movement. _____

  _____

- Briefly describe the two types of muscle contractions.

  a. Isotonic: _____

  _____

  b. Isometric: _____

  _____

- Define *leverage*. _____

  _____

- Briefly explain how posture and movement are coordinated and regulated. _____

  _____

Nervous System

- Briefly describe how movement and posture are regulated by the nervous system. _____

  _____

Pathological Influences on Mobility

- Briefly explain how the following pathological conditions affect mobility.

  a. Postural abnormalities: _____

  _____

  b. Impaired muscle development: _____

  _____

c. Damage to the central nervous system:

_____

_____

d. Direct trauma to the musculoskeletal system: _____

_____

Nursing Knowledge Base

Mobility-Immobility

- Define *bed rest.* _____

_____

- *Impaired physical mobility* is defined as: _____

_____

Systemic Effects of Immobility

- When there is an alteration in mobility, each body system is at risk. Identify at least two hazards of immobility for each area.

  a. Metabolic changes:

  1. _____

  2. _____

  b. Respiratory changes:

  1. _____

  2. _____

  c. Cardiovascular changes:

  1. _____

  2. _____

  d. Musculoskeletal changes:

  1. _____

  2. _____

  e. Urinary elimination changes:

  1. _____

  2. _____

  f. Integumentary changes:

  1. _____

  2. _____

Developmental Changes

- Identify the descriptive characteristics of body alignment and mobility related to the following developmental stages.

  a. Infants: _____

  b. Toddlers: _____

  c. Preschool children: _____

  d. Adolescents: _____

  e. Adults: _____

  f. Older adults: _____

Nursing Process for Impaired Body Alignment and Mobility

Assessment

- Briefly describe the four major areas for assessment of client mobility.

  a. Range of motion: _____

  _____

  b. Gait: _____

  _____

  c. Exercise and activity tolerance: _____

  _____

  d. Body alignment: _____

  _____

- Briefly describe the physiological hazards of immobility in relation to the following systems.

  a. Metabolic: _____

  _____

  b. Respiratory: _____

  _____

  c. Cardiovascular: _____

  _____

  d. Musculoskeletal: _____

  _____

  e. Integumentary: _____

  _____

  f. Elimination: _____

  _____

Nursing Diagnosis

- List six actual or potential nursing diagnoses related to an immobilized or partially immobilized client.

  a. _____

  b. _____

  c. _____

  d. _____

  e. _____

  f. _____

Planning

- The nurse plans therapies according to severity of risks to the client, and the plan is individualized according to the client's _____, _____, and _____.

Implementation

Health Promotion

- Many health care agencies have a "no-lift" policy, whereby manual lifting of the whole or a large part of the weight of the client by a health care worker is prohibited except for in exceptional or life-threatening situations. Therefore, the nurse should not attempt to lift a client without assistance unless the client is a _____ or _____.

- List alternatives to manual lifting.

  a. _____

  b. _____

  c. _____

- Briefly explain the benefits of exercise. _____

  _____

Acute Care

- Identify two nursing interventions to meet each of the following goals for the immobilized client.

  a. Maintain optimal nutritional (metabolic) state:

  1. _____

  2. _____

  b. Promote expansion of chest and lungs:

  1. _____

  2. _____

  c. Prevent stasis of pulmonary secretions:

  1. _____

  2. _____

  d. Maintain patent airway:

  1. _____

  2. _____

  e. Reduce orthostatic hypotension:

  1. _____

  2. _____

  f. Reduce cardiac workload:

  1. _____

  2. _____

  g. Prevent thrombus formation:

  1. _____

  2. _____

  h. Maintain muscle strength and joint mobility:

  1. _____

  2. _____

  i. Maintain normal elimination patterns:

  1. _____

  2. _____

  j. Prevent pressure ulcers:

  1. _____

  2. _____

  k. Maintain usual psychosocial state:

  1. _____

  2. _____

- Identify two nursing interventions for the immobilized child.

    a. _____

    b. _____

Positioning Techniques

- Indicate the correct use for each positioning device listed in the following table.

Device	Uses
Pillow	
Abductor pillow	
Bed board	
Footboard	
Footboot	
Trochanter roll	
Sandbag	
Hand roll	
Hand-wrist splint	
Trapeze bar	

- List the common trouble areas for clients in the following positions.

Positions (Give a brief description of the position)	Trouble Areas
Fowler's	a.
	b.
	c.
	d.
	e.
	f.
	g.
Supine	a.
	b.
	c.
	d.
	e.
	f.
	g.
	h.
Prone	a.
	b.
	c.
	d.
Side-lying	a.
	b.
	c.
	d.
	e.
Sims'	a.
	b.
	c.
	d.

- List some general guidelines to apply in any transfer procedure. _____

_____

- List four areas the nurse needs to consider in determining if assistance is required when moving a client in bed.

  a. _____

  b. _____

c. _____

d. _____

Restorative Care

- The goal of restorative care for the immobile client is to: _____

_____

- Instrumental activities of daily living (IADLs) are: _____

  _____

Joint Mobility

- Indicate the type of joint and range-of-motion exercises for the body parts listed in the table below.

Body Part	Type of Joint	Type of Movement
Neck		
Shoulder		
Elbow		
Forearm		
Wrist		
Fingers and thumb		
Hip		
Knee		
Ankle and foot		
Toes		

Walking

- Identify the steps the nurse should take to prepare to assist a client to walk. _____

_____

- Describe how the nurse assists clients with hemiplegia or hemiparesis in walking. _____

_____

Evaluation

Client Care

- To evaluate outcomes, the nurse measures the effectiveness of all interventions. The actual outcomes are compared with the outcomes selected during planning.

- The optimal outcomes are the client's ability to maintain or improve body alignment and joint mobility.

Client Expectations

- Client expectations evaluate care from the client's perspective.

Review Questions

The student should select the appropriate answer and cite the rationale for choosing that particular answer.

1. The nurse would expect all of the following physiological effects of exercise on the body systems *except:*
   a. Decreased cardiac output
   b. Increased respiratory rate and depth
   c. Increased muscle tone, size, and strength
   d. Change in metabolic rate

Answer: _____ Rationale: _____

_____

_____

2. Which of the following is a potential hazard that the nurse should assess when the client is in the prone position?
   a. Unprotected pressure points at the sacrum and heels
   b. Internal rotation of the shoulder
   c. Increased cervical flexion
   d. Plantar flexion

Answer: _____ Rationale: _____

_____

_____

3. Which of the following is a physiological effect of prolonged bed rest?
   a. A decrease in urinary excretion of nitrogen
   b. An increase in cardiac output
   c. A decrease in lean body mass
   d. A decrease in lung expansion

Answer: _____ Rationale: _____

_____

_____

4. All of the following measures are used to assess for deep vein thrombosis *except:*
   a. Measuring the circumference of each leg daily, placing the tape measure at the midpoint of the knee
   b. Observing the dorsal aspect of lower extremities for redness, warmth, and tenderness
   c. Asking the client about the presence of calf pain
   d. Checking for a positive Homans' sign, if not contraindicated

Answer: _____ Rationale: _____

_____

_____

5. Which of the following is an appropriate intervention to maintain the respiratory system of the immobilized client?

a. Turn the client every 4 hours.

b. Maintain a maximum fluid intake of 1500 mL per day.

c. Apply an abdominal binder continuously while in bed.

d. Encourage the use of an incentive spirometer.

Answer: _____ Rationale: _____
_____
_____

Critical Thinking for Nursing Care Plan for Impaired Physical Mobility

Imagine that you are the student nurse in the Care Plan on page 1460 of your text. Complete the *evaluation phase* of the critical thinking model by writing your answers in the appropriate boxes of the model shown. Think about the following:

- What knowledge did you apply in evaluating Ms. Adams' care?

- In what way might your previous experience influence your evaluation of Ms. Adams?

- During evaluation, what intellectual and professional standards were applied to Ms. Adams' care?

- In what ways do critical thinking attitudes play a role in how you approach evaluation of Ms. Adams' care?

- How might you adjust Ms. Adams' care?

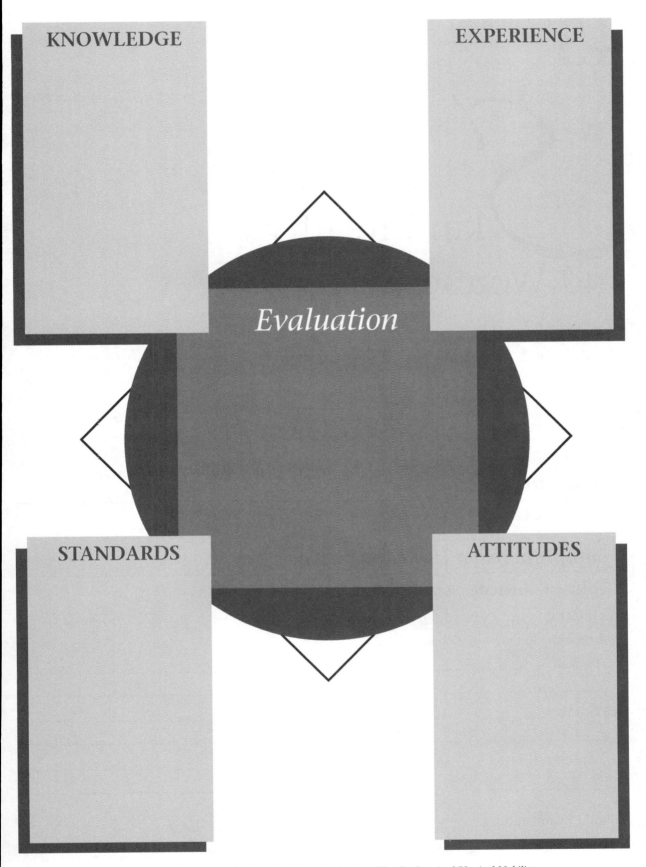

KNOWLEDGE

EXPERIENCE

Evaluation

STANDARDS

ATTITUDES

CHAPTER 42   Critical Thinking Model for Nursing Care Plan for *Impaired Physical Mobility*

See answers on page 601.

43

$\mathcal{S}$kin Integrity and Wound Care

Adapted by Deborah Mings, RN, MHSc, ACNP, GNC(C), St. Peter's Hospital

$\mathcal{P}$reliminary Reading

Chapter 43, pp. 1497-1571

$\mathcal{C}$omprehensive Understanding

Scientific Knowledge Base

Skin Integrity

- Describe the function of each of the following layers of skin.

  a. Epidermis: _____

  _____

  b. Dermis: _____

  _____

  c. Subcutaneous tissue: _____

  _____

Wound Classifications

- Briefly explain the following criteria used to classify wounds.

  a. Cause:_____

  _____

b. Intactness of the skin:_____

_____

c. Depth: _____

_____

d. Cleanliness: _____

_____

e. Duration (acute versus chronic): _____

_____

Pressure Ulcers

- Define *pressure ulcer*.

_____

_____

- Define the following terms that are related to the causes of pressure ulcers.

  a. Tissue ischemia: _____

  _____

  b. Necrosis: _____

  _____

  c. Pressure points:_____

  _____

- Pressure is the greatest factor causing pressure ulcers. Explain how the following factors also contribute.

  a. Friction: _____

  _____

  b. Shearing: _____

  _____

  c. Moisture: _____

  _____

- Briefly explain how the following factors contribute to an increased risk for pressure ulcers.

  a. Impaired mobility: _____

  _____

  b. Altered level of awareness: _____

  _____

c. Impaired sensory perception: _____

_____

_____

d. Chronic vascular disease:_____

_____

e. Malnutrition: _____

_____

f. Advanced age:_____

_____

Stages of Pressure Ulcer Formation

- A pressure ulcer is classified in stages according to its severity. Briefly describe the staging system devised by the National Pressure Ulcer Advisory Panel.

  a. Stage I: _____

  b. Stage II: _____

  c. Stage III: _____

  d. Stage IV: _____

Wound Healing

- Depending on the nature of the wound, wounds heal by either primary intention or secondary intention. Explain.

  a. Primary intention:_____

  _____

  b. Secondary intention: _____

  _____

- Explain the three phases of the wound healing process.

  a. Inflammatory phase: _____

  _____

  b. Proliferative phase: _____

  _____

  c. Remodelling phase: _____

  _____

- List 10 factors that can impair wound healing.

  a. _____

  b. _____

c. _____

d. _____

e. _____

f. _____

g. _____

h. _____

i. _____

j. _____

Wound Drainage

- Describe the four major types of wound drainage (exudate).

  a. _____
  _____

  b. _____
  _____

  c. _____
  _____

  d. _____
  _____

Nursing Knowledge Base

Complications Related to Wound Healing

- Briefly explain the following complications related to wound healing.

  a. Hemorrhage: _____
  _____

  b. Infection: _____
  _____

  c. Dehiscence: _____
  _____

  d. Evisceration: _____
  _____

  e. Fistulas: _____
  _____

- List 10 signs or symptoms of wound infection.

  a. _____

  b. _____

  c. _____

  d. _____

  e. _____

  f. _____

  g. _____

  h. _____

  i. _____

  j. _____

Psychosocial Impact of Wounds

- Identify the factors that may affect the client's perception of the wound. _____
  _____

Nursing Process

𝒩𝒫 Assessment

Assessing for Risk of Pressure Ulcers

- Explain the Braden scale used for assessing pressure ulcer risk. _____
  _____
  _____

Assessing the Skin for Signs of Pressure Ulcers

- The nurse should assess the skin for signs of pressure ulcers at least _____; however, high-risk clients will need more frequent skin assessments, such as _____.

- Define the following.

  a. Erythema: _____
  _____

  b. Blanching: _____
  _____

- Explain the difference between normal reactive hyperemia and abnormal reactive hyperemia. Indicate which of the two is a sign of deep tissue damage. _____ _____

Assessing Wounds

- Briefly explain how wound assessment differs under the following conditions.

  a. In the emergency setting: _____ _____

  b. In the stable setting: _____ _____

- Explain how the nurse assesses the following.

  a. Wound appearance: _____ _____

  b. Drainage: _____ _____

  c. Drains: _____ _____

  d. Wound closure: _____ _____

  e. Wound edges (palpation of wounds): _____ _____

  f. Wound cultures: _____ _____

  g. Pain: _____ _____

🕮 Nursing Diagnosis

- List three nursing diagnoses related to impaired skin integrity.

  a. _____

  b. _____

  c. _____

🕮 Planning

- List six possible goals for the client at risk for pressure ulcers.

  a. _____

  b. _____

  c. _____

  d. _____

  e. _____

  f. _____

Continuity of Care

- List information that should be provided when a client moves to another care setting.

  a. _____

  b. _____

  c. _____

  d. _____

  e. _____

  f. _____

  g. _____

  h. _____

  i. _____

🕮 Implementation

Health Promotion

- Briefly explain the following nursing interventions for the prevention of pressure ulcers.

  a. Topical skin care: _____ _____

  b. Positioning: _____ _____

  c. Therapeutic beds and mattresses: _____ _____

Emergency Care

- Briefly explain the following first aid measures for wounds.

  a. Hemostasis: _____ _____

b. Emergency cleansing: _____

_____

c. Protection: _____

_____

Acute Care

- Aspects of pressure ulcer treatment include local care of the wound and supportive measures such as adequate nutrition and relief of pressure.

Preventing Infections

- Prevention of wound infection includes wound cleansing and removal of non-viable tissue (debridement).

- List and explain three principles to follow when cleansing a wound or the area around a drain.

    a. _____

    b. _____

    c. _____

- _____ is a common method of delivering the wound cleansing solution to the wound and removing debris.

- Irrigation of an open wound requires _____ technique.

- Describe the following methods of debridement.

    a. Mechanical: _____

    b. Autolytic: _____

    c. Enzymatic: _____

    d. Surgical: _____

Dressings

- List the purposes for dressings.

    a. _____

    b. _____

    c. _____

    d. _____

e. _____

f. _____

g. _____

- List the clinical guidelines to use when selecting the appropriate dressing.

    a. _____

    b. _____

    c. _____

    d. _____

    e. _____

    f. _____

    g. _____

- Briefly describe the following types of dressings and their uses.

    a. Gauze: _____

    _____

    b. Self-adhesive, transparent film: _____

    _____

    d. Hydrocolloid: _____

    _____

    e. Hydrogel: _____

    _____

    f. Alginate: _____

    _____

- To prepare for a dressing change, the nurse must know _____, _____, and _____.

- The physician's order for changing a dressing should indicate the _____, _____, and _____ to the wound.

- Dressings over closed wounds should be removed or changed when _____, _____, and _____.

302   Chapter 43: Skin Integrity and Wound Care

- List the activities done by the nurse to prepare a client for a dressing change.

  a. _____

  b. _____

  c. _____

  d. _____

  e. _____

- The first step in packing a wound is to assess

  the _____, _____, and

  _____ of the wound.

- Summarize the principles of packing a wound.

  _____

  _____

- Briefly describe how the wound vacuum-assisted closure device works. _____

  _____

- A dressing may be secured by _____,

  _____, _____, or

  _____.

Suture Care

- Summarize the nursing responsibilities for suture care. _____

  _____

- The most important principle in suture removal is to: _____

  _____

Drainage Evacuation

- Explain the purpose for drainage evacuation.

  _____

  _____

Bandages and Binders

- Explain how bandages and binders applied over or around dressings provide extra protection and therapeutic benefits.

  a. _____

  _____

  b. _____

  _____

  c. _____

  _____

  d. _____

  _____

  e. _____

  _____

  f. _____

  _____

- List the nursing responsibilities when applying a bandage or binder.

  a. _____

  b. _____

  c. _____

  d. _____

- Describe the abdominal binder: _____

  _____

- Sling supports are used for: _____

  _____

Heat and Cold Therapy

- Prior to applying heat or cold therapies, the nurse assesses for temperature tolerance by:

- Cold therapy is contraindicated for: _____

  _____

- Summarize the body's responses to heat and cold. _____

  _____

Chapter 43: Skin Integrity and Wound Care   303

- Describe the physiologic responses to the following.

  a. Heat applications: _____

  _____

  b. Cold applications: _____

  _____

- List the factors that influence heat and cold tolerance.

  a. _____

  b. _____

  c. _____

  d. _____

  e. _____

  f. _____

  g. _____

  h. _____

  i. _____

- Heat and cold applications can be administered in _____ or _____ forms.

- Explain the following types of heat and cold applications, and give the nursing implications for each.

  a. Moist or dry: _____

  _____

  b. Warm, moist compresses: _____

  _____

  c. Warm soaks: _____

  _____

  d. Sitz baths:_____

  _____

  e. Commercial hot packs:_____

  _____

  f. Cold, moist, and dry compresses: _____

  _____

g. Cold soaks:_____

_____

h. Ice bags or collars: _____

_____

Evaluation

Client Care

- Nursing interventions for wound care and reducing the risk of pressure ulcers are evaluated by determining the client's response to nursing therapies and by determining whether each goal was achieved.

- The optimal outcomes are to _____, _____, and _____.

Client Expectations

- Clients with chronic wounds are often cared for in the home and have certain expectations about their level of _____ _____, _____, and _____.

Review Questions

The student should select the appropriate answer and cite the rationale for choosing that particular answer.

1. Ischemia is defined as:
   a. Increased tissue buildup during the healing process
   b. A deficiency of blood supply to tissue
   c. Decreased fluid to the tissues
   d. Increased irritability of nerves

Answer: _____   Rationale: _____

_____

_____

2. Mr. Prada is in a Fowler's position to improve his oxygenation status. The nurse notes that he frequently slides down in the bed and needs to be repositioned. Mr. Prada is at risk for developing a pressure ulcer on his coccyx because of:
   a. Friction
   b. Shearing force
   c. Maceration
   d. Impaired peripheral circulation

Answer: _____ Rationale: _____

_____

_____

3. Which of the following is not a sub-scale on the Braden scale for predicting pressure ulcer risk?
   a. Age
   b. Sensory perception
   c. Moisture
   d. Activity

Answer: _____ Rationale: _____

_____

_____

4. Which of these clients has a nutritional risk for pressure ulcer development?
   a. Client A has a serum albumin level of 37 g/L.
   b. Client B has a lymphocyte count of 2,000/mm³.
   c. Client C has a body mass index of 17.
   d. Client D has a body weight that is 5% greater than his ideal weight.

Answer: _____ Rationale: _____

_____

_____

5. Mrs. Tootoosis is an immobilized client. Which of the following will not increase her risk of pressure development?
   a. She has unrelieved pressure to her hip of greater than 32 mm Hg.
   b. She displays normal reactive hyperemia on her coccyx that lasts for 5 minutes after being turned to her side.
   c. She has low-intensity pressure over a long period to her heels as a result of elastic stockings.
   d. She is positioned so that she has an unequal distribution of body weight.

Answer: _____ Rationale: _____

_____

_____

6. Mr. Wong has a stage II ulcer of his right heel. What would be the most appropriate treatment for this ulcer?
   a. Apply a thick layer of enzymatic ointment to the ulcer and the surrounding skin.
   b. Apply a calcium alginate dressing and change when strike-through is noted.
   c. Apply a heat lamp to the area for 20 minutes twice daily.
   d. Apply a hydrocolloid dressing and change it as necessary.

Answer: _____ Rationale: _____

_____

_____

Critical Thinking for Nursing Care Plan for Impaired Skin Integrity

Imagine that you are the student nurse in the Care Plan on page 1525 of your text. Complete the *assessment phase* of the critical thinking model by writing your answers in the appropriate boxes of the model shown. Think about the following:

- What knowledge base was applied to Mrs. Stein?

- In what way might your previous experience assist you in this case?

- What intellectual or professional standards were applied to Mrs. Stein?

- What critical thinking attitudes did you use in assessing Mrs. Stein?

- As you review your assessment, what key areas did you cover?

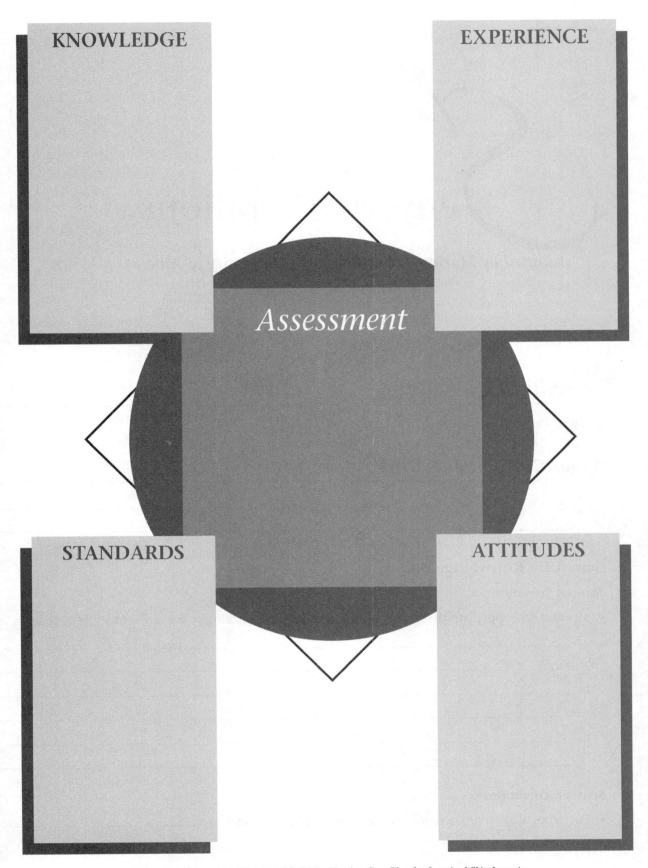

KNOWLEDGE

EXPERIENCE

Assessment

STANDARDS

ATTITUDES

CHAPTER *43* Critical Thinking Model for Nursing Care Plan for *Impaired Skin Integrity*

See answers on page 602.

44

$\mathcal{S}$ensory Alterations

Adapted by Marion Allen, RN, PhD, University of Alberta

$\mathcal{P}$reliminary Reading

Chapter 44, pp. 1572-1599

$\mathcal{C}$omprehensive Understanding

- Define *stereognosis*: _____

_____

Scientific Knowledge Base

Normal Sensation

- List and briefly explain the three functional components necessary for any sensory experience.

    a. _____

    _____

    b. _____

    _____

    c. _____

    _____

Sensory Alterations

- The types of sensory alterations commonly seen by the nurse are _____, _____, and _____.

- Define *sensory deficit*. _____

_____

- For each of the following, describe a disease or condition that may cause it.

  a. Visual deficit: _____

  _____

  b. Hearing deficit: _____

  _____

  c. Balance deficit: _____

  _____

  d. Taste deficit: _____

  _____

  e. Neurological deficit: _____

  _____

- List the three major types of sensory deprivation and give an example of each.

  a. _____

  b. _____

  c. _____

- Define *sensory overload*. _____

_____

- Identify the behavioural changes that are associated with sensory overload. _____

_____

Nursing Knowledge Base

Factors Affecting Sensory Function

- Explain how and why the following factors affect sensory function.

  a. Age: _____

  _____

  b. Quality of stimuli: _____

  _____

  c. Quantity of stimuli: _____

  _____

  d. Social interaction: _____

  _____

  e. Family factors: _____

  _____

  f. Environmental factors: _____

  _____

Nursing Process

Assessment

- The nurse collects a history that assesses the client's current sensory status and the degree to which a sensory deficit affects the client's

  _____, _____,

  _____, _____, and

  _____.

- When assessing the client's mental status the nurse needs to evaluate each of the following. Give an example of each.

  a. Physical appearance and behaviour: _____

  _____

  b. Cognitive ability: _____

  _____

  c. Emotional stability: _____

  _____

- Complete the grid that follows by describing at least one assessment technique for the identified sensory function and the behaviours for an adult and child that would indicate a sensory deficit.

Sense	Assessment Technique	Child Behaviour	Adult Behaviour
Vision			
Hearing			
Touch			
Smell			
Taste			
Position sense			

- Give an example of an assessment for the following that might assist the nurse in deciding if the client has a sensory alteration.

  a. Ability to perform self-care: _____

  b. Health promotion habits: _____

  c. Hazards: _____

- Define the following types of aphasia.

  a. Expressive: _____

  _____

  b. Receptive: _____

  _____

  c. Global: _____

  _____

Nursing Diagnosis

- List six actual or potential nursing diagnoses that might apply to a client with sensory alterations.

  a. _____

  b. _____

c. _____

d. _____

e. _____

f. _____

Planning

- List an example of a goal and four associated outcomes appropriate for a client with a sensory alteration.

  a. _____

  b. _____

  c. _____

  d. _____

  e. _____

ℳℬ Implementation

Health Promotion

- List the three recommended vision screening interventions.

  a. _____

  b. _____

  c. _____

- The most common visual problem is: _____
  _____

- Explain how hearing loss occurs from loud
  noises. _____
  _____

- Identify the common trauma injuries that
  result in hearing or vision loss in both adults
  and children.

  a. Adults: _____
  _____

  b. Children: _____
  _____

- Explain the measures to take to ensure that
  assistive devices being used help maintain
  sensory function at the highest level. _____
  _____

- Briefly explain how the nurse can promote
  meaningful stimulation for clients with sensory alterations in the following areas.

  a. Vision: _____
  _____

  b. Hearing: _____
  _____

  c. Taste and smell: _____
  _____

  d. Touch: _____
  _____

- List three methods of establishing a safe environment with regard to the following adapta-
  tions.

  a. Visual loss:

     1. _____

     2. _____

     3. _____

  b. Reduced hearing:

     1. _____

     2. _____

     3. _____

  c. Reduced olfaction:

     1. _____

     2. _____

     3. _____

  d. Reduced tactile sensation:

     1. _____

     2. _____

     3. _____

- Describe 10 communication methods that are
  appropriate for clients with a hearing impairment.

  a. _____

  b. _____

  c. _____

  d. _____

  e. _____

  f. _____

  g. _____

  h. _____

  i. _____

  j. _____

Acute Care

- When clients enter acute care settings for therapeutic management of sensory deficits or as a result of traumatic injury, the following approaches are used to maximize sensory function. Briefly explain each.

    a. Orientation to the environment: _____

    _____

    b. Communication: _____

    _____

    c. Controlling sensory stimuli: _____

    _____

    d. Safety measures: _____

    _____

Restorative and Continuing Care

- After a client experiences a sensory loss, it becomes important to understand the implications of the loss and to make the adjustments needed to continue a normal lifestyle. Briefly explain.

    a. Understanding sensory loss: _____

    _____

    b. Socialization: _____

    _____

    c. Promoting self-care: _____

    _____

ℳℰ Evaluation

Client Care

- The client is the only one who will know if his or her sensory abilities are improved and which specific interventions or therapies are most successful in facilitating a change in performance.

Client Expectations

- Client expectations are one of the evaluative criteria used by the nurse. What questions might the nurse ask to determine if client expectations have been met? _____

    _____

    _____

ℛeview Questions

The student should select the appropriate answer and cite the rationale for choosing that particular answer.

1. All of the following are true of age-related factors that influence sensory function *except:*
    a. Refractive errors are the most common types of visual disorders in children.
    b. Visual changes in adulthood include presbyopia.
    c. Older adults hear high-pitched sounds best.
    d. Neonates are unable to discriminate sensory stimuli.

Answer: _____ Rationale: _____

_____

_____

2. Mr. McDonald, a 62-year-old farmer, has been hospitalized for 2 weeks for thrombophlebitis. He has no visitors, and the nurse notices that he appears bored, restless, and anxious. The type of alteration occurring because of sensory deprivation is:
    a. Affective
    b. Cognitive
    c. Perceptual
    d. Receptual

Answer: _____ Rationale: _____

_____

_____

3. Which of the following would not provide meaningful stimuli for a client?
   a. A clock or calendar with large numbers
   b. A television that is kept on all day at a low volume
   c. Family pictures and personal possessions
   d. Interesting magazines and books

Answer: _____ Rationale: _____

_____

_____

4. Clients with existing sensory loss must be protected from injury. What determines the safety precautions taken?
   a. The existing dangers in the environment
   b. The financial means to make needed safety changes
   c. The nature of the client's actual or potential sensory loss
   d. The availability of a support system to enable the client to exist in his or her present environment

Answer: _____ Rationale: _____

_____

_____

5. A client who is unable to name common objects or express simple ideas in words or writing suffers from:
   a. Expressive aphasia
   b. Receptive aphasia
   c. Global aphasia
   d. Intellectual disability

Answer: _____ Rationale: _____

_____

_____

Critical Thinking for Nursing Care Plan for Disturbed Sensory Perception

Imagine that you are the community health nurse in the Care Plan on page 1586 of your text. Complete the *planning phase* of the critical thinking model by writing your answers in the appropriate boxes of the model shown. Think about the following:

- In developing Judy's plan of care, what knowledge did you apply?

- In what way might your previous experience assist in developing a plan of care?

- When developing a plan of care, what intellectual and professional standards were applied?

- What critical thinking attitudes might have been applied in developing Judy's plan?

- How will you accomplish the goals?

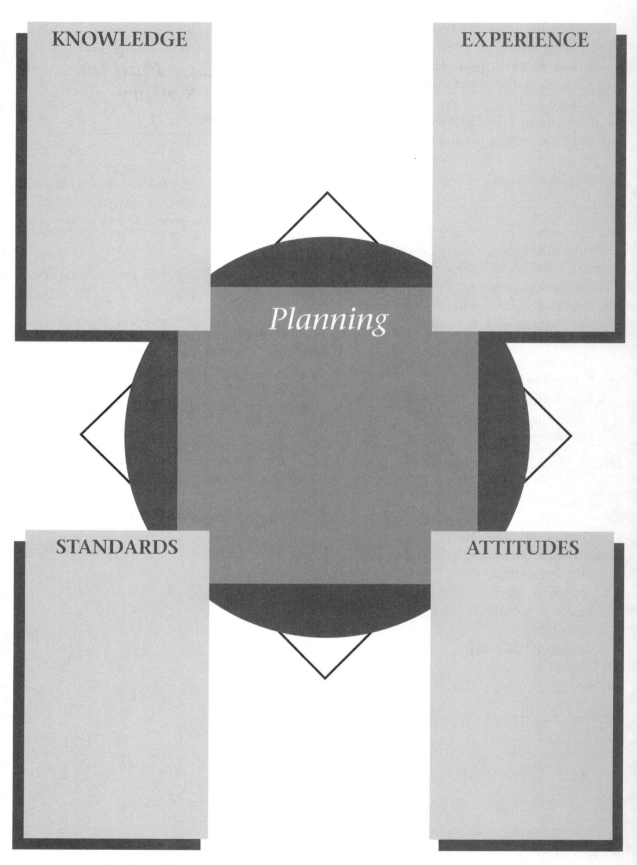

KNOWLEDGE

EXPERIENCE

Planning

STANDARDS

ATTITUDES

CHAPTER 44 Critical Thinking Model for Nursing Care Plan for *Disturbed Sensory Perception*

See answers on page 603.

45

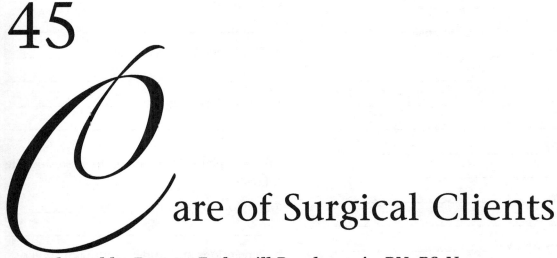

*C*are of Surgical Clients

Adapted by Frances Fothergill-Bourbonnais, RN, BScN,
MN, PhD, University of Ottawa

*P*reliminary Reading

Chapter 45, pp. 1600-1652

*C*omprehensive Understanding

History of Surgical Nursing

- Summarize the historical changes that have occurred in surgical nursing. _____
_____
_____

Ambulatory Surgery

- List the benefits of ambulatory surgery.

    a. _____

    b. _____

    c. _____

    d. _____

Scientific Knowledge Base

Classification of Surgery

- Define the following surgical procedure classifications.

    a. Palliative: _____
    _____

b. Ablative: _____

_____

c. Emergency: _____

_____

d. Minor: _____

_____

e. Urgent: _____

_____

f. Major: _____

_____

g. Reconstructive: _____

_____

h. Constructive: _____

_____

i. Elective: _____

_____

j. Procurement for transplant: _____

_____

k. Diagnostic: _____

_____

The Nursing Process in the Preoperative Surgical Phase

Assessment

- Identify the data the nurse would collect from the client's medical history. _____

_____

- Briefly explain the following factors that increase the client's risk in surgery.
  a. Age: _____

  _____

  b. Nutrition: _____

  _____

  c. Obesity: _____

  _____

d. Immunocompetence: _____

_____

e. Fluid and electrolyte balance: _____

_____

f. Pregnancy: _____

_____

- Briefly explain the rationale for assessing the following.
  a. Previous surgeries: _____

  _____

  b. Perceptions and understanding of surgery:

  _____

  _____

  c. Medication history: _____

  _____

  d. Allergies: _____

  _____

  e. Smoking habits: _____

  _____

  f. Alcohol ingestion and substance use and abuse: _____

  _____

  g. Family support: _____

  _____

  h. Occupation: _____

  _____

  i. Pain: _____

  _____

- Briefly explain each of the following factors that need to be assessed in order to understand the impact of surgery on a client's and family's emotional health.
  a. Body image: _____

  _____

  b. Coping resources: _____

  _____

- Cultural differences influence the surgical experience. Give an example. _____
_____

- Briefly describe the findings on which the nurse would focus related to the physical examination of the following body systems.

  a. General survey: _____
  _____

  b. Head and neck: _____
  _____

  c. Integument: _____
  _____

  d. Thorax and lungs: _____
  _____

  e. Heart and vascular system: _____
  _____

  f. Abdomen: _____
  _____

  g. Neurological status: _____
  _____

- Describe the following routine screening tests for surgical clients.

  a. CBC: _____
  _____

  b. Serum electrolytes: _____
  _____

  c. Coagulation studies: _____
  _____

  d. Serum creatinine: _____
  _____

  e. BUN: _____
  _____

  f. Glucose: _____
  _____

Nursing Diagnosis

- List 10 potential or actual nursing diagnoses appropriate for the preoperative client.

  a. _____
  b. _____
  c. _____
  d. _____
  e. _____
  f. _____
  g. _____
  h. _____
  i. _____
  j. _____

Planning

- Give an example of a goal of care for the perioperative client and associated outcomes.

  a. _____
  _____

  b. _____
  _____

  c. _____
  _____

  d. _____
  _____

Implementation

- Surgery cannot be performed until a client understands the _____, _____, _____, _____, and _____.

- Preparatory information helps clients anticipate the steps of a procedure and thus helps them form realistic images of the surgical experience. When events occur as predicted, clients are better able to cope and attend to the experiences.

- Describe the criteria that may demonstrate the client's understanding of the surgical procedure.

  a. _____

  _____

  b. _____

  _____

  c. _____

  _____

  d. _____

  _____

  e. _____

  _____

  f. _____

  _____

  g. _____

  _____

  h. _____

  _____

Acute Care

Physical Preparation

- Briefly describe the following preoperative preparations.

  a. Maintenance of normal fluid and electrolyte balance: _____

  _____

  b. Reduction of risk of surgical wound infection: _____

  _____

  c. Prevention of bowel and bladder incontinence: _____

  _____

  d. Promotion of rest and comfort: _____

  _____

Preparation on the Day of Surgery

- List nine responsibilities of a nurse caring for a client the day of surgery.

  a. _____

  b. _____

  c. _____

  d. _____

  e. _____

  f. _____

  g. _____

  h. _____

  i. _____

- The signs and symptoms of a latex reaction are: _____

  _____

- Describe methods to eliminate wrong site and wrong procedure surgery. _____

  _____

  _____

Evaluation

Client Care

- The nurse in the preoperative area will be the source for evaluating client outcomes in the preoperative period.

Client Expectations

- Explain the difficulty in determining a client's expectations regarding preoperative teaching.

  _____

  _____

Transport to the Operating Room

- After the client leaves the nursing division, the nurse prepares the bed and room for the client's return if the client is returning to the same nursing division. List 10 pieces of equipment that should be present in the post-operative bedside unit.

  a. _____

  b. _____

  c. _____

  d. _____

  e. _____

  f. _____

  g. _____

  h. _____

  i. _____

  j. _____

Intraoperative Surgical Phase

Assessment

- In the holding area, the nursing responsibilities include: _____

  _____

Implementation

Acute Care

Introduction of Anaesthesia

- Describe general anaesthesia and its risks.

  _____

  _____

  _____

- Regional anaesthesia results in: _____

  _____

- Local anaesthesia involves: _____

  _____

- Describe conscious sedation and identify its advantages. _____

  _____

Positioning the Client for Surgery

- Explain the principles of positioning the client for surgery. _____

  _____

- During the intraoperative phase, the nursing staff continues the preoperative plan. Documentation of intraoperative care provides useful data for the nurse who cares for the client post-operatively.

Post-operative Surgical Phase

- Identify the two phases of the post-operative period and describe the usual time frame for ambulatory and hospitalized clients.

  a. _____

  _____

  b. _____

  _____

Immediate Post-operative Recovery

- Describe the responsibilities of the nurse in the post-anaesthesia care unit (PACU). _____

  _____

Discharge From the Post-Anaesthesia Care Unit

- Identify the criteria for discharge from the PACU. _____

  _____

Recovery in Ambulatory Surgery

- Describe the two phases of post-anaesthesia recovery.

  a. Phase I: _____

  _____

  b. Phase II: _____

  _____

Post-operative Convalescence

- Identify the criteria for discharging ambulatory surgical clients. _____

  _____

The Nursing Process in Post-operative Care

🖋 Assessment

- Explain the frequency of assessments needed during the post-operative period. _____

  _____

- List four major causes of airway obstruction in the post-operative client.

  a. _____

  b. _____

  c. _____

  d. _____

- List four areas to assess in order to determine a post-operative client's circulatory status.

  a. _____

  b. _____

  c. _____

  d. _____

- Describe the characteristic findings associated with post-operative hemorrhage. _____

  _____

- Explain why clients awakening from surgery often complain of feeling cold. _____

  _____

- Define *malignant hyperthermia*. _____

  _____

- List three areas the nurse assesses to determine fluid and electrolyte alterations.

  a. _____

  b. _____

  c. _____

- List the areas of assessment that help to determine a post-operative client's neurological status.

  a. _____

  b. _____

  c. _____

  d. _____

- The nurse assesses the condition of the skin for _____, _____, _____, and _____.

- Describe how the nurse would assess the amount of drainage from a wound. _____

  _____

- Depending on the surgery, a client may not regain voluntary control over urinary function for _____ hours after anaesthesia.

- Normally during the immediate recovery phase, faint or absent bowel sounds are auscultated in all four quadrants. _____ loud gurgles per minute over each quadrant indicate that peristalsis has returned.

- Distention may occur in the client who develops a _____.

- Pain can be perceived before full consciousness is regained. Acute incisional pain causes clients to become _____ and may be responsible for temporary changes in _____.

- Assessment of the client's discomfort and evaluation of pain relief therapies are essential nursing functions.

𝒩𝒫 Nursing Diagnosis

- Identify two actual or potential nursing diagnoses that are appropriate for a post-operative client.

  a. _____
  _____

  b. _____
  _____

𝒩𝒫 Planning

- List the typical post-operative orders prescribed by surgeons.

  a. _____
  b. _____
  c. _____
  d. _____
  e. _____
  f. _____
  g. _____
  h. _____
  i. _____
  j. _____

- Give an example of a goal of care and associated outcomes for a post-operative client.

  a. _____
  _____

  b. _____
  _____

  c. _____
  _____

  d. _____
  _____

  e. _____
  _____

𝒩𝒫 Implementation

Health Promotion

- To prevent respiratory complications, the nurse begins pulmonary interventions early. Describe measures that will promote the following.

  a. Airway patency: _____
  _____

  b. Expansion of the lungs: _____
  _____

  c. Removal of pulmonary secretions: _____
  _____

- Briefly describe measures to promote normal venous return and circulatory blood flow.

  a. _____
  _____

  b. _____
  _____

  c. _____
  _____

  d. _____
  _____

  e. _____
  _____

  f. _____
  _____

- List some non-pharmaceutical pain-relief measures. _____
  _____

Acute Care

- Complete the grid below. Identify three nursing interventions for each area of need in the post-operative client.

Area of Need	Nursing Intervention
Temperature regulation	
Maintaining neurological function	
Maintaining fluid and electrolyte function	
Promoting normal bowel elimination and adequate nutrition	
Promoting urinary elimination	
Promoting wound healing	
Maintaining/enhancing self-concept	

Evaluation

Client Care

- The nurse evaluates the effectiveness of care provided to the surgical client on the basis of expected outcomes following nursing interventions.

- Describe how the nurse would evaluate the ambulatory surgical client. _____

_____

Client Expectations

- With short hospital stays and ambulatory surgery, it is important to evaluate the client's expectations early in the post-operative process.

Review Questions

The student should select the appropriate answer and cite the rationale for choosing that particular answer.

1. Mrs. Yong-Hing, a 45-year-old client with diabetes, is having a hysterectomy in the morning. Because of her history, the nurse would expect:
   a. An increased risk of hemorrhaging
   b. Fluid and electrolyte imbalances
   c. Altered elimination of anaesthetic agents
   d. Impaired wound healing

   Answer: _____ Rationale: _____
   _____
   _____

2. The purposes of the health history for the client who is to have surgery include all of the following except:
   a. Identifying the client's perception and expectations about surgery
   b. Obtaining information about the client's past experience with surgery
   c. Deciding whether surgery is indicated
   d. Understanding the impact surgery has on the client's and family's emotional health

   Answer: _____ Rationale: _____
   _____
   _____

3. All of the following clients are at risk for developing serious fluid and electrolyte imbalances during and after surgery, except:
   a. Client E, who is 81 years old and having emergency surgery for a bowel obstruction following 4 days of vomiting and diarrhea
   b. Client F, who is 1 year old and having a cleft palate repair
   c. Client G, who is 55 years old and has a history of chronic respiratory disease
   d. Client H, who is 79 years old and has a history of congestive heart failure

   Answer: _____ Rationale: _____
   _____
   _____

4. The primary purpose of post-operative leg exercises is to:
   a. Promote venous return
   b. Maintain muscle tone
   c. Assess range of motion
   d. Exercise fatigued muscles

   Answer: _____ Rationale: _____
   _____
   _____

5. The PACU nurse notices that the client is shivering. This is most commonly caused by:
   a. The use of a reflective blanket on the operating room table
   b. Side effects of certain anaesthetic agents
   c. Cold irrigations used during surgery
   d. Malignant hypothermia, a serious condition

   Answer: _____ Rationale: _____
   _____
   _____

Critical Thinking for Nursing Care Plan for Deficient Knowledge Regarding Preoperative and Post-operative Care Requirements

Imagine that you are Joe, the nurse in the Care Plan on page 1617 of your text. Complete the *evaluation phase* of the critical thinking model by writing your answers in the appropriate boxes of the model shown. Think about the following:

- During evaluation, what intellectual and professional standards were applied to Mrs. Campana's care?

- In what way might Joe's previous experience influence his evaluation of Mrs. Campana's care?

- In what way do critical thinking attitudes play a role in how you approach evaluation of Mrs. Campana's care?

- How might Joe adjust Mrs. Campana's care?

- What knowledge did Joe apply in evaluating Mrs. Campana's care?

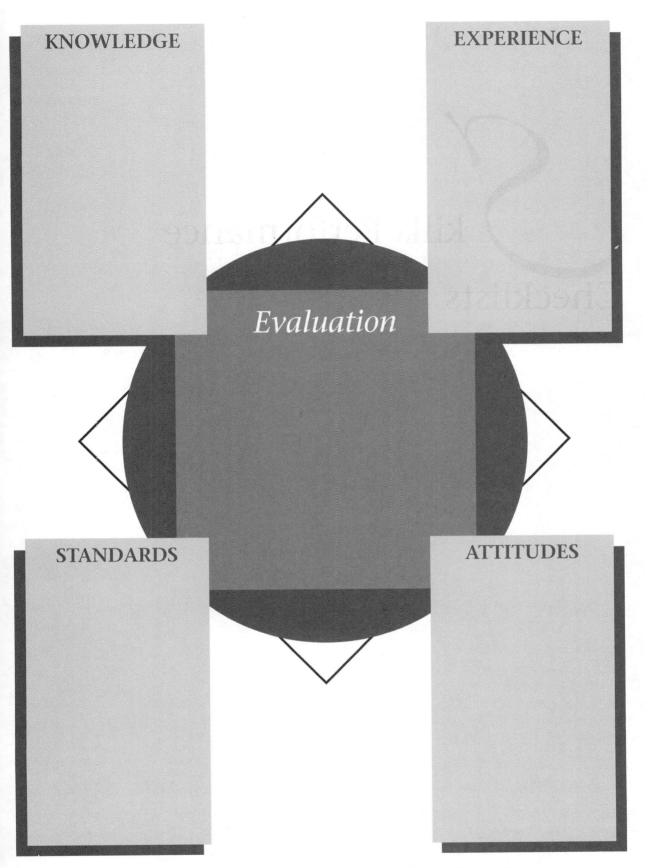

KNOWLEDGE

EXPERIENCE

Evaluation

STANDARDS

ATTITUDES

CHAPTER 45 Critical Thinking Model for Nursing Care Plan for *Deficient Knowledge Regarding Preoperative and Post-operative Care Requirements*

See answers on page 604.

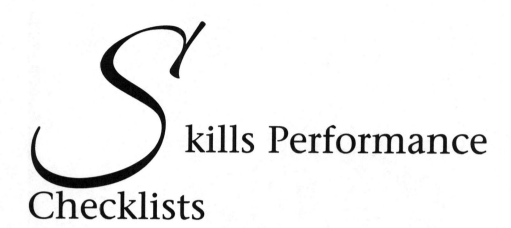

STUDENT: _____ DATE: _____

INSTRUCTOR: _____ DATE: _____

Skill 27-1 Measuring Body Temperature

	S	U	NP	Comments
1. Assess for temperature alterations and factors that influence body temperature.	___	___	___	_____
2. Determine any activity that may interfere with accuracy of temperature measurement.	___	___	___	_____
3. Determine appropriate site and measurement device to be used.	___	___	___	_____
4. Explain to client how temperature will be taken and importance of maintaining proper position.	___	___	___	_____
5. Perform hand hygiene.	___	___	___	_____
6. Obtain temperature reading:				
A. Oral temperature measurement with electronic thermometer:				
(1) Apply disposable gloves (optional).	___	___	___	_____
(2) Remove thermometer pack from charging unit. Attach oral probe (blue tip) to thermometer unit. Grasp top of probe stem, being careful not to apply pressure on the ejection button.	___	___	___	_____
(3) Slide disposable plastic probe cover over thermometer probe until it locks in place.	___	___	___	_____
(4) Have client sit or lie in bed. Ask client to open mouth, then place thermometer probe under tongue in posterior sublingual pocket lateral to centre of lower jaw.	___	___	___	_____
(5) Ask client to hold thermometer probe with lips closed.	___	___	___	_____
(6) Leave thermometer probe in place until audible signal occurs and temperature appears on digital display. Remove thermometer probe from client's mouth.	___	___	___	_____
(7) Push ejection button on thermometer stem to discard plastic probe cover into appropriate receptacle.	___	___	___	_____
(8) Return thermometer stem to storage well of recording unit.	___	___	___	_____
(9) If gloves were worn, remove and dispose of them in appropriate receptacle. Perform hand hygiene.	___	___	___	_____
(10) Return thermometer to charger.	___	___	___	_____

Continued

327

	S	U	NP	Comments

B. Rectal temperature measurement with electronic thermometer:

(1) Provide privacy and assist client to Sims' position. Drape client. ____ ____ ____ _____

(2) Apply disposable gloves. ____ ____ ____ _____

(3) Remove thermometer pack from charging unit. Attach rectal probe (red tip) to thermometer unit. Grasp top of probe stem. ____ ____ ____ _____

(4) Slide disposable plastic probe cover over thermometer probe until it locks in place. ____ ____ ____ _____

(5) Lubricate 2.5 to 3.5 cm of probe for an adult. ____ ____ ____ _____

(6) With non-dominant hand, separate buttocks to expose anus. Ask client to breathe slowly and relax. ____ ____ ____ _____

(7) Gently insert thermometer 3.5 cm for adult. ____ ____ ____ _____

(8) If resistance is felt, withdraw thermometer immediately. Never force thermometer. ____ ____ ____ _____

(9) Leave thermometer probe in place until audible signal occurs and temperature appears on digital display. Remove thermometer probe from client's anus. ____ ____ ____ _____

(10) Push ejection button on thermometer stem to discard plastic probe cover. Wipe probe with alcohol swab. ____ ____ ____ _____

(11) Return thermometer stem to storage well of recording unit. ____ ____ ____ _____

(12) Wipe client's anal area with soft tissue and discard tissue. Assist client to a comfortable position. ____ ____ ____ _____

(13) Remove and dispose of gloves. Perform hand hygiene. ____ ____ ____ _____

(14) Return thermometer to charger. ____ ____ ____ _____

C. Axillary temperature measurement with electronic thermometer:

(1) Provide privacy. ____ ____ ____ _____

(2) Assist client to supine or sitting position. ____ ____ ____ _____

(3) Move client's clothing or gown away from his or her shoulder and arm. ____ ____ ____ _____

(4) Remove thermometer pack from charging unit. Be sure oral probe (blue tip) is attached to thermometer unit. Grasp top of probe stem. ____ ____ ____ _____

Continued

328

	S	U	NP	Comments
(5) Slide disposable plastic probe cover over thermometer probe until it locks in place.	___	___	___	_____
(6) Raise client's arm away from torso and inspect for skin lesions and excessive perspiration. Insert probe into centre of client's axilla, lower arm over probe, and place arm across chest.	___	___	___	_____
(7) Hold probe in place until audible signal occurs and temperature appears on digital display.	___	___	___	_____
(8) Remove probe from axilla.	___	___	___	_____
(9) Push ejection button on probe to discard plastic probe cover.	___	___	___	_____
(10) Return probe to storage well of recording unit.	___	___	___	_____
(11) Assist client to a comfortable position.	___	___	___	_____
(12) Perform hand hygiene.	___	___	___	_____
(13) Return thermometer to charger.	___	___	___	_____

D. Tympanic membrane temperature with electronic thermometer:

	S	U	NP	Comments
(1) Assist client to a comfortable position with head turned toward the side, away from nurse.	___	___	___	_____
(2) Note if there is obvious cerumen in the ear canal.	___	___	___	_____
(3) Remove handheld thermometer unit from charging base, being careful to not apply pressure on the ejection button.	___	___	___	_____
(4) Slide disposable speculum cover over tip until it locks into place.	___	___	___	_____
(5) Insert speculum into ear canal following manufacturer's instructions for tympanic probe positioning:	___	___	___	_____
(a) Pull ear pinna backward, up, and out for adult.	___	___	___	_____
(b) Move thermometer in a figure-eight pattern.	___	___	___	_____
(c) Fit probe gently in ear canal and do not move it.	___	___	___	_____
(d) Point probe toward client's nose.	___	___	___	_____
(6) Depress scan button on handheld unit. Leave thermometer probe in place until audible signal occurs and client's temperature appears on digital display.	___	___	___	_____
(7) Carefully remove speculum from client's auditory canal.	___	___	___	_____

Continued

	S	U	NP	Comments
(8) Push ejection button on handheld unit to discard plastic probe cover.	___	___	___	_____
(9) If second reading is required, replace probe cover and wait 2 to 3 minutes.	___	___	___	_____
(10) Return handheld unit to charging base.	___	___	___	_____
(11) Assist client to a comfortable position.	___	___	___	_____
7. Perform hand hygiene.	___	___	___	_____
8. Discuss findings with client as needed.	___	___	___	_____
9. If temperature is being assessed for the first time, establish temperature as baseline if within normal range.	___	___	___	_____
10. Compare temperature reading with previous baseline and normal temperature range for client's age group.	___	___	___	_____
11. Record temperature and report abnormal findings.	___	___	___	_____

STUDENT: _____ DATE: _____

INSTRUCTOR: _____ DATE: _____

<small>SKILL PERFORMANCE CHECKLIST</small>
Skill 27-2 Assessing the Radial and Apical Pulses

	S	U	NP	Comments
1. Determine need to assess radial or apical pulse.	——	——	——	————————
2. Assess for factors that influence pulse rate.	——	——	——	————————
3. Determine previous baseline apical rate (if available) from client's record.	——	——	——	————————
4. Explain that pulse or heart rate is to be assessed. Encourage client to relax and not speak.	——	——	——	————————
5. Perform hand hygiene.	——	——	——	————————
6. Provide privacy.	——	——	——	————————
7. Obtain pulse measurement:				
A. Radial pulse:				
(1) Assist client to supine or sitting position.	——	——	——	————————
(2) If client is supine, place client's forearm straight alongside the body or across lower chest or upper abdomen with wrist extended straight. If client is sitting, bend client's elbow 90 degrees and support his or her lower arm on a chair or on your arm. Slightly flex client's wrist, with palm down.	——	——	——	————————
(3) Place tips of first two fingers of hand over groove along radial or thumb side of client's inner wrist.	——	——	——	————————
(4) Lightly compress against client's radius, obliterate pulse initially, then relax pressure.	——	——	——	————————
(5) Determine strength of pulse.	——	——	——	————————
(6) After pulse can be felt regularly, look at watch's second hand and begin to count rate.	——	——	——	————————
(7) If pulse is regular, count rate for 30 seconds and multiply total by 2.	——	——	——	————————
(8) If pulse is irregular, count rate for 60 seconds. Assess frequency and pattern of irregularity.	——	——	——	————————
B. Apical pulse:				
(1) Assist client to supine or sitting position. Expose client's sternum and left side of chest.	——	——	——	————————

Continued

(2) Locate anatomical landmarks to identify the point of maximal impulse.

(3) Place diaphragm of stethoscope in palm of your hand for 5 to 10 seconds.

(4) Place diaphragm of stethoscope over point of maximal impulse at the fifth intercostal space at the left midclavicular line and auscultate for normal S_1 and S_2 heart sounds.

(5) When S_1 and S_2 are heard with regularity, look at watch's second hand and begin to count rate.

(6) If apical rate is regular, count for 30 seconds and multiply by 2.

(7) If rate is irregular or client is receiving cardiovascular medication, count for 60 seconds.

(8) Note regularity of any dysrhythmia.

(9) Replace client's gown and bed linen; assist client to a comfortable position.

(10) Clean earpieces and diaphragm of stethoscope with alcohol swab as needed.

8. Perform hand hygiene.

9. Discuss findings with client as needed.

10. Compare readings with client's previous baseline and/or acceptable range of heart rate for client's age group.

11. Compare peripheral pulse rate with apical rate and note discrepancy.

12. Compare radial pulse equality and note discrepancy.

13. Correlate pulse rate with data obtained from blood pressure and related signs and symptoms.

STUDENT: _____ DATE: _____

INSTRUCTOR: _____ DATE: _____

Skill 27-3 Assessing Respirations

	S	U	NP	Comments
1. Determine need to assess client's respirations.	——	——	——	_____
2. Assess pertinent laboratory values.	——	——	——	_____
3. Determine previous baseline respiratory rate (if available) from client's record.	——	——	——	_____
4. Perform hand hygiene. Provide privacy.	——	——	——	_____
5. Assist client to a comfortable position, preferably sitting or lying with the head of the bed elevated 45 to 60 degrees. Be sure client's chest is visible. If necessary, move client's bed linen or gown.	——	——	——	_____
6. Place client's arm in relaxed position across the abdomen or lower chest, or place nurse's hand directly over client's upper abdomen.	——	——	——	_____
7. Observe complete respiratory cycle (one inspiration and one expiration).	——	——	——	_____
8. After cycle is observed, look at watch's second hand and begin to count rate.	——	——	——	_____
9. If rhythm is regular, count number of respirations in 30 seconds and multiply by 2. If rhythm is irregular, less than 12, or greater than 20, count respirations for 60 seconds.	——	——	——	_____
10. Note depth of respirations.	——	——	——	_____
11. Note rhythm of ventilatory cycle.	——	——	——	_____
12. Replace client's bed linen and gown.	——	——	——	_____
13. Perform hand hygiene.	——	——	——	_____
14. Discuss findings with client as needed.	——	——	——	_____
15. If respirations are being assessed for the first time, establish rate, rhythm, and depth as baseline if within normal range.	——	——	——	_____
16. Compare respirations with client's previous baseline and normal rate, rhythm, and depth.	——	——	——	_____
17. Record respiratory rate and character and any use of oxygen, and report abnormal findings.	——	——	——	_____

SKILL PERFORMANCE CHECKLIST

Skill 27-4 Measuring Oxygen Saturation (Pulse Oximetry)

	S	U	NP	Comments
1. Determine need to measure client's oxygen saturation.	——	——	——	_____
2. Assess for factors that influence measurement of SpO_2.	——	——	——	_____
3. Review client's record for prescriber's order.	——	——	——	_____
4. Determine previous baseline SpO_2 (if available) from client's record.	——	——	——	_____
5. Perform hand hygiene.	——	——	——	_____
6. Explain purpose and method of procedure to client.	——	——	——	_____
7. Assess site for sensor probe placement.	——	——	——	_____
8. Assist client to a comfortable position. If client's finger is chosen as monitoring site, support client's lower arm.	——	——	——	_____
9. Instruct client to breathe normally.	——	——	——	_____
10. Use acetone to remove any fingernail polish from digit to be assessed.	——	——	——	_____
11. Attach sensor probe to monitoring site. Tell client that clip-on probe will feel like a clothespin on the finger and will not hurt.	——	——	——	_____
12. Turn on oximeter by activating power. Observe pulse waveform/intensity display and audible beep. Correlate oximeter pulse rate with client's radial pulse.	——	——	——	_____
13. Leave probe in place until oximeter readout reaches constant value and pulse display reaches full strength during each cardiac cycle. Read SpO_2 on digital display.	——	——	——	_____
14. Verify SpO_2 alarm limits and alarm volume for continuous monitoring. Verify that alarms are on. Assess skin integrity under sensor probe and relocate sensor probe at least every 4 hours.	——	——	——	_____
15. Assist client in returning to a comfortable position.	——	——	——	_____
16. Perform hand hygiene.	——	——	——	_____
17. Discuss findings with client as needed.	——	——	——	_____
18. Remove probe and turn oximeter power off after intermittent measurements. Store probe in appropriate location.	——	——	——	_____
19. Compare SpO_2 reading with client baseline and acceptable values.	——	——	——	_____

Continued

	S	U	NP	Comments
20. Correlate SpO$_2$ reading with SaO$_2$ reading obtained from arterial blood gas measurements, if available.	___	___	___	_____
21. Correlate SpO$_2$ reading with data obtained from respiratory assessment.	___	___	___	_____

SKILL PERFORMANCE CHECKLIST
Skill 27-5 Measuring Blood Pressure

	S	U	NP	Comments
1. Determine need to assess client's blood pressure (BP).	___	___	___	_____
2. Determine best site for BP assessment.	___	___	___	_____
3. Select appropriate cuff size.	___	___	___	_____
4. Determine previous baseline BP (if available) from client's record.	___	___	___	_____
5. Encourage client to avoid exercise and smoking for 30 minutes, and ingestion of caffeine for 60 minutes, before assessment of BP.	___	___	___	_____
6. Perform hand hygiene. Assist client to sitting or lying position. Make sure room is warm, quiet, and relaxing.	___	___	___	_____
7. Explain to client that BP is to be assessed and have client rest at least 5 minutes before measurement is taken. Ask client not to speak while BP is being measured.	___	___	___	_____
8. With client sitting or lying, position client's forearm or thigh and provide support if needed.	___	___	___	_____
9. Expose extremity by removing constricting clothing.	___	___	___	_____
10. Palpate brachial artery or popliteal artery. Position cuff 2.5 cm above site of pulsation.	___	___	___	_____
11. Centre bladder of cuff above artery. With cuff fully deflated, wrap cuff evenly and snugly around extremity.	___	___	___	_____
12. To determine BP (two-step method), palpate artery distal to cuff with fingertips of one hand while inflating cuff rapidly to pressure 30 mm Hg above point at which pulse disappears. Slowly deflate cuff and note point when pulse reappears. Deflate cuff fully and wait 30 seconds.	___	___	___	_____
13. Place stethoscope earpieces in ears.	___	___	___	_____
14. Relocate brachial or popliteal artery and place bell or diaphragm chestpiece of stethoscope over it.	___	___	___	_____
15. Close valve of pressure bulb clockwise until tight. Inflate cuff to 30 mm Hg above palpated systolic pressure.	___	___	___	_____
16. Slowly release valve and allow mercury to fall at rate of 2 mm Hg/second.	___	___	___	_____

Continued

	S	U	NP	Comments
17. Note point on manometer when first clear sound is heard.	___	___	___	_____
18. Continue to deflate cuff, noting point at which muffled or dampened sound appears.	___	___	___	_____
19. Continue to deflate cuff gradually, noting point at which sound disappears in adults. Listen for 10 to 20 mm Hg after the last sound, then allow remaining air to escape quickly.	___	___	___	_____
20. Remove cuff from client's extremity unless measurement must be repeated. If this is the first assessment of the client, repeat procedure on other extremity.	___	___	___	_____
21. Assist client in returning to a comfortable position and cover upper arm if previously clothed.	___	___	___	_____
22. Perform hand hygiene.	___	___	___	_____
23. Discuss findings with client as needed.	___	___	___	_____
24. Compare reading with previous baseline and/or acceptable BP for client's age group.	___	___	___	_____
25. Compare BP in both of client's arms or legs.	___	___	___	_____
26. Correlate BP with data obtained from pulse assessment and related cardiovascular signs and symptoms.	___	___	___	_____
27. Inform client of value of and need for periodic reassessment of BP.	___	___	___	_____

STUDENT: _____ DATE: _____

INSTRUCTOR: _____ DATE: _____

Procedure 28-1 Critical Components of Indirect Percussion Techniques

	S	U	NP	Comments
1. Trim the fingernail short on the plexor finger.	___	___	___	_____
2. Place pleximeter finger (finger being struck) on the skin surface over the area to be percussed.	___	___	___	_____
3. Place pleximeter firmly.	___	___	___	_____
4. Do not move pleximeter.	___	___	___	_____
5. Limit contact of pleximeter to one small area on the skin; preferably only the distal interphalangeal joint (DIP) touches the skin surface.	___	___	___	_____
6. Strike a sharp, perpendicular blow to the DIP joint of the stationary pleximeter with the plexor finger (striking finger).	___	___	___	_____
7. Use brisk arc-like wrist action with relaxed wrist.	___	___	___	_____
8. Limit movement to wrist action, avoiding movement at elbow.	___	___	___	_____
9. Limit percussion to one or two sharp blows.	___	___	___	_____
10. Select the appropriate force of blow to achieve a clear percussion note.	___	___	___	_____
11. Use the lightest blow possible to achieve a clear percussion note.	___	___	___	_____

Adapted from *A Primer on Physical Examination Techniques* [WebCT], by D. L. Skillen, 2004a, Edmonton, AB: Faculty of Nursing, University of Alberta.

STUDENT: _____ DATE: _____

INSTRUCTOR: _____ DATE: _____

SKILL PERFORMANCE CHECKLIST
Procedure 28-2 Assessing the Face

	S	U	NP	Comments

INSPECTION: Skin, face, lips

1. Inspect skin, face, and lips. _____ _____ _____ _____

PALPATION: Temporal arteries

1. Palpate temporal arteries with fingertips or pads. _____ _____ _____ _____

Temporomandibular joint

2. Position index fingertips in front of each tragus. _____ _____ _____ _____

3. Instruct client to open and close jaw with fingertips in position. _____ _____ _____ _____

CRANIAL NERVE (CN)

1. Instruct client to clench teeth. _____ _____ _____ _____

V (trigeminal); Motor function

2. Palpate temporal and masseter muscles with fingertips or pads. _____ _____ _____ _____

3. Note strength and symmetry of contraction. _____ _____ _____ _____

Sensory function

1. Demonstrate how sharp, dull, and light touch feels before beginning tests. _____ _____ _____ _____

2. Instruct client to close eyes and indicate when touched. _____ _____ _____ _____

3. Test side to side, varying rhythm, touching ophthalmic, maxillary, and mandibular regions lightly with cotton ball. _____ _____ _____ _____

4. Repeat with splintered tongue blade. Use dull to check client's reliability at least once. _____ _____ _____ _____

5. Compare sides. _____ _____ _____ _____

CN VII (facial): Motor function

1. Instruct client to:
   A. show upper and lower teeth _____ _____ _____ _____
   B. puff out cheeks _____ _____ _____ _____
   C. smile _____ _____ _____ _____

2. Observe for symmetry. _____ _____ _____ _____

3. Instruct client to:
   A. frown _____ _____ _____ _____
   B. raise eyebrows _____ _____ _____ _____
   C. close eyes tight and resist opening by examiner _____ _____ _____ _____

Continued

	S	U	NP	Comments
4. Attempt to open client's closed eyes, exerting pressure on bony orbit, avoiding pressure on eye.	___	___	___	_____
5. Observe for symmetry and strength of motion.	___	___	___	_____

From *A Syllabus for Adult Health Assessment* (pp. 31, 34–35), edited by D. L. Skillen and R. A. Day, 2004, Edmonton, AB: Faculty of Nursing, University of Alberta.

STUDENT: _____ DATE: _____

INSTRUCTOR: _____ DATE: _____

Procedure 28-3 Inspecting the External Structures of the Eyes

	S	U	NP	Comments
INSPECTION:				
Eyebrows, lids, lashes				
1. Inspect eyebrows, lids, lashes.	___	___	___	_____
Cornea				
1. Use tangential lighting, with penlight, to inspect cornea.	___	___	___	_____
Lens, iris, pupils				
1. Inspect:				
• lens from anterior view	___	___	___	_____
• iris of each eye	___	___	___	_____
• size, shape, equality of pupils	___	___	___	_____
Sclera, conjunctiva				
1. Instruct client to look up while gently retracting lower lid to inspect sclera and conjunctiva.	___	___	___	_____
2. Instruct client to look down and side to side while gently retracting upper lid to view sclera and possibly lacrimal gland.	___	___	___	_____
Lacrimal sacs/glands				
1. Inspect lacrimal sac puncta/gland regions bilaterally.	___	___	___	_____
PUPILLARY REACTION CN II, III (optic, oculomotor)				
Test each eye separately.				
1. Instruct client to look past examiner.	___	___	___	_____
Pupillary reaction to light; direct, consensual reactions				
2. Shine a bright light from temporal region on each pupil in turn.	___	___	___	_____
3. Inspect for direct and consensual reactions.	___	___	___	_____
NEAR REACTION (accommodation)				
Test each eye separately.				
Dilatation				
1. Instruct client to look into distance with each eye.	___	___	___	_____
2. Observe pupil for dilatation.	___	___	___	_____
Constriction				
3. Instruct client to look at examiner's finger held 10 cm from client's eye.	___	___	___	_____

Continued

	S	U	NP	Comments

4. Observe for pupillary constriction while client focuses on finger. ___ ___ ___ _____

5. Repeat for other eye. ___ ___ ___ _____

CONVERGENCE CN III, IV (oculomotor, trochlear)

1. Instruct client to follow finger. ___ ___ ___ _____

Convergence

2. From directly in front of client, move finger to within 5 to 8 cm from bridge of client's nose. ___ ___ ___ _____

3. Observe convergence. ___ ___ ___ _____

CORNEAL REFLEX

Test each eye separately.

CN V, VII (trigeminal, facial)

1. Ask client if wearing contact lenses. ___ ___ ___ _____

2. Instruct client to look up and away from examiner. ___ ___ ___ _____

3. Approach from side with fine wisp of cotton. ___ ___ ___ _____

4. Touch cornea, avoiding eyelashes and sclera. ___ ___ ___ _____

Bilateral blink

5. Observe for bilateral blink. ___ ___ ___ _____

From *A Syllabus for Adult Health Assessment* (pp. 29–31), edited by D. L. Skillen and R. A. Day, 2004, Edmonton, AB: Faculty of Nursing, University of Alberta.

SKILL PERFORMANCE CHECKLIST
Procedure 28-4 Assessing Visual Fields and Extraocular Movements

	S	U	NP	Comments

VISUAL FIELDS BY CONFRONTATION

1. Position self 60 cm away from client with eyes level. ___ ___ ___ _____

CNII (optic); Visual fields

2. Instruct client to cover one eye and to look at examiner's eye directly opposite. ___ ___ ___ _____

3. Cover own eye opposite to client's covered eye. ___ ___ ___ _____

4. Instruct client to indicate when wiggling finger seen. ___ ___ ___ _____

5. Test temporal, inferotemporal, and superotemporal fields of vision by placing wiggling finger somewhat behind client and slowly moving it within client's visual field. ___ ___ ___ _____

6. Test nasal, superior, and inferior fields of vision in turn by maintaining wiggling finger equidistant between client and self. Test eight different positions for each eye. ___ ___ ___ _____

7. Slowly move wiggling finger within visual fields. ___ ___ ___ _____

8. Compare client's visual field against own. ___ ___ ___ _____

Extraocular muscles and movements

1. Inspect extraocular muscle function by performing:
   A. Cardinal directions test AND ___ ___ ___ _____
   B. Cover test OR ___ ___ ___ _____
   C. Corneal reflection test ___ ___ ___ _____

CN III, IV, VI (oculomotor, trochlear, abducens)

A. Cardinal directions (extraocular movements)
   1. Ask client if wearing contact lenses ___ ___ ___ _____
   2. Position self so client can focus. ___ ___ ___ _____
   3. Instruct client to follow finger or pen (consider age) without moving head. ___ ___ ___ _____
   4. Move finger slowly avoiding straight up and down midline position to client's (R) in line with shoulder, upward to (R) of midline, downward to (R) of midline, to client's (L) in line with shoulder, upward to (L) of midline, downward to (L) of midline. ___ ___ ___ _____

Continued

	S	U	NP	Comments

Parallel tracking, nystagmus, lid lag

    5. Avoid fixation of extreme lateral points. ____ ____ ____ _____

    6. Observe for parallel tracking (conjugate ____ ____ ____ _____
       movements), nystagmus, and lid lag.

 B. Cover test ____ ____ ____ _____

    1. Keep eyes level with those of client. ____ ____ ____ _____

    2. Instruct client to look at examiner. ____ ____ ____ _____

    3. Hold opaque cover over one eye for 5 to ____ ____ ____ _____
       10 seconds before removing it quickly,
       without warning and without touching.

    4. Observe eye that was covered. ____ ____ ____ _____

    5. Repeat with other eye. ____ ____ ____ _____

 C. Corneal reflections ____ ____ ____ _____

    1. Stand at least 0.6 m away from client. ____ ____ ____ _____

    2. Shine penlight from midline of ____ ____ ____ _____
       examiner directly onto bridge of client's
       nose; ask client to look directly at light.

    3. Observe site on each cornea from which ____ ____ ____ _____
       light is reflected.

From *A Syllabus for Adult Health Assessment* (p. 32), edited by D. L. Skillen and R. A. Day, 2004, Edmonton, AB: Faculty of Nursing, University of Alberta.

STUDENT: _____ DATE: _____

INSTRUCTOR: _____ DATE: _____

Procedure 28-5 Assessing the Internal Structures of the Eyes

	S	U	NP	Comments
FUNDUS: INSPECTION BY OPHTHALMOSCOPE				
Both eyes:				
1. Instruct client to look slightly up and over examiner's shoulder at specific point on wall.	___	___	___	_____
2. Turn lens disc of ophthalmoscope to 0 diopters.	___	___	___	_____
3. Maintain index finger on lens disc for refocusing during examination.	___	___	___	_____
4. Use (R) hand, (R) eye for client's (R) eye.	___	___	___	_____
5. Use (L) hand, (L) eye for client's (L) eye.	___	___	___	_____
6. Shine small light beam on pupil from about 40 cm away from client and 15 degrees lateral to midline.	___	___	___	_____
7. Place hand on client's forehead above eye being examined with thumb extended.	___	___	___	_____
Red reflex				
8. Observe for red reflex.	___	___	___	_____
9. Move in toward client while maintaining focus on pupil and until eyelashes almost touch.	___	___	___	_____
Disc, cups, arterioles				
10. Inspect disc, cup, arterioles, veins, crossings, adjusting lens disc if necessary.	___	___	___	_____
Veins, crossings				
11. Move head and ophthalmoscope as one unit and follow vessels peripherally in four directions.	___	___	___	_____
Macula				
12. Instruct client to briefly look directly at the light.	___	___	___	_____
13. Inspect macula and fovea.	___	___	___	_____

From *A Syllabus for Adult Health Assessment* (p. 33), edited by D.L. Skillen and R.A. Day, 2004, Edmonton, AB: Faculty of Nursing, University of Alberta.

STUDENT: _____ DATE: _____

INSTRUCTOR: _____ DATE: _____

Procedure 28-6 Inspecting and Palpating the Ears

	S	U	NP	Comments

INSPECTION: Ears fully exposed

Auricle, mastoid surface

1. Inspect auricle and mastoid bilaterally, adjusting hair where necessary for clear vision.   _____ _____ _____ _____

Alignment

1. Inspect alignment of ears from anterior and lateral views (angle of attachment, horizontal, vertical).   _____ _____ _____ _____

PALPATION:

1. Inquire about tenderness during palpation.   _____ _____ _____ _____

Mastoid surface

2. Palpate both mastoid surfaces of temporal bones with pads of fingers.   _____ _____ _____ _____

Auricle

3. Pull up on each auricle.   _____ _____ _____ _____

Tragus

4. Press on each tragus with fingertip.   _____ _____ _____ _____

From *A Syllabus for Adult Health Assessment* (p. 28), edited by D.L. Skillen and R.A. Day, 2004, Edmonton, AB: Faculty of Nursing, University of Alberta.

STUDENT: _____ DATE: _____

INSTRUCTOR: _____ DATE: _____

SKILL PERFORMANCE CHECKLIST
Procedure 28-7 Assessing Hearing Acuity

	S	U	NP	Comments
CN VIII (acoustic): Test hearing; Gross hearing; Cranial nerve VIII				
Each ear separately.				
1. Mask hearing in one ear by moving fingertip in client's auditory canal.	____	____	____	_____
2. Stand 0.3 to 0.6 m from client (ensuring that client cannot lip-read).	____	____	____	_____
3. Exhale fully and direct whisper toward ear being tested.	____	____	____	_____
4. Start with three low whispered, two-syllable, equally accented numbers or words. *Only if* client does not identify first numbers or words in low whispers, gradually increase intensity of whispering (while changing numbers or words) to spoken voice.	____	____	____	_____
Weber test				
1. Select tuning fork of 512 or 1024 Hz.	____	____	____	_____
2. Activate tuning fork using:				
A. thumb and finger OR	____	____	____	_____
B. reflex hammer OR	____	____	____	_____
C. other part of hand	____	____	____	_____
3. Hold base of vibrating tuning fork.	____	____	____	_____
4. Press end of base of vibrating tuning fork firmly on:				
A. midline of skull OR	____	____	____	_____
B. midline of forehead	____	____	____	_____
5. Ask client, "Where do you hear the sound?"	____	____	____	_____
Rinné test				
1. Select tuning fork of 512 or 1024 Hz.	____	____	____	_____
2. Activate tuning fork using:				
A. thumb and finger OR	____	____	____	_____
B. reflex hammer OR	____	____	____	_____
C. other part of hand	____	____	____	_____
3. Hold base of vibrating tuning fork and place end on mastoid surface level with ear canal.	____	____	____	_____
4. Request client to indicate when sound is no longer heard.	____	____	____	_____

Continued

	S	U	NP	Comments
5. Following client response, place vibrating tuning fork about 2.54 cm from auditory meatus of same ear with "U" facing forward (anteriorly).	____	____	____	_____
6. Ask client if sound is heard.	____	____	____	_____

From *A Syllabus for Adult Health Assessment* (pp. 28–29), edited by D.L. Skillen and R.A. Day, 2004, Edmonton, AB: Faculty of Nursing, University of Alberta.

STUDENT: _____ DATE: _____

INSTRUCTOR: _____ DATE: _____

Procedure 28-8 Otoscopy

	S	U	NP	Comments

INSPECTION BY OTOSCOPY:

Otoscopic examination (each ear, tender ear last)
1. Select largest ear speculum that fits in canal. ___ ___ ___ _____
2. Brace hand against head when holding otoscope. ___ ___ ___ _____
3. Lift auricle upward, backward, and slightly out from head *before inserting* speculum. ___ ___ ___ _____
4. Instruct client to tilt head slightly toward other shoulder. ___ ___ ___ _____
5. Insert speculum gently and not deeply. ___ ___ ___ _____

Auditory canal
6. Inspect auditory canal. ___ ___ ___ _____

Tympanic membrane, cone of light, umbo, handle of the malleus, short process
7. Inspect tympanic membrane, handle of malleus, umbo, cone of light, short process (structures and vascularity). ___ ___ ___ _____
8. Adjust position of speculum in order to visualize drum entirely. ___ ___ ___ _____
9. Remove speculum before releasing auricle. ___ ___ ___ _____

From *A Syllabus for Adult Health Assessment* (p. 29), edited by D.L. Skillen and R.A. Day, 2004, Edmonton, AB: Faculty of Nursing, University of Alberta.

SKILL PERFORMANCE CHECKLIST
Procedure 28-9 Assessing the Nose and Paranasal Sinuses

	S	U	NP	Comments

INSPECTION: Nose
1. Inspect nose from anterior view and profile.   ___ ___ ___ _____

Frontal and maxillary sinuses
2. Inspect frontal and maxillary sinus regions.   ___ ___ ___ _____

PALPATION: Nose
1. Palpate entire length of nose with finger pads.   ___ ___ ___ _____
2. Inquire of tenderness.   ___ ___ ___ _____

Frontal, maxillary sinuses
3. Palpate maxillary sinuses simultaneously by pressing upward on maxillae with thumbs and ask about tenderness.   ___ ___ ___ _____
4. Palpate frontal sinuses by pressing upward, inferior to the supraorbital ridge, from medial border of eyebrow to mideyebrow, using thumbs and ask about tenderness   ___ ___ ___ _____

Test for patency:
1. Occlude each nostril in turn.   ___ ___ ___ _____
2. Instruct client to breathe with mouth closed.   ___ ___ ___ _____
3. Listen to complete inspiration for each nostril.   ___ ___ ___ _____

Test of smell (Cranial nerve): CNI
1. Instruct client to close eyes.   ___ ___ ___ _____
2. Occlude one nostril (naris).   ___ ___ ___ _____
3. Hold pungent odour for client identification at opposite nostril. Ask client what odour is.   ___ ___ ___ _____
4. Change pungent odour and repeat on other side.   ___ ___ ___ _____

INSPECTION WITH NASAL SPECULUM:
Nose
1. Instruct to tilt head back slightly.   ___ ___ ___ _____
2. Insert nasal speculum posteriorly in horizontal plane into vestibule of nares.   ___ ___ ___ _____
3. Stabilize speculum with index finger.   ___ ___ ___ _____
4. Avoid touching septum.   ___ ___ ___ _____

Mucous membrane, septum, inferior and middle turbinates
5. Inspect mucous membrane, septum, and inferior turbinates moving speculum slowly upward.   ___ ___ ___ _____

Continued

	S	U	NP	Comments
6. Inspect middle turbinates and mucous membranes.	____	____	____	_____
7. Offer client a tissue if needed.	____	____	____	_____

From *A Syllabus for Adult Health Assessment* (pp. 33–34), edited by D.L. Skillen and R.A. Day, 2004, Edmonton, AB: Faculty of Nursing, University of Alberta.

STUDENT: _____ DATE: _____

INSTRUCTOR: _____ DATE: _____

Procedure 28-10 Assessing the Mouth and Pharynx

	S	U	NP	Comments

INSPECTION:

Mouth

1. Ask client to remove dentures. ___ ___ ___ _____

2. Instruct client to sip some water. ___ ___ ___ _____

Gums, teeth, tongue, floor of mouth uvula, palates tonsils, tonsillar pillars posterior pharynx

3. Use penlight and tongue blade to inspect: ___ ___ ___ _____
   - buccal mucosa bilaterally
   - upper and lower gums
   - upper and lower teeth
   - dorsal and ventral surfaces and sides of tongue
   - floor of mouth
   - uvula, soft and hard palates
   - tonsils, tonsillar pillars
   - posterior pharyngeal wall

4. If lesion present, palpate with gloved hand. ___ ___ ___ _____

Cranial nerve (CN) IX, X (glossopharyngeal, vagus); Motor and sensory

1. Depress tongue with tongue blade and instruct client to say "ah." ___ ___ ___ _____

2. Watch uvula and soft palate rise during "ah." ___ ___ ___ _____

Uvula, soft palate, gag reflex

3. Touch each side of posterior pharyngeal wall to elicit gag reflex (ability to swallow is tested during examination of the thyroid). ___ ___ ___ _____

CN XII (hypoglossal)

1. Observe tongue at rest on floor of mouth. ___ ___ ___ _____

Motor function

2. Instruct client to protrude tongue and observe. ___ ___ ___ _____

Symmetry and strength

3. Instruct client to
   A. wag tongue laterally ___ ___ ___ _____
   B. stick tongue into each cheek ___ ___ ___ _____

4. Palpate for strength in each cheek. ___ ___ ___ _____

From *A Syllabus for Adult Health Assessment* (pp. 35–36), edited by D.L. Skillen and R.A. Day, 2004, Edmonton, AB: Faculty of Nursing, University of Alberta.

STUDENT: _____ DATE: _____

INSTRUCTOR: _____ DATE: _____

SKILL PERFORMANCE CHECKLIST

Procedure 28-11 Assessing Neck Veins and Arteries and Range of Motion

	S	U	NP	Comments
INSPECTION: Neck fully exposed. Sitting position or supine at 30-degree angle				
Neck, carotid arteries, jugular veins				
1. Use tangential lighting on neck.	___	___	___	_____
2. Inspect neck.	___	___	___	_____
3. Inspect carotid arteries and jugular veins.	___	___	___	_____
PALPATION: Carotid arteries				
1. Palpate each carotid artery separately (at the level of the cricoid cartilage), using thumb or index and middle fingers.	___	___	___	_____
2. Assess amplitude, contour, and presence of thrills (humming vibrations).	___	___	___	_____
3. Avoid carotid sinus.	___	___	___	_____
AUSCULTATION: Carotid arteries				
1. Instruct client to hold breath while holding own breath.	___	___	___	_____
2. Use diaphragm of stethoscope to auscultate over each carotid artery.	___	___	___	_____
INSPECTION: Jugular veins: Neck and upper thorax exposed. Client in supine position with head on pillow and elevated 45 degrees.				
1. Use tangential lighting on neck.	___	___	___	_____
2. Locate external jugular first and then the internal jugular veins.	___	___	___	_____
3. Repeat on other side.	___	___	___	_____
4. Locate sternal angle (angle of Louis).	___	___	___	_____
5. Use (R) internal jugular vein to measure jugular venous pressure.	___	___	___	_____
6. Line up bottom edge of ruler with the top of the highest point of pulsations of the (R) internal jugular vein, holding it horizontal.	___	___	___	_____
7. Stand a second ruler on end on the sternal angle (angle of Louis), perpendicular to the first ruler.	___	___	___	_____
8. Measure the vertical distance between the sternal angle and the second ruler and the highest level of internal jugular vein pulsation (first ruler).	___	___	___	_____
9. Repeat on other side.	___	___	___	_____

Continued

	S	U	NP	Comments

INSPECTION: Range of motion of neck

Client in sitting or standing position.

1. Inspect range of motion of cervical vertebrae by instructing client to:

   A. touch chin to chest (flexion) ____ ____ ____ _____

   B. look up at ceiling (extension) ____ ____ ____ _____

   C. touch ear to shoulder bilaterally (lateral flexion) while examiner restricts shoulder movement ____ ____ ____ _____

   D. turn head to each side, looking over shoulder (rotation) ____ ____ ____ _____

From *A Syllabus for Adult Health Assessment* (pp. 36–37), edited by D.L. Skillen and R.A. Day, 2004, Edmonton, AB: Faculty of Nursing, University of Alberta.

SKILL PERFORMANCE CHECKLIST
Procedure 28-12 Assessing Lymph Nodes of the Neck, Trachea, and Thyroid Gland

	S	U	NP	Comments
INSPECTION: Lymph nodes				
1. Inspect area of each set of lymph nodes.	___	___	___	_____
PALPATION: Lymph nodes				
1. Palpate lymph nodes (bilaterally) using finger pads in circular (rotary) motion to move the skin over the underlying structure. May palpate simultaneously: • preauricular • postauricular • occipital • tonsillar • submaxillary • submental (braces top of head with one hand) • superficial cervical • deep cervical • posterior cervical • supraclavicular	___	___	___	_____
PALPATION: Trachea; Client sitting or supine.				
1. Locate trachea above suprasternal notch with index finger and compare spacing from sternomastoid on each side.	___	___	___	_____
INSPECTION: Cricoid cartilage and below thyroid				
1. Instruct client to extend head slightly.	___	___	___	_____
2. Direct tangential lighting from tip of chin toward thyroid region.	___	___	___	_____
3. Inspect region below cricoid cartilage at rest.	___	___	___	_____
4. Ask client to hold water in mouth.	___	___	___	_____
5. Instruct client to extend head slightly again.	___	___	___	_____
INSPECTION: Thyroid gland; Movement; Cranial nerve (CN) IX, X				
6. Inspect for isthmus and thyroid gland movement during swallowing.	___	___	___	_____
PALPATION: Thyroid				
1. From the front, palpate down midline to identify each structure.	___	___	___	_____
2. From behind, place index fingers just below cricoid cartilage on neck.	___	___	___	_____
3. Instruct client to flex head *slightly* toward the side being examined.	___	___	___	_____

Continued

	S	U	NP	Comments

4. Instruct client to swallow water while palpating for glandular tissues (isthmus and lobes) first on one side and then the other.

AUSCULTATION: Thyroid gland
1. Place bell of stethoscope lightly over thyroid lobe.
2. Ask client to hold breath while holding own breath.
3. Listen for bruit.
4. Let client breathe and then ask to hold breath again.
5. Repeat auscultation on other side.

Test motor function of CN XI (spinal accessory)
Client in sitting position.
1. Observe client shrug shoulders.
2. Instruct client to shrug shoulders which applying resistance with hands on client's shoulders.
3. Instruct client to look straight ahead.
4. Place hand on side of face, then instruct client to turn head to the same side against resistance. Observe opposite sternomastoid contraction and force against hand.
5. Repeat on other side.

From *A Syllabus for Adult Health Assessment* (pp. 36–37), edited by D.L. Skillen and R.A. Day, 2004, Edmonton, AB: Faculty of Nursing, University of Alberta.

STUDENT: _____ DATE: _____

INSTRUCTOR: _____ DATE: _____

Skip Performance Checklist

SKILL PERFORMANCE CHECKLIST

SKILL PERFORMANCE CHECKLIST
Procedure 28-13 Assessing the Spine

	S	U	NP	Comments
Spine Inspection: Client standing, loosely draped, feet together. Pants should rest just below sacroiliac joints.				
Curvatures				
1. Inspect from side (profile).	___	___	___	_____
2. Inspect from back, midline.	___	___	___	_____
Vertical alignment				
1. Inspect symmetry of shoulders, scapulae, iliac crests, sacroiliac joints, and gluteal folds.	___	___	___	_____
PALPATION:				
2. Palpate structures to confirm symmetry.	___	___	___	_____
INSPECTION: Range of motion				
1. Instruct client to touch toes (flexion).	___	___	___	_____
2. Place hand on posterior superior iliac spine, fingers pointing toward midline.	___	___	___	_____
3. Instruct client to bend backward as far as possible (extension).	___	___	___	_____
4. Place hands on client's hips.	___	___	___	_____
5. Instruct client to bend sideways as far as possible (lateral bending).	___	___	___	_____
6. Repeat on other side.	___	___	___	_____
7. Place hand on client's hip and other hand on opposite shoulder.	___	___	___	_____
8. Rotate trunk by pulling shoulder, then hip (rotation).	___	___	___	_____
9. Repeat on other side.	___	___	___	_____
Palpation: Spinous processes; Client standing.				
1. Palpate spinous processes from C1 to L5.	___	___	___	_____
2. Use finger pads or thumbs in rotary motion.	___	___	___	_____
3. Inquire about tenderness.	___	___	___	_____
4. Assess alignment by running two fingers down spine C1 to L5.	___	___	___	_____
Paravertebral muscles				
1. Palpate paravertebral muscles bilaterally from level of C1 to L5.	___	___	___	_____
2. Use finger pads or thumbs.	___	___	___	_____
3. Inquire about tenderness.	___	___	___	_____

From *A Syllabus for Adult Health Assessment* (p. 38), edited by D.L. Skillen and R.A. Day, 2004, Edmonton, AB: Faculty of Nursing, University of Alberta.

STUDENT: _____ DATE: _____

INSTRUCTOR: _____ DATE: _____

Procedure 28-14 Examination of the Posterior Thorax and Lungs

	S	U	NP	Comments

Thorax Inspection: Anteroposterior/Lateral (AP/lateral); Posterior lung fields; Client sitting disrobed to waist.

1. Inspect from side (profile). ____ ____ ____ _____
2. Inspect posterior thorax from midline. ____ ____ ____ _____

Palpation: Chest Expansion

1. Place thumbs at level of and parallel to 10th ribs. ____ ____ ____ _____
2. Wrap hands loosely around lateral rib cage. ____ ____ ____ _____
3. Slide hands medially to raise skin folds between thumb and spine. ____ ____ ____ _____
4. Instruct client to inhale deeply and exhale. ____ ____ ____ _____
5. Compare sides. ____ ____ ____ _____

Tactile fremitus

1. Instruct client to round shoulders with arms folded across chest, hands on shoulders. ____ ____ ____ _____
2. Palpate and compare symmetrical areas: ____ ____ ____ _____
   - Upper (apices and interscapular)
   - Lower
   - Lateral (in midaxillary line)
3. Ask client to repeat "99" OR words (blue moon) in a deep voice. ____ ____ ____ _____
4. Use ball of hand (palm at base of fingers) OR ulnar aspect of hand. ____ ____ ____ _____
5. Use one OR two hands to assess fremitus in symmetrical areas (upper, lower, and lateral). ____ ____ ____ _____

Percussion: Posterior chest

1. Instruct client to continue rounding shoulders. ____ ____ ____ _____
2. Percuss and compare symmetrical areas at 5-cm intervals over: ____ ____ ____ _____
   - upper (apices and interscapular)
   - lower
   - lateral (in midaxillary line)
3. Press distal phalanx and joint of middle (pleximeter) finger firmly over intercostals space (avoiding contact with other fingers). ____ ____ ____ _____
4. Aim at distal phalanx or interphalangeal joint. ____ ____ ____ _____
5. Strike pleximeter a sharp perpendicular blow with tip of middle (plexor) finger (may support plexor finger with thumb). ____ ____ ____ _____
6. Use wrist action only. ____ ____ ____ _____

Continued

	S	U	NP	Comments

Auscultation: Posterior lung fields

1. Instruct client to continue rounding shoulders.   ____ ____ ____ _____
2. Auscultate with diaphragm of stethoscope.   ____ ____ ____ _____
3. Instruct client to breathe through open mouth, more deeply than usual, and inform if dizzy.   ____ ____ ____ _____
4. Listen to at least ONE full breath in each area.   ____ ____ ____ _____
5. Listen to and compare symmetrical areas: ____ ____ ____ _____
   - upper (apices and interscapular)
   - lower
   - lateral (in midaxillary line)

From *A Syllabus for Adult Health Assessment* (pp. 39–40), edited by D.L. Skillen and R.A. Day, 2004, Edmonton, AB: Faculty of Nursing, University of Alberta.

STUDENT: _____ DATE: _____
INSTRUCTOR: _____ DATE: _____

Procedure 28-15 Assessing the Heart

	S	U	NP	Comments

INSPECTION: Client in supine position with head elevated 30 degrees, anterior thorax and epigastric area exposed, examiner at client's right side   ____ ____ ____ _____

Precordium
1. Inspect precordium tangentially using penlight.   ____ ____ ____ _____

PALPATION:
1. Landmark using sternal angle.   ____ ____ ____ _____
2. Palpate, proceeding from the apex to the base OR the base to the apex.   ____ ____ ____ _____

Apical area
1. Use finger pads to palpate 5th interspace medial to (L) MCL.   ____ ____ ____ _____
2. Ask client to exhale and hold if unable to locate apical area in 1 above.   ____ ____ ____ _____
3. Analyze impulses in apical area using fingertips, then one finger.   ____ ____ ____ _____

Right ventricular area
1. Place tips of curved fingers in (L) 3rd, 4th, and 5th interspaces close to sternum.   ____ ____ ____ _____
2. Ask client to exhale and hold breath.   ____ ____ ____ _____

Epigastric area (subxiphoid)
1. Press index finger of flattened hand under (L) costal margin and up toward left shoulder.   ____ ____ ____ _____
2. Ask client to inhale and hold.   ____ ____ ____ _____

Left 2nd interspace (pulmonic area)
1. Place index finger pad in 2nd (L) interspace.   ____ ____ ____ _____
2. Ask client to exhale and hold breath, palpate firmly.   ____ ____ ____ _____

Right 2nd interspace (aortic area)
1. Place index finger pad in 2nd (R) interspace.   ____ ____ ____ _____
2. Ask client to exhale and hold breath, palpate firmly.   ____ ____ ____ _____

Auscultation:
1. Use diaphragm and bell to listen to all six areas.   ____ ____ ____ _____
2. Apply bell lightly to the chest wall.   ____ ____ ____ _____
3. Auscultate proceeding from apex to base OR base to apex.   ____ ____ ____ _____

Continued

	S	U	NP	Comments

4. Listen for 5 seconds in each area with diaphragm and bell.

Right 2nd interspace; Left 2nd, 3rd, 4th, 5th interspace; Apex; Apical rate

5. Auscultate:
   - right 2nd interspace close to sternum
   - left 2nd interspace close to sternum
   - left 3rd interspace close to sternum
   - left 4th interspace close to sternum
   - left 5th interspace close to sternum
   - apex

6. Listen for 1 minute at apex for rate, using diaphragm.

STUDENT: _____ DATE: _____

INSTRUCTOR: _____ DATE: _____

Procedure 28-16 Assessing Breasts and Axillae

	S	U	NP	Comments

Inspection: Breast, areola, nipple; Client in sitting position, disrobed to waist.

1. Inspect breast, areola, and nipple bilaterally from anterior and lateral view: ___ ___ ___ _____
   - with arms at side
   - with arms raised over head
   - with hands pressed against hips OR with hands pressed together, not obstructing view of breasts.
2. Inspect with client leaning forward, and then with breasts lifted. ___ ___ ___ _____

Palpation: Large breasts

1. With the client leaning forward, palpate breast tissue between the examiner's hands. ___ ___ ___ _____

Inspection: Axillae

1. Inspect skin of axillae with arms raised over head. ___ ___ ___ _____
2. *Only* if signs of infection, put on gloves for palpation. ___ ___ ___ _____

Palpation:

Axillary lymph nodes

1. Assist client to dry axillae. ___ ___ ___ _____
2. Support client's (L) hand and wrist with examiner's (L) hand to examine (L) axilla and reverses for (R) axilla. ___ ___ ___ _____
3. Instruct client to relax arm. ___ ___ ___ _____

Central lymph nodes

4. Cup fingers together. ___ ___ ___ _____
5. Reach as high as possible into apex of (L) axilla. ___ ___ ___ _____
6. Press fingers against chest wall. ___ ___ ___ _____
7. Bring finger pads down over ribs and feel for central nodes ___ ___ ___ _____

Pectoral lymph nodes

8. Slide fingers under anterior axillary fold, palpating chest wall with finger pads for pectoral nodes. ___ ___ ___ _____
9. Grasp anterior axillary folds (pectoral) and palpate with finger pads, using thumbs as anchor. ___ ___ ___ _____

Continued

	S	U	NP	Comments

10. Slide fingers under posterior axillary fold, palpating chest wall with finger pads for subscapular nodes.

Subscapular lymph nodes
11. Turn hands and feels inside posterior axillary folds with finger pads (subscapular)

Lateral lymph nodes
12. Feel along upper humerus with finger pads (lateral).
13. Repeat on (R) side.

Palpation: Infraclavicular lymph nodes
1. Palpate bilaterally for infraclavicular nodes below clavicle in 1st interspace with finger pads.

Palpation: Supraclavicular lymph nodes
1. Palpate bilaterally for supraclavicular nodes above clavicle with finger pads.

Inspection: Breast, areola, nipple; Client supine, with pillow removed from under head. Uses small pillow under client's shoulder on side examined *only if breasts are large.*
1. Inspect breasts bilaterally.

Palpation: Breast, areola, nipple, and tail of Spence; Ask client to move arm away from chest on side being examined.
1. Palpate each breast.
2. Use flat of 2nd, 3rd, and 4th fingers in a rotary motion to compress breast tissue.
3. Flex from the wrist, not the fingers.
4. Apply moderate pressure, keeping constant contact with skin.
5. Move back and forth across breast in straight lines, making constant small circles.
6. Slide hand down one finger width for each pass.
7. Cover full area from below clavicle to 3 cm below breast, from mid-axillary line to mid-sternal line:
   • glandular tissue
   • areolar area
   • nipple
   • tail of Spence

From *A Syllabus for Adult Health Assessment* (pp. 43–44), edited by D.L. Skillen and R.A. Day, 2004, Edmonton, AB: Faculty of Nursing, University of Alberta.

STUDENT: _____ DATE: _____

INSTRUCTOR: _____ DATE: _____

Procedure 28-17 Inspecting the Abdomen

	S	U	NP	Comments
Inspection: Abdomen; Abdomen fully exposed, bladder empty, draped; client with arms at sides OR folded across chest.				
1. Inspect tangentially from "R" side and from foot of table.	___	___	___	_____
2. Inspect across abdomen.	___	___	___	_____
3. Ask client to inhale deeply and hold breath.	___	___	___	_____
4. Inspect for symmetry.	___	___	___	_____

From *A Syllabus for Adult Health Assessment* (p. 45), edited by D.L. Skillen and R.A. Day, 2004, Edmonton, AB: Faculty of Nursing, University of Alberta.

STUDENT: _____ DATE: _____

INSTRUCTOR: _____ DATE: _____

Procedure 28-18 Auscultating the Abdomen

	S	U	NP	Comments
Auscultation: Bowel sounds				
1. Inquire about abdominal tenderness and ask to indicate area.	___	___	___	_____
2. Auscultate prior to percussion and palpation.	___	___	___	_____
3. Place diaphragm gently.	___	___	___	_____
4. Listen in all four quadrants.	___	___	___	_____
Auscultation:				
1. Press diaphragm **gently** against abdomen.	___	___	___	_____
Aorta				
2. Listen slightly "L" of midline in epigastric region (aorta).	___	___	___	_____
Renal arteries				
3. Listen to "L" and "R" of midline just superior to umbilicus (renal).	___	___	___	_____
Iliac arteries				
4. Listen just above inguinal ligament midway between anterior superior iliac spine and symphysis pubis (iliac).	___	___	___	_____

From *A Syllabus for Adult Health Assessment* (p. 45), edited by D.L. Skillen and R.A. Day, 2004, Edmonton, AB: Faculty of Nursing, University of Alberta.

STUDENT: _____ DATE: _____

INSTRUCTOR: _____ DATE: _____

SKILL PERFORMANCE CHECKLIST
Procedure 28-19 Percussing the Abdomen

	S	U	NP	Comments

Percussion: Abdomen

1. Place distal phalanx and joint of middle (pleximeter) finger on abdominal wall (avoiding contact with other fingers). | ____ | ____ | ____ | _____
2. Aim at distal phalanx or interphalangeal joint. | ____ | ____ | ____ | _____
3. Strike pleximeter a sharp, light blow with tip of middle (plexor) finger. | ____ | ____ | ____ | _____
4. Percuss lightly over entire abdomen. | ____ | ____ | ____ | _____
5. Inquire about areas of tenderness. | ____ | ____ | ____ | _____
6. Observe client's facial reactions during percussion. | ____ | ____ | ____ | _____

Percussion: Liver

1. Percuss in right midclavicular line from lung resonance to liver dullness (upper border); mark level. | ____ | ____ | ____ | _____
2. Start at level below umbilicus in right midclavicular line and percuss upward to liver dullness (lower border); mark level. | ____ | ____ | | _____
3. Measure vertical span of liver dullness in centimetres. | ____ | ____ | ____ | _____
4. Request client to inhale deeply. | ____ | ____ | ____ | _____
5. Percuss upward toward lower border. | ____ | ____ | ____ | _____

Splenic percussion sign

1. Percuss lowest interspace in left anterior axillary line. | ____ | ____ | ____ | _____
2. Instruct client to take a deep breath, and repeat percussion in lowest interspace of left anterior axillary line. | ____ | ____ | ____ | _____
3. Note any change in percussion. | ____ | ____ | ____ | _____

Percussion: Bladder; Percuss downward in midline from umbilicus to the pelvic brim.

Percussion: Kidney; Client sitting or standing. Inform client of procedure.

1. Inquire about kidney tenderness. | ____ | ____ | ____ | _____
2. If tender, press in each costovertebral angle in turn with fingertips. | ____ | ____ | ____ | _____
3. Inquire about tenderness. | ____ | ____ | ____ | _____
4. If not tender, place palm (fingers not touching client) of non-dominate hand over each costovertebral angle in turn. | ____ | ____ | ____ | _____

Continued

	S	U	NP	Comments
5. Strike dorsum of hand with ulnar surface of fist.	____	____	____	_____
6. Inquire about tenderness.	____	____	____	_____

From *A Syllabus for Adult Health Assessment* (pp. 38–39, 45–46), edited by D.L. Skillen and R.A. Day, 2004, Edmonton, AB: Faculty of Nursing, University of Alberta.

SKILL PERFORMANCE CHECKLIST
Procedure 28-20 Palpating the Abdomen

	S	U	NP	Comments
PALPATION				
1. Use flat of four fingers held together, in a light dipping motion.	___	___	___	_____
Light abdominal palpation				
2. Palpate over entire abdomen, more than once in each of four quadrants.	___	___	___	_____
3. Inquire about tenderness.	___	___	___	_____
Deep abdominal palpation				
1. Palpate deeply after light palpation.	___	___	___	_____
2. Palpate over entire abdomen, more than once in each quadrant. Use flat of four fingers of one hand OR use two hands, one placed on top of the other and pressure exerted with top hand.	___	___	___	_____
3. Inquire about tenderness.	___	___	___	_____
4. Observe client's facial reactions during palpation.	___	___	___	_____
Palpation: Liver				
1. Place (L) hand behind client parallel to and supporting 11th and 12th ribs and soft tissue below.	___	___	___	_____
2. Press (L) hand forward while client relaxes.	___	___	___	_____
3. Place (R) hand on client's abdomen:	___	___	___	_____
• below lower border of liver dullness percussed upon deep inspiration				
• lateral to rectus muscle with hand held parallel or obliquely to midline of body OR parallel to costal margin.				
4. Palpate deeply with flat of four fingers.	___	___	___	_____
5. Instruct client to take a deep breath and try to feel liver edge as it comes down to meet fingertips OR lateral edge of index finger.	___	___	___	_____
6. If liver not palpable,	___	___	___	_____
• inch hand closer to (R) costal margin and repeat procedure				
• exert more pressure inward upon expiration and repeat procedure				
PALPATION: Inguina nodes; horizontal				
1. Palpate inferior to inguinal ligament from symphysis pubis to anterior superior iliac spine.	___	___	___	_____

Continued

	S	U	NP	Comments

Palpation: Inguinal nodes; vertical

2. Palpate medial to femoral canal from superior ramus to an area 5 cm distally.   ____ ____ ____ _____

From *A Syllabus for Adult Health Assessment* (p. 46), edited by D.L. Skillen and R.A. Day, 2004, Edmonton, AB: Faculty of Nursing, University of Alberta.

SKILL PERFORMANCE CHECKLIST
Procedure 28-21 Assessing the External Female Genitalia

	S	U	NP	Comments
Client in lithotomy position, with feet in stirrups, draped with pubis and genitalia exposed, nurse gloved, and light coming over nurse's shoulder.				

Inspection: Pubic hair

	S	U	NP	Comments
1. Inspect hair, hair distribution and skin of pubis.	____	____	____	_____

Inspection: Labia majora

	S	U	NP	Comments
1. Inspect labia majora.	____	____	____	_____
2. Use thumb and index finger of non-dominant hand inside labia minora to gently but firmly retract tissues forward.	____	____	____	_____
3. Inspect labia minora.	____	____	____	_____

Palpation: Labia minora

	S	U	NP	Comments
1. With other hand, palpate labia minora between thumb and index finger on one side.	____	____	____	_____
2. Repeat on other side.	____	____	____	_____

Inspection: Clitoris

	S	U	NP	Comments
1. Inspect clitoris.	____	____	____	_____

Inspection: Urethral meatus

	S	U	NP	Comments
1. Locate urethral meatus above vaginal canal.	____	____	____	_____
2. Inspect meatus.	____	____	____	_____

Inspection: Vaginal orifice (introitus)

	S	U	NP	Comments
1. With the labia minora still retracted, inspect the introitus.	____	____	____	_____
2. With the labia minora still retracted, and using the dominant hand, first dip the index finger into a basin of warm water for lubrication.	____	____	____	_____
3. With the palm facing upward, insert index finger into the vagina as far as the proximal interphalangeal joint (second finger joint).	____	____	____	_____

Palpation: Skene's glands

	S	U	NP	Comments
4. Exert upward pressure by moving fingers outward (milking action) on either side of urethra and directly over the urethra.	____	____	____	_____
5. Inquire about tenderness.	____	____	____	_____
6. Culture any discharge.	____	____	____	_____
7. Remove retracting hand.	____	____	____	_____

Continued

		S	U	NP	Comments

8. Insert index finger into posterior vaginal opening toward the (L) side and palpate the posterior labia majora between the index finger and the thumb.

9. Repeat on other side.

10. Culture any discharge.

11. Change gloves.

Palpation: Bartholin's glands, Perineum, vaginal orifice

1. Insert first two fingers into vagina and instruct client to squeeze examiner's fingers.

2. Instruct client to strain downward as if voiding. Determine if any structures touch examining fingers.

3. Remove fingers from vagina and use first two fingers of both hands to separate the vaginal orifice.

4. Instruct client to bear down.

5. Inspect vaginal orifice.

Inspection: Anus
See Procedure 28-24, "Inspecting the Anus, Rectum, and Prostate"

From "Female External and Internal Genital Examination," by R.A. Day, 2004a, in *A Syllabus for Adult Health Assessment* (pp. 92–95), edited by D.L. Skillen and R.A. Day, 2004, Edmonton, AB: Faculty of Nursing, University of Alberta.

STUDENT: _____ DATE: _____
INSTRUCTOR: _____ DATE: _____

Procedure 28-22 Assessing the Internal Female Genitalia

	S	U	NP	Comments

Client continues in lithotomy position, with feet in stirrups, draped with pubis and genitalia exposed, nurse newly gloved, in a sitting position and with light coming over nurse's shoulder.

Inspection: Cervix

	S	U	NP	Comments
1. Select appropriate size speculum and lubricate with warm water.	___	___	___	_____
2. Hold speculum in dominant hand, with blades closed.	___	___	___	_____
3. Insert first two fingers of non-dominant hand into vagina and press downward.	___	___	___	_____
4. Insert speculum obliquely.	___	___	___	_____
5. Instruct client to bear down.	___	___	___	_____
6. When the speculum has passed the inserted fingers, continue to insert downward toward the table at a 45-degree angle.	___	___	___	_____
7. Rotate speculum blades to horizontal position.	___	___	___	_____
8. After full insertion, open blades slowly and move to visualize cervix.	___	___	___	_____
9. Lock blades in open position.	___	___	___	_____

Papanicolaou (Pap) smear

	S	U	NP	Comments
1. Inspect cervix and os. If blood is visible, delay taking specimens.	___	___	___	_____
2. Use a spatula or cotton-tipped applicator rotated 360 degrees against the surface of the cervix (endocervix).	___	___	___	_____
3. Remove and gently spread specimen on glass slide.	___	___	___	_____
4. Spray specimen with cytological fixative immediately and label.	___	___	___	_____

Other specimens

	S	U	NP	Comments
5. Use cotton-tipped applicator or cytobrush to collect a specimen from inside the cervical os (endocervix). (Rotate one or two full turns).	___	___	___	_____
6. Spread specimen gently on glass slide.	___	___	___	_____
7. Spray specimen with cytological fixative immediately and label. If unusual vaginal discharge is present, collect specimens for culture and test specifically for sexually transmitted infections.	___	___	___	_____
8. Inspect walls of vagina while slowly withdrawing speculum.	___	___	___	_____

Continued

	S	U	NP	Comments

9. After passing the cervix, loosen thumbscrew on speculum but keep blades open with thumb. _____ _____ _____ _____

10. As speculum approaches the vaginal opening, close blades carefully. _____ _____ _____ _____

11. Turn blades obliquely and remove speculum. _____ _____ _____ _____

Bimanual exam: Examiner in standing position.

Vagina

1. Make the 'obstetric' position with the first two fingers extended, the last two flexed into palm and the thumb abducted _____ _____ _____ _____

2. Use water-based lubricant on first two fingers of dominant hand. _____ _____ _____ _____

3. Insert fingers into vagina and again press downward. _____ _____ _____ _____

4. Allow time for walls of vagina to relax, then insert fingers completely. _____ _____ _____ _____

5. Palpate vaginal walls in all directions. _____ _____ _____ _____

Cervix

1. Palpate cervix. _____ _____ _____ _____

2. Place fingers on either side of cervix and move it gently from side to side. _____ _____ _____ _____

Uterus

Place other hand on abdomen, halfway between the umbilicus and symphysis pubis. Press down firmly to push the pelvic organs closer to the examining fingers.

1. Palpate to determine position. _____ _____ _____ _____

2. Palpate walls of uterus with fingers in fornices. _____ _____ _____ _____

3. Move the uterus carefully between abdominal hand and intravaginal hand. _____ _____ _____ _____

4. Attempt to feel the ovaries between the abdominal hand and the intravaginal hand. _____ _____ _____ _____

Other manoeuvres

1. In the rectovaginal examination, insert one finger into the vagina and one into the rectum and repeat from 1 (obstetric position) above. _____ _____ _____ _____

2. If stool is present when removing gloved finger, test for occult (hidden) blood. _____ _____ _____ _____

Completion of examination

1. Provide client with tissues to clean areas examined. _____ _____ _____ _____

2. Assist client to move upward on examining table. _____ _____ _____ _____

3. Assist client to sit up. _____ _____ _____ _____

From "Female External and Internal Genital Examination," by R.A. Day, 2004a, in *A Syllabus for Adult Health Assessment* (pp. 92–95), edited by D.L. Skillen and R.A. Day, 2004, Edmonton, AB: Faculty of Nursing, University of Alberta.

SKILL PERFORMANCE CHECKLIST
Procedure 28-23 Assessing the Male Genitalia and Inguinal Regions

	S	U	NP	Comments
Inspection: Client standing or supine, pubis and genitalia exposed, nurse gloved.				
Pubic hair				
1. Inspect hair and skin of pubis.	___	___	___	_____
Penis				
1. Inspect shaft of penis.	___	___	___	_____
Skin, prepuce, glans, corona, urethral meatus				
2. Ask client to retract prepuce (foreskin) if present.	___	___	___	_____
3. Inspect glans and corona.	___	___	___	_____
4. Inspect location of meatus.	___	___	___	_____
5. Compress glans gently.	___	___	___	_____
6. Inspect meatus.	___	___	___	_____
7. Replace prepuce if retracted.	___	___	___	_____
Palpation: Shaft				
1. Palpate shaft between thumb and first two fingers.	___	___	___	_____
2. Inquire about tenderness.	___	___	___	_____
Inspection: Scrotum				
1. Inspect anterior and lateral surfaces.	___	___	___	_____
2. Lift scrotum gently to inspect posterior surface.	___	___	___	_____
Palpation:				
1. Use thumb and first two fingers of examining hand.	___	___	___	_____
2. Palpate one side in sequence:				
A. testis	___	___	___	_____
B. epididymis	___	___	___	_____
C. spermatic cord (and vas deferens)	___	___	___	_____
3. Repeat on other side.	___	___	___	_____
Inspection: Client standing.				
Inguinal region; Pubic tubercle to anterior superior iliac spine (inguinal canal)				
1. Inspect (L) (R) inguinal regions.	___	___	___	_____
2. Instruct client to strain or bear down.	___	___	___	_____
3. Inspect regions using tangential lighting.	___	___	___	_____
4. Compare regions.	___	___	___	_____
Femoral canal				
1. Inspect (L) (R) femoral regions.	___	___	___	_____
2. Use tangential lighting.	___	___	___	_____

Continued

	S	U	NP	Comments

Palpation:

3. Instruct client to cough or strain down (R) (L). _____ _____ _____ _____
4. Use tangential lighting. _____ _____ _____ _____
5. Compare regions. _____ _____ _____ _____

Inguinal ring, inguinal canal

Client remains standing.

1. Stand on (R) side of client. _____ _____ _____ _____
2. Place index finger of (R) hand against scrotal skin on (R) side. _____ _____ _____ _____
3. Place finger low on scrotum. _____ _____ _____ _____
4. Move finger toward inguinal ring by invaginating scrotal skin over finger. _____ _____ _____ _____
5. Assess possibility of passage through inguinal ring. _____ _____ _____ _____
6. Insert index finger superiorly and obliquely along vas deferens into inguinal canal, following spermatic cord. _____ _____ _____ _____
7. When index finger can not move further, instruct client to cough and strain down. _____ _____ _____ _____
8. Assess for bulging pressure against finger. _____ _____ _____ _____
9. Observe relationship to pubic tubercle. _____ _____ _____ _____
10. Repeat on (L) side with (L) index finger. _____ _____ _____ _____

Femoral canal

1. Place finger pads on anterior thigh in region of femoral canal. _____ _____ _____ _____
2. Instruct client to cough and strain down. _____ _____ _____ _____
3. Assess for bulge or impulse against fingers. _____ _____ _____ _____
4. Observe relationship to pubic tubercle. _____ _____ _____ _____
5. Repeat on opposite thigh. _____ _____ _____ _____

Inguinal lymph nodes

See Procedure 28-20

From "Male Genitalia Examination," by D.L. Skillen, in *A Syllabus for Adult Health Assessment* (pp. 89–90), edited by D.L. Skillen and R.A. Day, 2004b, Edmonton, AB: Faculty of Nursing, University of Alberta.

STUDENT: _____   DATE: _____

INSTRUCTOR: _____   DATE: _____

SKILL PERFORMANCE CHECKLIST
Procedure 28-24 Assessing the Anus, Rectum, Prostate, and Cervix

	S	U	NP	Comments

Inspection: Client forward bending or in Sims' position

Palpation: Anus: Anal area exposed. Nurse gloved.
1. Spread buttocks apart. ____ ____ ____ _____
2. Inspect perianal and sacrococcygeal regions. ____ ____ ____ _____
3. Lubricate index finger of dominant hand by dropping lubricant onto gloved finger. ____ ____ ____ _____
4. Place finger pad across anus. ____ ____ ____ _____
5. Instruct client to bear down. ____ ____ ____ _____
6. Assess tone of anal sphincter. ____ ____ ____ _____

Palpation: Rectum
1. Flex fingertip and insert gently into anal canal. ____ ____ ____ _____
2. Insert finger in direction of umbilicus. ____ ____ ____ _____

Palpation: Prostate (male)
1. Turn the hand to position finger for assessing all rectal surfaces. ____ ____ ____ _____
2. Instruct client to bear down. ____ ____ ____ _____
3. Reposition hand so that finger palpates anterior rectal surface. ____ ____ ____ _____
4. Locate median groove (sulcus) of prostate gland. ____ ____ ____ _____
5. Sweep index finger across prostate lobe from superior to inferior surface. ____ ____ ____ _____
6. Repeat on other lobe beginning at superior surface. ____ ____ ____ _____
7. Withdraw finger. ____ ____ ____ _____
8. Examine colour of material on glove. ____ ____ ____ _____
9. Make smear to test for occult blood. ____ ____ ____ _____
10. Offer client tissues. ____ ____ ____ _____

Palpation: Cervix (female)
1. Reposition hand so that finger palpates anterior rectal surface. ____ ____ ____ _____
2. Locate rounded protrusion of cervix. ____ ____ ____ _____
3. Sweep index finger across protrusion. ____ ____ ____ _____
4. Withdraw finger. ____ ____ ____ _____
5. Examine colour of material on glove. ____ ____ ____ _____

Continued

	S	U	NP	Comments
6. Make smear to test for occult blood.	___	___	___	_____
7. Offer client tissues.	___	___	___	_____

Adapted from "Anus, Rectum, and Prostate Examination," by D.L. Skillen, in *A Syllabus for Adult Health Assessment* (p. 96), edited by D.L. Skillen and R.A. Day, 2004, Edmonton, AB: Faculty of Nursing, University of Alberta.

SKILL PERFORMANCE CHECKLIST

Procedure 28-25 Inspecting the Upper Extremities

	S	U	NP	Comments

Skin, nails, hair, symmetry

1. Fully expose the hands and arms of the seated or supine client.
2. Inspect skin, nails, and symmetry of both arms and hands.

Range of motion (ROM)
The examiner inspects the ROM. Each arm is tested, either separately or simultaneously, and compared. Only if the client is unable to perform active ROM does the examiner attempt passive ROM.

Thumbs

1. Instruct client to supinate hands and
2. Touch base of 5th finger with thumb (flexion).
3. Move thumb back and forth away from fingers (extension).
4. Move thumb anteriorly away from palm (abduction).
5. Move thumb back down (adduction).
6. Touch tip of thumb to each fingertip (opposition).

Fingers

1. Instruct client to make a fist (flexion), thumb across knuckles.
2. Straighten fingers (extension).
3. Spread extended fingers (abduction).
4. Close extended fingers together (adduction).

Wrists

1. Instruct client to flex wrist and
2. Extend wrist.
3. Stabilize client's forearm and hand in supination and instruct client to
4. Move hand medially (ulnar deviation).
5. Move hand laterally (radial deviation).

Elbows

1. Instruct client to bend elbows (flexion) and
2. Straighten elbows (extension).
3. Instruct client to hold flexed elbows close to sides and turn palms upward (supination), and
4. Turn palms downward (pronation).

Continued

	S	U	NP	Comments

Shoulders

1. Instruct client to extend arms forward (flexion), and   ___ ___ ___ _____

2. Extend straightened arms as far back as possible (extension).   ___ ___ ___ _____

3. Instruct client to bring straightened arms across anterior midline (adduction).   ___ ___ ___ _____

4. Instruct client to lift arms laterally in an arc starting from sides and ending with both arms extended above head, palms facing (abduction).   ___ ___ ___ _____

5. Instruct client to place hands behind own neck (external rotation), and   ___ ___ ___ _____

6. Place hands behind small of back (internal rotation).   ___ ___ ___ _____

From *A Syllabus for Adult Health Assessment* (pp. 47–48), edited by D.L. Skillen and R.A. Day, 2004, Edmonton, AB: Faculty of Nursing, University of Alberta.

SKILL PERFORMANCE CHECKLIST

Procedure 28-26 Palpating Temperature and Joints of the Upper Extremities

	S	U	NP	Comments

Palpation: Temperature

1. Use dorsum of hands or fingers to compare temperature of each hand with forearm and upper arm above it.
2. Compare sides.

Palpation: Joints: Examiner instructs the client to indicate if there is any tenderness during joint palpation. Both limbs are palpated separately and compared.

Fingers: Interphalangeal (IP) joints

1. Palpate with thumb and index finger of one hand all of the distal and proximal IP joints of fingers and thumb of both hands at the medial and lateral aspects of each joint.

Fingers: Metacarpophalangeal (MCP) joints

1. Palpate with thumbs of both hands the MCP joints of both hands just distal to and on each side of the knuckle.

Wrists

1. Palpate medial and lateral surfaces of each wrist (distal radius and ulna).
2. Palpate each wrist with thumbs dorsally and fingers ventrally.

Elbows

1. Support the left slightly flexed arm with the left hand and forearm.
2. Palpate
   A. The olecranon process
   B. The groove on either side of the olecranon process
   C. The lateral and medial epicondyles.
3. Inquire about tenderness.
4. Repeat on the right side.

Shoulders

1. Cup a hand over each of the client's exposed shoulders and
2. Feel for crepitus during adduction, abduction, external and internal rotation.
3. Palpate the sternoclavicular (SC) joint.
4. Palpate the acromioclavicular (AC) joint.

Continued

	S	U	NP	Comments
5. Palpate the biceps groove for long head of biceps tendon.	____	____	____	_____
6. Inquire about tenderness during 3, 4, 5 above.	____	____	____	_____

From *A Syllabus for Adult Health Assessment,* edited by D.L. Skillen and R.A. Day, 2004, Edmonton, AB: Faculty of Nursing, University of Alberta.

STUDENT: _____   DATE: _____

INSTRUCTOR: _____   DATE: _____

Procedure 28-27 Assessing Muscle Tone and Strength of Upper Extremities

	S	U	NP	Comments

Palpation: Muscle tone
1. Support the relaxed arm at the hand and elbow.   ____ ____ ____ _____
2. Move each arm (fingers, wrist, elbow, shoulder) through a modified passive range of motion (ROM).   ____ ____ ____ _____
3. Attend to the resistance offered.   ____ ____ ____ _____
4. Test muscle tone prior to testing muscle strength.   ____ ____ ____ _____

Muscle strength: Fingers
1. Place two crossed fingers in each hand of client.   ____ ____ ____ _____
2. Instruct client to squeeze firmly (grip).   ____ ____ ____ _____
3. Compare sides; may test simultaneously.   ____ ____ ____ _____
4. Try, against resistance, to force client's outspread fingers of each hand together (abduction).   ____ ____ ____ _____
5. Instruct client to touch thumb to little fingertip.   ____ ____ ____ _____
6. Resist pull of examiner's thumb against client's thumb (opposition).   ____ ____ ____ _____
7. Compare sides; may test simultaneously.   ____ ____ ____ _____

Muscle strength: Wrists
1. Instruct client to hold flexed elbows close to sides with forearm in pronation.   ____ ____ ____ _____
2. Instruct client to make a fist and flex wrists.   ____ ____ ____ _____
3. Try to pull client's fist up against resistance (flexion).   ____ ____ ____ _____
4. Instruct client to make a fist and extend wrist.   ____ ____ ____ _____
5. Try to pull client's fist down against resistance (extension).   ____ ____ ____ _____
6. Compare sides; may test simultaneously.   ____ ____ ____ _____

Muscle Strength: Elbows
1. Instruct client to flex arm at the elbow.   ____ ____ ____ _____
2. Try, against resistance, to extend client's flexed elbows (biceps).   ____ ____ ____ _____
3. Instruct client to flex arm at the elbow.   ____ ____ ____ _____
4. Try, against resistance, to further flex client's elbows (triceps).   ____ ____ ____ _____
5. Compare sides; may test simultaneously.   ____ ____ ____ _____

Continued

	S	U	NP	Comments
Muscle Strength: Shoulders				
1. Instruct client to raise both extended arms above the head.	____	____	____	_____
2. Try, against resistance, to force client's arms to sides.	____	____	____	_____
3. Compare sides; may test simultaneously.	____	____	____	_____

From *A Syllabus for Adult Health Assessment* (pp. 49–50), edited by D.L. Skillen and R.A. Day, 2004, Edmonton, AB: Faculty of Nursing, University of Alberta.

STUDENT: _____ DATE: _____

INSTRUCTOR: _____ DATE: _____

Procedure 28-28 Palpating Pulses and Epitrochlear Nodes in Upper Extremities

	S	U	NP	Comments
Palpation: Brachial pulse				
1. Palpate brachial artery with finger pads or thumbs at the antecubital crease (fossa) **OR** above elbow in groove between biceps and triceps muscles.	___	___	___	_____
2. Compare sides.	___	___	___	_____
Palpation: Radial pulse				
1. Palpate radial artery with finger pads on the lateral flexor surface of wrist.	___	___	___	_____
2. Compare sides.	___	___	___	_____
Palpation: Epitrochlear nodes				
1. Support client's right forearm with examiner right hand as client flexes elbow about 90 degrees.	___	___	___	_____
2. Palpate for epitrochlear node in groove between biceps and triceps muscles with finger pads of the left hand medially and approximately 3 cm above the medial epicondyle.	___	___	___	_____
3. Reverse hand position to examine client's left arm.	___	___	___	_____

From *A Syllabus for Adult Health Assessment* (p. 50), edited by D.L. Skillen and R.A. Day, 2004, Edmonton, AB: Faculty of Nursing, University of Alberta.

STUDENT: _____ DATE: _____

INSTRUCTOR: _____ DATE: _____

SKILL PERFORMANCE CHECKLIST

Procedure 28-29 Inspecting Coordination in the Upper Extremities

	S	U	NP	Comments
Coordination: Test each hand separately.				
Rapid alternating testing:				
1. Instruct client to pat thigh as rapidly as possible, alternating between palm and dorsum of hand.	____	____	____	_____
2. Compare sides.	____	____	____	_____
3. Instruct client to touch distal joint of thumb with index fingertip repeatedly as rapidly as possible.	____	____	____	_____
4. Compare sides.	____	____	____	_____
Point-to-point testing:				
1. Instruct client to extend arm.	____	____	____	_____
2. Instruct client to alternately touch client's nose, then examiner's finger with fully extended arm.	____	____	____	_____
3. Alter finger position.	____	____	____	_____
4. Hold finger in one place	____	____	____	_____
5. Instruct client to raise extended arm over head and lower it to touch finger.	____	____	____	_____
6. After several tries, instruct client to close eyes and repeat.	____	____	____	_____
7. Repeat 5 and 6 with other arm.	____	____	____	_____

From *A Syllabus for Adult Health Assessment* (p. 50), edited by D.L. Skillen and R.A. Day, 2004, Edmonton, AB: Faculty of Nursing, University of Alberta.

STUDENT: _____ DATE: _____

INSTRUCTOR: _____ DATE: _____

Procedure 28-30 Assessing Sensation of the Upper Extremities

	S	U	NP	Comments

Inspection and palpation: Both arms are tested. The examiner demonstrates how sharp, dull, and light touch feel before beginning tests.

Sensation: Superficial pain

1. Instruct client to close eyes and report with each touch whether it is "sharp" or "dull." ____ ____ ____ _____
2. Touch client's arms lightly and alternately in corresponding areas with sharp end of splintered tongue blade (occasionally using blunt end), covering C4 to C8 and T1 dermatomes in upper arms, forearms, and hands. ____ ____ ____ _____
3. Compare sides. ____ ____ ____ _____

Sensation: Light touch

1. Instruct client to close eyes and report each time touch of the cotton wisp is perceived. ____ ____ ____ _____
2. Touch client's arms lightly, avoiding pressure, alternately in corresponding areas with cotton wisp, testing C4 to C8 and T1 dermatomes in upper arms, forearms, and hands. ____ ____ ____ _____
3. Vary the intervals between touches. ____ ____ ____ _____
4. Compare sides. ____ ____ ____ _____

Sensation: Vibration

1. Instruct client to close eyes and describe the sensation felt. ____ ____ ____ _____
2. Place vibrating 128 Hz tuning fork firmly over distal interphalangeal (DIP) joint of one finger and proceed proximally to proximal interphalangeal (PIP) and metacarpophalangeal (MCP) joints, etc., until vibrations are felt and reported. ____ ____ ____ _____
3. Stop vibration and ask what is felt. ____ ____ ____ _____
4. Compare sides. ____ ____ ____ _____

Sensation: Position sense

1. Demonstrate "up" and "down" position of a finger. ____ ____ ____ _____
2. Instruct client to close eyes and identify position of finger. ____ ____ ____ _____
3. Grasp distal phalanx by medial and lateral aspects and move it "up" or "down." Ensure that adjacent digits are not involved. ____ ____ ____ _____
4. Compare sides. ____ ____ ____ _____

Continued

	S	U	NP	Comments

Inspection and palpation: Tactile discrimination: Both sides are tested.

Stereognosis

1. Instruct client to close eyes and identify object placed in palm. ___ ___ ___ _____
2. Place a small familiar object in each palm in turn. The object can only be manipulated by the hand being tested. ___ ___ ___ _____
3. Compare sides. ___ ___ ___ _____

Graphesthesia

1. Instruct client to close eyes and identify what number is drawn on the skin. ___ ___ ___ _____
2. With palm facing client, draw number with a blunt object on palm of hand. ___ ___ ___ _____
3. Compare sides. ___ ___ ___ _____

Extinction

1. Instruct client to close eyes and identify where touched. ___ ___ ___ _____
2. Touch client in corresponding area of both arms simultaneously. ___ ___ ___ _____
3. Ask client where touched. ___ ___ ___ _____

From *A Syllabus for Adult Health Assessment* (pp. 50–52), edited by D.L. Skillen and R.A. Day, 2004, Edmonton, AB: Faculty of Nursing, University of Alberta.

SKILL PERFORMANCE CHECKLIST

Procedure 28-31 Assessing Deep Tendon Reflexes of the Upper Extremities

	S	U	NP	Comments

Inspection and percussion: Deep tendon reflexes: Both sides are tested and compared. **Only if** responses are symmetrically diminished or absent does examiner use reinforcement (augmentation). The examiner strikes the slightly stretched tendon briskly with reflex hammer held loosely and swung freely in an arc.

Biceps reflex

1. Position client with arm supported and relaxed, elbow flexed and palm downward on thigh (seated client) or abdomen (supine client).   ____ ____ ____ _____

2. Use hammer to tap own thumb placed over biceps tendon at antecubital fossa (crease).   ____ ____ ____ _____

3. Compare flexion of forearm on each side.   ____ ____ ____ _____

Triceps reflex

1. Position client with arm supported and relaxed, elbow flexed OR abducted and flexed in a right angle, in "hang-to-dry" position.   ____ ____ ____ _____

2. Use hammer to tap the triceps tendon 2 to 5 cm above elbow.   ____ ____ ____ _____

3. Compare extension of forearm on each side.   ____ ____ ____ _____

Brachioradialis reflex

1. Position client with arm resting on lap (sitting) or abdomen (supine) and palm down.   ____ ____ ____ _____

2. Use hammer to tap the brachioradialis tendon 2 to 5 cm above wrist.   ____ ____ ____ _____

3. Compare flexion and supination of hand on each side.   ____ ____ ____ _____

From *A Syllabus for Adult Health Assessment* (pp. 50–52), edited by D.L. Skillen and R.A. Day, 2004, Edmonton, AB: Faculty of Nursing, University of Alberta.

STUDENT: _____ DATE: _____
INSTRUCTOR: _____ DATE: _____

Procedure 28-32 Inspecting the Lower Extremities Including Range of Motion

	S	U	NP	Comments

Skin, nails, hair, symmetry
1. Fully expose legs and feet of supine client. ____ ____ ____ _____
2. Inspect skin, nails, muscle mass, and symmetry of both legs and feet. ____ ____ ____ _____
3. Inspect knee for expected depressions on either side of patella. ____ ____ ____ _____

Range of motion (ROM): Test each leg either separately or simultaneously and compare. Only if client is unable to perform active ROM does the examiner attempt passive ROM.

Toes
1. Instruct client to bend toes downward (flexion). ____ ____ ____ _____
2. Instruct client to straighten toes and point upward (extension). ____ ____ ____ _____

Ankles
1. Instruct client to bring foot upward toward shin (dorsiflexion). ____ ____ ____ _____
2. Instruct client to bend foot downward away from shin (plantar-flexion). ____ ____ ____ _____
3. Stabilize ankle and hold heel and instruct client to tilt foot inward with sole toward midline (inversion). ____ ____ ____ _____
4. Stabilize ankle and hold heel and instruct client to tilt foot outward with sole facing laterally (eversion). ____ ____ ____ _____
5. Repeat on other foot. ____ ____ ____ _____

Hips and knees
1. Place hand under lumbar spine. ____ ____ ____ _____
2. Instruct client to bring each knee in turn up toward chest and press firmly onto the abdomen (flexion at hip and knee). ____ ____ ____ _____
3. Note when back touches hand. ____ ____ ____ _____
4. Observe that opposite thigh remains flat on table. ____ ____ ____ _____
5. Instruct client to straighten leg (extension). ____ ____ ____ _____

Hips
1. Stabilize pelvis by pressing on one anterior superior iliac crest with left hand. ____ ____ ____ _____
2. Grasp opposite ankle with right hand and move leg over other leg (adduction). ____ ____ ____ _____

Continued

	S	U	NP	Comments
3. Repeat on other side.	____	____	____	_____
4. Stabilize pelvis by pressing on one anterior superior iliac crest with left hand.	____	____	____	_____
5. Grasp opposite leg at ankle and abduct leg until iliac spine moves (abduction).	____	____	____	_____
6. Repeat on other side.	____	____	____	_____
7. Flex leg at hip and knee to 90 degrees.	____	____	____	_____
8. Support thigh with left hand and ankle with right hand.	____	____	____	_____
9. Turn lower leg medially (external rotation), then laterally (internal rotation).	____	____	____	_____
10. Repeat on other side.	____	____	____	_____

From *A Syllabus for Adult Health Assessment* (pp. 52–53), edited by D.L. Skillen and R.A. Day, 2004, Edmonton, AB: Faculty of Nursing, University of Alberta.

SKILL PERFORMANCE CHECKLIST
Procedure 28-33 Palpating Joints and Skin Surface for Temperature and Edema

	S	U	NP	Comments

Temperature:
1. Use dorsum of hands or fingers to compare temperature of each foot with lower leg and thigh above it.
2. Compare sides.

Edema:
1. Press firmly and gently with thumb for 5 seconds over dorsum of each foot and/or medial malleolus.
2. Assess for extent of depression in the skin.
3. Press firmly and gently with thumb for 5 seconds over each shin.
4. Assess for extent of depression in the skin.

Feet:
Interphalangeal (IP) joints
1. Palpate with thumb and index finger of one hand all of the distal and proximal interphalangeal (IP) joints of the toes.

Metatarsophalangeal (MTP) joints
2. Compress each forefoot just proximal to MTP joints with thumb and fingers placed on medial and lateral surfaces.

Heel
3. Palpate each heel.

Ankles: Ankle joint and Achilles tendon
1. Place thumbs dorsally and fingers ventrally.
2. Palpate anterior aspect of each ankle joint.
3. Palpate along each Achilles tendon with thumb and fingers.

Knees:
Knees
1. Instruct client to bend knees (flexion).
2. Cup hands over each knee in turn as client returns leg to resting position (extension).

Suprapatellar pouch
3. Note any crepitations.
4. Palpate each side of quadriceps in progressive steps, from 10 cm above superior border of patella to patellar pouch.

Continued

	S	U	NP	Comments

Patella

5. Continue palpation along sides of patella.   _____ _____ _____ _____

Tibiofemoral joint

6. Instruct client to slightly flex knee.   _____ _____ _____ _____
7. Palpate tibiofemoral joints (inferior, medial, and lateral to patella).   _____ _____ _____ _____

From *A Syllabus for Adult Health Assessment* (pp. 53–54), edited by D.L. Skillen and R.A. Day, 2004, Edmonton, AB: Faculty of Nursing, University of Alberta

STUDENT: _____ DATE: _____

INSTRUCTOR: _____ DATE: _____

Procedure 28-34 Assessing Muscle Tone and Muscle Strength of the Lower Extremities

	S	U	NP	Comments
Muscle tone: Legs				
1. Support the leg at the foot and lower thigh.	___	___	___	_____
2. Move each leg (ankle, knee, hip) through a modified range of motion (ROM).	___	___	___	_____
3. Assess resistance offered.	___	___	___	_____
4. Test muscle tone prior to testing muscle strength.	___	___	___	_____
Muscle strength: Feet				
1. May test separately or simultaneously.	___	___	___	_____
2. Place hands on client's soles of feet.	___	___	___	_____
3. Ask client to plantar-flex foot against the resistance offered.	___	___	___	_____
4. Compare sides.	___	___	___	_____
5. Place hands on dorsum of client's feet.	___	___	___	_____
6. Ask client to dorsiflex feet against resistance offered.	___	___	___	_____
7. Compare sides.	___	___	___	_____
Muscle strength: Legs				
1. Instruct client to flex knee.	___	___	___	_____
2. Place left hand at knee and grasp client's ankle with right hand.	___	___	___	_____
3. Instruct client to keep foot in contact with table as you attempt to straighten client's leg (flexion at knee).	___	___	___	_____
4. Compare sides.	___	___	___	_____
5. Instruct client to flex knee.	___	___	___	_____
6. Support client's flexed knee with left hand and push against lower shin with right hand as client attempts to straighten leg (extension at knee).	___	___	___	_____
7. Compare sides.	___	___	___	_____
Muscle strength: Hip				
1. Place both hands on client's thigh.	___	___	___	_____
2. Try to force thigh downward as client raises leg against hand (flexion).	___	___	___	_____
3. Place hand under client's thigh.	___	___	___	_____
4. Instruct client to force thigh downward on examiner's hand (extension).	___	___	___	_____
5. Compares sides.	___	___	___	_____
6. Place both hands firmly on surface between client's knees, and	___	___	___	_____

Continued

	S	U	NP	Comments
7. Instruct client to bring legs together (adduction).	___	___	___	_____
8. Place hands firmly on surface at lateral aspect of client's knees, and	___	___	___	_____
9. Instruct client to spread legs (abduction).	___	___	___	_____
10. Compare sides.	___	___	___	_____

From *A Syllabus for Adult Health Assessment* (pp. 54–55), edited by D.L. Skillen and R.A. Day, 2004, Edmonton, AB: Faculty of Nursing, University of Alberta.

STUDENT: _____ DATE: _____

INSTRUCTOR: _____ DATE: _____

SKILL PERFORMANCE CHECKLIST
Procedure 28-35 Assessing Pulses in the Lower Extremities

	S	U	NP	Comments
Popliteal pulses				
1. Instruct client to flex leg slightly and relax muscles.	___	___	___	_____
2. Palpate popliteal artery with fingertips of both hands midline in popliteal fossa, pressing deeply.	___	___	___	_____
3. Compare sides.	___	___	___	_____
4. If unable to palpate, ask client to lie prone on examining surface with legs flexed at knee and palpate.	___	___	___	_____
Posterior tibial pulses				
1. Palpate posterior tibial artery behind and below medial malleolus with finger pads.	___	___	___	_____
2. Compare sides. May palpate simultaneously.	___	___	___	_____
Dorsalis pedis pulses				
1. Palpate dorsalis pedis artery with finger pads on dorsum of foot just lateral to extensor tendon of great toe.	___	___	___	_____
2. Compare sides. May palpate simultaneously.	___	___	___	_____

From *A Syllabus for Adult Health Assessment* (p. 55), edited by D.L. Skillen and R.A. Day, 2004, Edmonton, AB: Faculty of Nursing, University of Alberta.

STUDENT: _____ DATE: _____

INSTRUCTOR: _____ DATE: _____

SKILL PERFORMANCE CHECKLIST
Procedure 28-36 Assessing Coordination of the Lower Extremities

	S	U	NP	Comments
Coordination: Test each leg separately.				
Rapid alternating movements				
1. Instruct client to pat foot against examiner's hand as rapidly as possible (rhythmic patting).	___	___	___	_____
Point-to-point test				
2. Instruct client to place heel on opposite knee and run heel down shin and off great toe.	___	___	___	_____
Position sense				
3. Repeat each side with eyes closed.	___	___	___	_____
4. Compare sides.	___	___	___	_____

From *A Syllabus for Adult Health Assessment* (p. 55), edited by D.L. Skillen and R.A. Day, 2004, Edmonton, AB: Faculty of Nursing, University of Alberta.

STUDENT: _____ DATE: _____

INSTRUCTOR: _____ DATE: _____

Procedure 28-37 Assessing Sensation and Tactile Discrimination of the Lower Extremities

	S	U	NP	Comments

Tests of sensation: Both sides are tested and compared. Demonstrate how sharp, dull, and light touch feels before beginning tests.

Superficial pain

1. Instruct client to close eyes and report with each touch whether it is "sharp" or "dull." ___ ___ ___ _____

2. Touch client's legs lightly and alternately in corresponding areas with sharp end of splintered tongue blade (occasionally using blunt end), covering L2 to S1 dermatomes in thighs, legs, and feet. ___ ___ ___ _____

3. Compare sides. ___ ___ ___ _____

Light touch

1. Instruct client to close eyes and report each time touch is perceived (avoids pressure). ___ ___ ___ _____

2. Touch client's legs lightly in turn in corresponding areas with cotton wisp, covering L2 to S1 dermatomes in thighs, legs, and feet. ___ ___ ___ _____

3. Compare sides. ___ ___ ___ _____

Vibration

1. Instruct client to close eyes and describe sensation felt. ___ ___ ___ _____

2. Place vibrating 128 Hz tuning fork firmly over distal interphalangeal (DIP) joint of great toe. ___ ___ ___ _____

3. Proceed proximally until vibrations felt. ___ ___ ___ _____

4. Stop vibrations and ask what is felt. ___ ___ ___ _____

5. Compare sides. ___ ___ ___ _____

Position sense

1. Demonstrate "up" and "down" position of great toe. ___ ___ ___ _____

2. Instruct client to close eyes and identify position of great toe. ___ ___ ___ _____

3. Grasp great toe by medial and lateral aspects and move it "up" or "down," avoiding contact with other toes. ___ ___ ___ _____

4. Proceed proximally if necessary. ___ ___ ___ _____

5. Compare sides. ___ ___ ___ _____

Continued

	S	U	NP	Comments

Test for tactile discrimination:

Extinction

1. Instruct client to close eyes and identify where touched.

2. Touch client in corresponding areas of legs simultaneously.

3. Ask client where touched.

From *A Syllabus for Adult Health Assessment* (pp. 55–56), edited by D.L. Skillen and R.A. Day, 2004, Edmonton, AB: Faculty of Nursing, University of Alberta.

STUDENT: _____ DATE: _____

INSTRUCTOR: _____ DATE: _____

Procedure 28-38 Assessing Deep Tendon and Superficial Reflexes of the Lower Extremities

	S	U	NP	Comments

Deep tendon reflexes: Both sides are tested. **Only if** responses are symmetrically diminished or absent does examiner use reinforcement (augmentation). Strike tendon briskly with hammer held loosely and swung freely in an arc.

Patellar reflex

1. Position client so that leg is relaxed and knee is flexed. ____ ____ ____ _____
2. Use hammer to tap patellar tendon just below patella. ____ ____ ____ _____
3. Compare extension on each side. ____ ____ ____ _____

Ankle reflex

1. Position client so that knee is flexed and foot is supported in dorsiflexed position by examiner. ____ ____ ____ _____
2. Use hammer to tap Achilles tendon just above the heel. ____ ____ ____ _____
3. Compare plantar flexion on each side. ____ ____ ____ _____

Superficial reflex:
Plantar reflex

1. Stroke the lateral aspect of sole with blunt pointed object beginning at heel, laterally along sole, and curving medially across ball of the foot. ____ ____ ____ _____
2. Compare toe movement on each side. ____ ____ ____ _____

From *A Syllabus for Adult Health Assessment* (p. 56), edited by D.L. Skillen and R.A. Day, 2004, Edmonton, AB: Faculty of Nursing, University of Alberta.

STUDENT: _____ DATE: _____

INSTRUCTOR: _____ DATE: _____

Procedure 28-39 Inspecting the Legs and Assessing Coordination in Standing Position

	S	U	NP	Comments
Legs and feet:				
Symmetry, veins, arches, and popliteal fossae				
1. Inspect both legs, noting symmetry, veins, arches, and popliteal fossae.	___	___	___	_____
2. Palpate popliteal fossae.	___	___	___	_____
Cerebellar tests, position sense				
1. Instruct client to stand without support, arms at sides and feet together, first with eyes open, then closed for 20 seconds (Romberg test).	___	___	___	_____
2. Protect client from falling.	___	___	___	_____
3. Instruct client to walk in straight line by placing heel of foot directly before toes of other foot (tandem walking).	___	___	___	_____
Muscle strength				
4. Instruct client to hop in place on one foot, then the other.	___	___	___	_____
Shallow knee bend				
5. Instruct client to stand on one foot and do a shallow knee bend, first on one leg, then the other.	___	___	___	_____
6. Support elbow if risk of falling.	___	___	___	_____
Heel walk				
7. Instruct client to walk on heels.	___	___	___	_____
Toe walk				
8. Instruct client to walk on toes.	___	___	___	_____
Gait, balance, and posture:				
1. Instruct client to walk away and then back toward examiner.	___	___	___	_____
2. Inspect during walking for posture, gait (stance and swing), balance, arm swing, leg movement, and position of head on turning.	___	___	___	_____

From *A Syllabus for Adult Health Assessment* (p. 57), edited by D.L. Skillen and R.A. Day, 2004, Edmonton, AB: Faculty of Nursing, University of Alberta.

STUDENT: _____ DATE: _____

INSTRUCTOR: _____ DATE: _____

SKILL PERFORMANCE CHECKLIST
Skill 29-1 Hand Hygiene

	S	U	NP	Comments
1. Inspect surfaces of hands for breaks or cuts in skin or cuticles. Report and cover lesions before providing client care.	____	____	____	_____
2. Inspect hands for heavy soiling.	____	____	____	_____
3. Inspect nails for length and presence of artificial acrylics or chipped nail polish.	____	____	____	_____
4. Assess client's risk for or extent of infection.	____	____	____	_____
5. Push wristwatch and long uniform sleeves above wrists. Remove rings during washing.	____	____	____	_____
6. If hands are visibly dirty or contaminated with protein-containing material, use plain or antimicrobial soap and water:	____	____	____	_____
A. Stand in front of sink, keeping hands and uniform away from sink surface.	____	____	____	_____
B. Turn on water. Turn faucet on or push knee pedals laterally or press foot pedals to regulate water flow and temperature.	____	____	____	_____
C. Avoid splashing water onto uniform.	____	____	____	_____
D. Regulate flow of water so that temperature is warm.	____	____	____	_____
E. Wet hands and wrists thoroughly under running water. Keep hands and forearms lower than elbows during washing.	____	____	____	_____
F. Apply a small amount of soap, lathering thoroughly.	____	____	____	_____
G. Wash hands using plenty of lather and friction for at least 10 to 15 seconds. Interlace fingers and rub palms and back of hands with circular motion at least 5 times each. Keep fingertips down. Rub knuckles of one hand into the palm of the other; repeat with other hand.	____	____	____	_____
H. Rub thumb on one hand with the palm of the other hand; repeat with other hand.	____	____	____	_____
I. Work the fingertips on one hand into the palm of the other. Massage soap into nail spaces. Repeat with other hand.	____	____	____	_____
J. Clean fingernails of both hands with additional soap or clean orangewood stick.	____	____	____	_____
K. Rinse hands and wrists thoroughly, keeping hands down and elbows up.	____	____	____	_____
L. Optional: Repeat steps a through j and extend period of washing if hands are heavily soiled.	____	____	____	_____

Continued

	S	U	NP	Comments

M. Dry hands thoroughly from fingers to wrists and forearms with paper towel, single-use cloth, or warm air dryer.

N. Discard paper towel, if used, in proper receptacle.

O. Turn off water with foot or knee pedals. To turn off hand faucet, use clean, dry paper towel. Avoid touching handles with hands.

P. If hands are dry or chapped, a small amount of lotion or barrier cream can be applied.

Q. Inspect surfaces of hands for obvious signs of soil or other contaminants.

R. Inspect hands for dermatitis or cracked skin.

7. If hands are not visibly soiled, use an alcohol-based waterless antiseptic for routine decontamination in all clinical situations.

A. Apply an ample amount of product to the palm of one hand.

B. Rub hands together, covering all surfaces.

C. Rub hands together until alcohol is dry. Allow hands to dry before applying gloves.

D. If hands are dry or chapped, a small amount of lotion or barrier cream can be applied.

Skill 29-2 Preparation of a Sterile Field

	S	U	NP	Comments
1. Prepare sterile field just before planned procedure.	___	___	___	_____
2. Select clean work surface above waist level.	___	___	___	_____
3. Assemble equipment.	___	___	___	_____
4. Check dates on supplies.	___	___	___	_____
5. Perform hand hygiene.	___	___	___	_____
6. Place pack with sterile drape on work surface and open pack.	___	___	___	_____
7. With fingertips of one hand, pick up folded top edge.	___	___	___	_____
8. Lift drape from its outer cover and let it unfold by itself without touching anything. Discard outer cover with other hand.	___	___	___	_____
9. With other hand, grasp adjacent corner of drape and hold it straight up and away from your body.	___	___	___	_____
10. Holding drape, first position and lay bottom half over intended work surface.	___	___	___	_____
11. Allow top half of drape to be placed over work surface last.	___	___	___	_____
12. Grasp 2.5-cm border around edge to position as needed.	___	___	___	_____

Adding Sterile Items:

	S	U	NP	Comments
13. Open sterile item.	___	___	___	_____
14. Peel wrapper.	___	___	___	_____
15. Being sure wrapper does not fall down on sterile field, place item onto field at angle. Do not hold arm over field.	___	___	___	_____
16. Dispose of wrapper.	___	___	___	_____
17. Perform procedure using sterile technique.	___	___	___	_____

STUDENT: _____ DATE: _____

INSTRUCTOR: _____ DATE: _____

SKILL PERFORMANCE CHECKLIST
Skill 29-3 Surgical Hand Hygiene: Preparing for Gowning

	S	U	NP	Comments
1. Consult agency policy for length of time for hand washing.	___	___	___	_____
2. Keep fingernails short, clean, and healthy. Remove artificial nails.	___	___	___	_____
3. Inspect hands for presence of abrasions, cuts, or open lesions.	___	___	___	_____
4. Apply surgical shoe covers, cap or hood, face mask, and protective eyewear.	___	___	___	_____
5. Surgical hand washing:				
A. Turn on water using knee or foot controls, and adjust water to comfortable temperature.	___	___	___	_____
B. Wet hands and arms under running lukewarm water and lather with detergent to 5 cm above elbows. Keep hands above elbows.	___	___	___	_____
C. Rinse hands and arms thoroughly under running water, keeping hands above elbows.	___	___	___	_____
D. Under running water, clean under nails of both hands with nail pick. Discard nail pick after use.	___	___	___	_____
E. Wet clean sponge and apply antimicrobial detergent. Scrub the nails of one hand with 15 strokes. Holding sponge perpendicular, scrub the palm, each side of the thumb and all fingers, and the posterior side of the hand with 10 strokes each. Scrub each section of the arm 10 times. Check manufacturers recommendations for the duration of the scrub, usually 2 to 6 minutes. Rinse sponge and repeat for other arm.	___	___	___	_____
F. Discard sponge and rinse hands and arms thoroughly. Turn off water with foot or knee controls and back into room entrance with hands elevated in front of and away from the body.	___	___	___	_____
G. Bend slightly forward at the waist to pick up a sterile towel. Dry one hand thoroughly, moving from fingers to elbow. Dry in a rotating motion from cleanest to least clean area.	___	___	___	_____

Continued

	S	U	NP	Comments

H. Repeat drying method for other hand, using a different area of the towel or a new sterile towel.

I. Discard towel.

J. Proceed with sterile gowning.

6. Alternate method of surgical hand hygiene using alcohol-based antiseptic:

A. Wash hands with soap and water for 10 to 15 seconds.

B. Clean nails of both hands under running water with nail pick. Discard nail pick after use and dry hands with a paper towel.

C. Apply enough alcohol-based waterless antiseptic to one palm to cover both hands thoroughly. Spread antiseptic over all hand and nail surfaces. Allow to air dry.

D. Repeat the process and allow hands to air dry before applying sterile gloves.

STUDENT: _____ DATE: _____

INSTRUCTOR: _____ DATE: _____

Skill 29-4 Applying a Sterile Gown and Performing Closed Gloving

	S	U	NP	Comments
1. Apply cap, face mask, eyewear, and foot covers.	____	____	____	_____
2. Perform surgical hand hygiene.	____	____	____	_____
3. Have circulating nurse open pack containing sterile gown.	____	____	____	_____
4. Have circulating nurse prepare glove package.	____	____	____	_____
5. Reach down to sterile gown package; lift gown directly upward and step back from table.	____	____	____	_____
6. Holding folded gown, locate neckband. Grasp inside front of gown just below neckband.	____	____	____	_____
7. Allow gown to unfold, keeping inside of gown toward body. Do not touch outside of gown.	____	____	____	_____
8. Insert each hand through armholes simultaneously. Ask circulating nurse to bring gown over shoulders, leaving sleeves covering hands.	____	____	____	_____
9. Have circulating nurse tie back of gown at neck and waist.	____	____	____	_____
10. Closed gloving procedure:				
A. With hands covered by sleeves, open glove package.	____	____	____	_____
B. With dominant hand inside gown cuff, pick up glove for non-dominant hand.	____	____	____	_____
C. Extend non-dominant forearm with palm up and place palm of glove against palm of non-dominant hand. Glove fingers will point toward elbow.	____	____	____	_____
D. Grasp back of glove cuff with covered dominant hand and turn glove cuff over end of non-dominant hand and gown cuff.	____	____	____	_____
E. Grasp top of glove and underlying gown sleeve with covered dominant hand. Carefully extend fingers into glove, being sure glove's cuff covers gown's cuff.	____	____	____	_____
F. Repeat steps a through e to glove dominant hand.	____	____	____	_____
G. Adjust fingers until fully extended into both gloves.	____	____	____	_____
11. For wraparound sterile gowns, release front fastener with gloved hand.	____	____	____	_____
12. Handing tie to stationary team member, turn 360 degrees to left and secure tie to gown.	____	____	____	_____

STUDENT: _____ DATE: _____

INSTRUCTOR: _____ DATE: _____

SKILL PERFORMANCE CHECKLIST
Skill 29-5 Open Gloving

	S	U	NP	Comments
1. Perform thorough hand hygiene.	——	——	——	_____
2. Peel apart sides of outer package of glove wrapper.	——	——	——	_____
3. Lay inner package on clean, flat surface just above waist level. Open package, keeping gloves on inside surface of wrapper.	——	——	——	_____
4. If gloves are not prepowdered, apply powder lightly to hands over sink or wastebasket.	——	——	——	_____
5. Identify right and left gloves.	——	——	——	_____
6. Start by applying glove to dominant hand. With thumb and first two fingers of non-dominant hand, grasp edge of cuff of glove for dominant hand, touching only inside surface.	——	——	——	_____
7. Carefully pull glove over dominant hand, ensuring cuff does not roll up wrist.	——	——	——	_____
8. With gloved dominant hand, slip fingers underneath second glove's cuff.	——	——	——	_____
9. Carefully pull second glove over non-dominant hand, and do not allow gloved hand to touch any part of exposed non-dominant hand.	——	——	——	_____
10. When both gloves are on, interlock fingers of both hands to secure gloves in position, being careful to touch only sterile sides.	——	——	——	_____

Glove disposal:

11. Without touching wrist, grasp outside of one cuff with other gloved hand.	——	——	——	_____
12. Pull glove off, turning it inside out. Discard in receptacle.	——	——	——	_____
13. Tuck fingers of bare hand inside remaining glove cuff. Peel glove off, inside out. Discard in receptacle.	——	——	——	_____

SKILL PERFORMANCE CHECKLIST
Skill 30-1 Administering Oral Medications

	S	U	NP	Comments
1. Assess for any contraindications to client receiving oral medication.	___	___	___	_____
2. Assess client's medical history, history of allergies, medication history, and diet history.	___	___	___	_____
3. Gather physical assessment and laboratory data that may influence medication administration.	___	___	___	_____
4. Assess client's knowledge regarding health and medication usage.	___	___	___	_____
5. Assess client's preferences for fluids.	___	___	___	_____
6. Check accuracy and completeness of each MAR with prescriber's written medication order.	___	___	___	_____
7. Prepare medications:				
A. Perform hand hygiene.	___	___	___	_____
B. If medication cart is used, move it outside client's room.	___	___	___	_____
C. Unlock medicine drawer or cart.				
D. Prepare medications for one client at a time. Keep all pages of MAR for one client together.	___	___	___	_____
E. Select correct medication from stock supply or unit-dose drawer. Compare label of medication with MAR. Check expiration date.	___	___	___	_____
F. Calculate medication dose as necessary. Double-check calculation.	___	___	___	_____
G. To prepare tablets or capsules from a floor stock bottle, pour required number into bottle cap and transfer medication to medication cup. Do not touch medication with fingers. Extra tablets or capsules may be returned to bottle.	___	___	___	_____
H. To prepare unit-dose tablets or capsules, place packaged tablet or capsule directly into medicine cup. (Do not remove wrapper.)	___	___	___	_____
I. Place tablets or capsules to be given to client at the same time in one medicine cup unless client requires pre-administration assessments.	___	___	___	_____

Continued

	S	U	NP	Comments

J. If client has difficulty swallowing
and liquid medications are not an option,
use a pill-crushing device. If a pill-crushing
device is not available, place tablet between
two medication cups and grind with a blunt
instrument. Mix ground tablet in small
amount of soft food (e.g., custard
or applesauce).

K. Prepare liquids:

    (1) Gently shake container. If medication
is in a unit dose container, no further
preparation is needed. If medication
is in a multidose bottle, remove bottle
cap from container and place cap
upside down.

    (2) Hold multidose bottle with label
against palm of hand while pouring.

    (3) Hold medication cup at eye level
and fill to desired level on scale.
Draw up volumes of liquid medication
of less than 10 mL in syringe
without needle.

    (4) Discard any excess liquid into sink.
Wipe lip and neck of bottle with
paper towel.

L. Compare MAR with prepared medication
and container.

M. Return stock containers or unused
unit-dose medications to shelf or drawer
and read label again.

N. Do not leave drugs unattended.

8. Administering medications:

A. Take medications to client at correct time.

B. Identify client by comparing name on
MAR with name on client's identification
bracelet. Ask client to state name.

C. Explain to client the purpose of each
medication and its action. Allow client
to ask any questions about medications.

D. Assist client to sitting position or to
side-lying position if sitting is
contraindicated.

E. Administer medications:

    (1) For tablets: Client may wish to hold
solid medications in hand or cup
before placing in mouth.

    (2) Offer water or juice to help client
swallow medications. Give client cold
carbonated water if available and not
contraindicated.

Continued

	S	U	NP	Comments

(3) For sublingual-administered
medications: Instruct client to place
medication under tongue and allow it
to dissolve completely. Caution client
against swallowing tablet.

(4) For drugs administered buccally,
instruct client to place medication in
mouth against mucous membranes of
the cheek until it dissolves. Avoid
administering liquids until medication
has dissolved.

(5) For powdered medications: Mix with
liquids at bedside and give to client
to drink.

(6) Caution client against chewing
or swallowing lozenges.

(7) Give effervescent powders and tablets
to client immediately after they
have dissolved.

F. If client is unable to hold medications,
place medication cup to client's lips
and gently introduce each drug into the
mouth, one at a time.

G. If tablet or capsule falls to the floor,
discard it and repeat preparation.

H. Stay in room until client has completely
swallowed each medication. Ask client to
open mouth if you are uncertain whether
medication has been swallowed.

I. For highly acidic medications, offer client
a non-fat snack if not contraindicated.

J. Assist client in returning to a comfortable
position.

K. Dispose of soiled supplies. Perform
hand hygiene.

9. Evaluate client's response to medication at
times that correlate with medication's onset,
peak, and duration.

10. Ask client or family member to identify drug
name and explain purpose, action, dosage
schedule, and potential side effects of drug.

11. Notify prescriber if the client exhibits a toxic
effect or allergic reaction or if there is an
onset of side effects. If either of these occurs,
withhold further doses of medication.

12. Record administration (or withholding)
of oral medications.

STUDENT: _____ DATE: _____

INSTRUCTOR: _____ DATE: _____

Skill 30-2 Administering Nasal Instillations

	S	U	NP	Comments
1. For nasal drops, determine which of client's sinuses is affected.	____	____	____	_____
2. Assess client's history of hypertension, heart disease, diabetes mellitus, and hyperthyroidism.	____	____	____	_____
3. Review prescriber's order.	____	____	____	_____
4. Determine if client has allergies to medication.	____	____	____	_____
5. Identify client.	____	____	____	_____
6. Perform hand hygiene. Inspect condition of client's nose and sinuses. Palpate sinuses for tenderness.	____ ____	____ ____	____ ____	_____ _____
7. Assess client's knowledge regarding use of and technique for instillation and willingness to learn self-administration.	____	____	____	_____
8. Explain procedure to client regarding positioning and sensations to expect.	____	____	____	_____
9. Arrange supplies and medications at bedside. Apply gloves if client has nasal drainage.	____	____	____	_____
10. Instruct client to clear or blow nose gently, unless contraindicated.	____	____	____	_____
11. Administer nasal drops:				
A. Assist client to supine position.	____	____	____	_____
B. Position client's head properly:				
(1) For access to posterior pharynx, tilt client's head backward.	____	____	____	_____
(2) For access to ethmoid or sphenoid sinus, tilt client's head back over edge of bed or place small pillow under client's shoulder and tilt head back.	____	____	____	_____
(3) For access to frontal and maxillary sinuses, tilt client's head back over edge of bed or pillow with head turned toward side to be treated.	____	____	____	_____
C. Support client's head with non-dominant hand.	____	____	____	_____
D. Instruct client to breathe through mouth.	____	____	____	_____
E. Hold dropper 1 cm above client's nares and instill prescribed number of drops toward midline of ethmoid bone.	____	____	____	_____
F. Have client remain in supine position 5 minutes.	____	____	____	_____
G. Offer facial tissue to client to blot runny nose, but caution client against blowing nose for several minutes.	____	____	____	_____

Continued

431

	S	U	NP	Comments
12. Assist client to a comfortable position after drug is absorbed.	___	___	___	_____
13. Dispose of soiled supplies in proper container and perform hand hygiene.	___	___	___	_____
14. Observe client for onset of side effects 15 to 30 minutes after administration.	___	___	___	_____
15. Ask if client is able to breathe through nose after decongestant administration.	___	___	___	_____
16. Reinspect condition of nasal passages between instillations.	___	___	___	_____
17. Ask client to review risks of overuse of decongestants and methods for administration.	___	___	___	_____
18. Have client demonstrate self-medication.	___	___	___	_____

STUDENT: _____ DATE: _____

INSTRUCTOR: _____ DATE: _____

SKILL PERFORMANCE CHECKLIST

Skill 30-3 Administering Ophthalmic Medications

	S	U	NP	Comments
1. Review prescriber's medication order.	___	___	___	_____
2. Identify client.	___	___	___	_____
3. Assess condition of client's external eye structures.	___	___	___	_____
4. Determine whether client has any known allergies to eye medications. Ask if client is allergic to latex.	___ ___	___ ___	___ ___	_____ _____
5. Determine whether client has any symptoms of visual alterations.	___	___	___	_____
6. Assess client's level of consciousness and ability to follow directions.	___	___	___	_____
7. Assess client's knowledge regarding medication therapy and desire to self-administer medication.	___	___	___	_____
8. Assess client's ability to manipulate and hold eye dropper.	___	___	___	_____
9. Explain procedure to client.	___	___	___	_____
10. Perform hand hygiene. Arrange supplies at client's bedside. Apply disposable gloves.	___	___	___	_____
11. Ask client to lie supine or to sit back in chair with head slightly hyperextended.	___	___	___	_____
12. Wash away any crusts or drainage along client's eyelid margins or inner canthus. Soak any crusts that are dried and difficult to remove by applying a damp washcloth or cotton ball over eye for a few minutes. Wipe from inner to outer canthus.	___	___	___	_____
13. Hold cotton ball or clean tissue in non-dominant hand on client's cheekbone just below lower eyelid.	___	___	___	_____
14. With tissue or cotton ball resting below lower lid, gently press downward with thumb or forefinger against bony orbit.	___	___	___	_____
15. Ask client to look at ceiling and explain steps to client.	___	___	___	_____
A. Instill eye drops:				
(1) With dominant hand resting on client's forehead, hold filled medication eye dropper or ophthalmic solution approximately 1 to 2 cm above conjunctival sac.	___	___	___	_____

Continued

	S	U	NP	Comments

(2) Drop prescribed number of medication drops into conjunctival sac.

(3) If client blinks or closes eye or if drops land on outer lid margins, repeat procedure.

(4) After instilling drops, ask client to close eye gently.

(5) For drugs that cause systemic effects, with a clean tissue apply gentle pressure with your finger on the client's nasolacrimal duct for 30 to 60 seconds.

B. Instill eye ointment:

(1) Holding ointment applicator above lower lid margin, apply thin stream of ointment evenly along inner edge of lower eyelid on conjunctiva from inner canthus to outer canthus.

(2) Have client close eye and rub lid gently in circular motion with cotton ball, if rubbing is not contraindicated.

C. Intraocular disk procedures:

(1) Application:

a. Open package containing disk. Gently press fingertip against disk so it adheres to finger. Position convex side of disk on fingertip.

b. With other hand, gently pull client's lower eyelid away from the eye. Ask client to look up.

c. Place disk in the conjunctival sac so that it floats on the sclera between the iris and lower eyelid.

d. Pull client's lower eyelid out and over disk.

(2) Removal:

a. Perform hand hygiene and apply gloves.

b. Explain procedure to client.

c. Gently pull on client's lower eyelid to expose disk.

d. Using forefinger and thumb of opposite hand, pinch disk and lift it out of client's eye.

16. If excess medication is on eyelid, gently wipe eyelid from inner to outer canthus.

Continued

434

	S	U	NP	Comments
17. If client has an eye patch, apply clean patch by placing it over affected eye so entire eye is covered. Tape securely without applying pressure to eye.	____	____	____	_____
18. Remove gloves. Dispose of soiled supplies in proper receptacle and perform hand hygiene.	____	____	____	_____
19. Note client's response to instillation. Ask if any discomfort was felt.	____	____	____	_____
20. Observe client's response to medication by assessing visual changes and noting any side effects.	____	____	____	_____
21. Ask client to discuss medication's purpose, action, side effects, and technique of administration.	____	____	____	_____
22. Have client demonstrate self-administration of next dose.	____	____	____	_____

STUDENT: _____ DATE: _____

INSTRUCTOR: _____ DATE: _____

SKILL PERFORMANCE CHECKLIST
Skill 30-4 Administering Vaginal Medications

	S	U	NP	Comments
1. Review physician's order.	___	___	___	_____
2. Review client's history of allergies, including latex.	___	___	___	_____
3. Perform hand hygiene.	___	___	___	_____
4. Identify client.	___	___	___	_____
5. Inspect client's external genitalia and vaginal canal.	___	___	___	_____
6. Assess client's ability to manipulate applicator or suppository and position herself.	___	___	___	_____
7. Explain procedure to client.	___	___	___	_____
8. Arrange supplies at bedside.	___	___	___	_____
9. Provide privacy.	___	___	___	_____
10. Assist client to dorsal recumbent position.	___	___	___	_____
11. Keep client's abdomen and lower extremities draped.	___	___	___	_____
12. Apply disposable gloves.	___	___	___	_____
13. Ensure adequate lighting. Cleanse vaginal area if necessary.	___	___	___	_____
14. Insert suppository with gloved hand:	___	___	___	_____
A. Take suppository from wrapper and lubricate smooth or rounded end. Lubricate gloved index finger of dominant hand.	___	___	___	_____
B. Gently retract client's labial folds with non-dominant gloved hand.	___	___	___	_____
C. Insert rounded end of suppository 7.5 to 10 cm along posterior wall of vaginal canal.	___	___	___	_____
D. Withdraw finger and wipe away lubricant from client's orifice and labia.	___	___	___	_____
15. Apply cream or foam:	___	___	___	_____
A. Fill applicator as directed.	___	___	___	_____
B. Retract client's labial folds with non-dominant gloved hand.	___	___	___	_____
C. With dominant gloved hand, insert applicator 5 to 7.5 cm; push plunger.	___	___	___	_____
D. Withdraw applicator and place it on paper towel. Wipe off residual cream from labia or vaginal orifice.	___	___	___	_____
16. Dispose of supplies. Remove and discard gloves. Perform hand hygiene.	___	___	___	_____
17. Instruct client to remain flat on her back for at least 10 minutes.	___	___	___	_____

Continued

	S	U	NP	Comments

18. Wash applicator (wearing gloves) and store for future use, if indicated.

19. Offer client perineal pad.

20. Inspect appearance of discharge from client's vaginal canal and condition of external genitalia between applications.

STUDENT: _____   DATE: _____
INSTRUCTOR: _____   DATE: _____

Skill 30-5 Administering Rectal Suppositories

	S	U	NP	Comments
1. Review prescriber's order.	____	____	____	_____
2. Review client's medical record for rectal surgery, bleeding, history of allergies.	____	____	____	_____
3. Perform hand hygiene.	____	____	____	_____
4. Apply disposable gloves.	____	____	____	_____
5. Identify client.	____	____	____	_____
6. Explain procedure to client.	____	____	____	_____
7. Arrange supplies at client's bedside.	____	____	____	_____
8. Provide privacy.	____	____	____	_____
9. Assist client to Sims' position. Keep client draped, with anal area exposed.	____	____	____	_____
10. Examine external condition of client's anus. Palpate rectal walls. Dispose of gloves if soiled.	____	____	____	_____
11. Apply disposable gloves (if previous gloves were discarded).	____	____	____	_____
12. Remove suppository from wrapper and lubricate rounded end. Lubricate gloved index finger of dominant hand.	____	____	____	_____
13. Ask client to take slow, deep breaths through mouth and to relax anal sphincter.	____	____	____	_____
14. Retract buttocks with non-dominant hand. Insert suppository through anus, past internal sphincter, and against rectal wall, 10 cm in adults, 5 cm in children and infants.	____	____	____	_____
15. Withdraw finger and wipe anal area clean.	____	____	____	_____
16. Discard gloves.	____	____	____	_____
17. Ask client to remain flat or on side for 5 minutes.	____	____	____	_____
18. If suppository contains a laxative or fecal softener, place call light within reach.	____	____	____	_____
19. Perform hand hygiene.	____	____	____	_____
20. Observe for effects of suppository at times that correlate with the medication's onset, peak, and duration.	____	____	____	_____
21. Record medication administration or client refusal.	____	____	____	_____

SKILL PERFORMANCE CHECKLIST
Skill 30-6 Using Metered-Dose or Dry Powder Inhalers

	S	U	NP	Comments
1. Review prescriber's order.	___	___	___	_____
2. Identify client.	___	___	___	_____
3. Assess client's ability to hold, manipulate, and depress canister and inhaler.	___	___	___	_____
4. Assess client's readiness and ability to learn.	___	___	___	_____
5. Assess client's ability to learn.	___	___	___	_____
6. Assess client's knowledge and understanding of disease and purpose of the action of prescribed medications.	___	___	___	_____
7. Determine medication schedule and number of inhalations prescribed for each dose.	___	___	___	_____
8. Assess client's technique for using an inhaler if he or she has been previously instructed in self-medication.	___	___	___	_____
9. Instruct client in a comfortable environment.	___	___	___	_____
10. Provide adequate time for teaching session.	___	___	___	_____
11. Perform hand hygiene. Arrange necessary equipment.	___	___	___	_____
12. Allow client the opportunity to manipulate inhaler, canister, and spacer device. Explain and demonstrate how canister fits into inhaler.	___	___	___	_____
13. Explain what metered dose is and warn client about overuse of the inhaler, including medication side effects.	___	___	___	_____
14. Explain steps for administering inhaled dose of medication of metered-dose inhaler (MDI; d demonstrate when possible):	___	___	___	_____
A. Insert MDI canister into the holder.	___	___	___	_____
B. Remove mouthpiece cover from inhaler.	___	___	___	_____
C. Shake inhaler vigorously 5 or 6 times.	___	___	___	_____
D. Have client take a deep breath and exhale.	___	___	___	_____
E. Instruct the client to position the inhaler in one of two ways:	___	___	___	_____
(1) Close mouth around MDI, with opening toward back of throat.	___	___	___	_____
(2) Position the device 2 to 4 cm in front of the mouth.	___	___	___	_____
F. With the inhaler properly positioned, have client hold it with thumb at the mouthpiece and the index and middle fingers at the top.	___	___	___	_____

Continued

	S	U	NP	Comments
G. Instruct client to tilt head back slightly, inhale deeply and slowly through mouth for 3 to 5 seconds while depressing canister fully.	____	____	____	_____
H. Instruct client to hold breath for approximately 10 seconds.	____	____	____	_____
I. Have client remove MDI from mouth and exhale through pursed lips.	____	____	____	_____
15. Explain steps to administer MDI using a spacer such as an Aerochamber (demonstrate when possible):	____	____	____	_____
A. Remove mouthpiece cover from MDI and mouthpiece of spacer. Inspect spacer.	____	____	____	_____
B. Insert MDI into end of spacer.	____	____	____	_____
C. Shake inhaler vigorously 5 or 6 times.	____	____	____	_____
D. Have client exhale completely before closing mouth around mouthpiece of the spacer. Avoid covering small exhalation slots with the lips.	____	____	____	_____
E. Have client depress medication canister, spraying one puff into spacer.	____	____	____	_____
F. Instruct client to breathe slowly and fully for 3 to 5 seconds.	____	____	____	_____
G. Have client hold a breath for 10 seconds.	____	____	____	_____
H. Remove MDI and spacer before exhaling.	____	____	____	_____
16. Explain steps to administer dry powder inhaler (DPI; demonstrate when possible):	____	____	____	_____
A. Remove cover from mouthpiece. Do not shake DPI.	____	____	____	_____
B. Hold inhaler upright and turn wheel to the right and left until click is heard.	____	____	____	_____
C. Exhale away from inhaler prior to inhalation.	____	____	____	_____
D. Position mouthpiece between the lips.	____	____	____	_____
E. Inhale deeply and forcefully through the mouth.	____	____	____	_____
F. Hold breath for 5 to 10 seconds.	____	____	____	_____
17. Instruct client to wait at least 20 to 30 seconds between inhalations or as ordered by prescriber.	____	____	____	_____
18. Instruct client against repeating inhalations before next scheduled dose.	____	____	____	_____
19. Explain that client may feel gagging sensation in throat caused by droplets of medication.	____	____	____	_____
20. Instruct client in cleaning inhaler hand mouthpiece. (Rinse inhaler and cap daily under warm water; wash mouthpiece twice weekly with mild soap and warm water.)	____	____	____	_____
21. Ask if client has any questions.	____	____	____	_____

Continued

	S	U	NP	Comments
22. Have client explain and demonstrate steps in use of inhaler.	____	____	____	_____
23. Ask client to explain medication schedule.	____	____	____	_____
24. Ask client to describe side effects of medication and criteria for calling physician.	____	____	____	_____
25. After medication instillation, assess client's respirations and auscultate lungs.	____	____	____	_____

STUDENT: _____ DATE: _____

INSTRUCTOR: _____ DATE: _____

Skill 30-7 Preparing Injections

	S	U	NP	Comments
1. Check client's name and medication order.	___	___	___	_____
2. Review pertinent information related to medication.	___	___	___	_____
3. Assess client's body build, muscle size, and weight.	___	___	___	_____
4. Perform hand hygiene and assemble supplies.	___	___	___	_____
5. Check medication order against MAR and check expiration date of vial or ampule.	___	___	___	_____
6. Prepare medication:				
A. Ampule preparation:				
(1) Tap top of ampule lightly and quickly with finger until fluid moves from neck of ampule.	___	___	___	_____
(2) Place small gauze pad or unopened alcohol swab around neck of ampule.	___	___	___	_____
(3) Snap neck of ampule quickly and firmly away from hands.	___	___	___	_____
(4) Draw up medication quickly, using filter needle long enough to reach bottom of ampule.	___	___	___	_____
(5) Hold ampule upside down or set it on a flat surface. Insert syringe or filter needle into centre of ampule opening. Do not allow needle tip or shaft to touch rim of ampule.	___	___	___	_____
(6) Aspirate medication into syringe by gently pulling back on plunger.	___	___	___	_____
(7) Keep needle tip under surface of liquid. Tip ampule to bring all fluid within reach of needle.	___	___	___	_____
(8) If air bubbles are aspirated, do not expel air into ampule.	___	___	___	_____
(9) To expel excess air bubbles, remove needle from ampule. Hold syringe with needle pointing up. Tap side of syringe to cause bubbles to rise toward needle. Draw back slightly on plunger, then push plunger upward to eject air. Do not eject fluid.	___	___	___	_____

Continued

	S	U	NP	Comments

(10) If syringe contains excess fluid, use sink for disposal. Hold syringe vertically with needle tip up and slanted slightly toward sink. Slowly eject excess fluid into sink. Recheck fluid level in syringe by holding it vertically.

(11) Cover needle with its safety sheath or cap. Replace filter needle with needle for injection.

B. Vial containing a solution:

(1) Remove cap covering top of unused vial to expose sterile rubber seal. If using a multidose vial that has been used before, firmly and briskly wipe surface of rubber seal with alcohol swab and allow it to dry.

(2) Pick up syringe and remove needle cap or cap covering needleless vial access device. Pull back on plunger to draw amount of air into syringe equivalent to volume of medication to be aspirated from vial.

(3) With vial on flat surface, insert tip of needle with bevelled tip entering first through centre of rubber seal. Apply pressure to tip of needle during insertion.

(4) Inject air into vial's airspace, holding on to plunger. Hold plunger with firm pressure; plunger may be forced backward by air pressure within the vial.

(5) Invert vial while keeping firm hold on syringe and plunger. Hold vial between thumb and middle fingers of non-dominant hand. Grasp end of syringe barrel and plunger with thumb and forefinger of dominant hand to counteract pressure in vial.

(6) Keep tip of needle below fluid level.

(7) Allow air pressure from vial to fill syringe gradually with medication. Pull back slightly on plunger to obtain correct amount of solution.

Continued

	S	U	NP	Comments

(8) When desired volume has been obtained, position needle into vial's airspace. Tap side of syringe barrel carefully to dislodge any air bubbles. Eject any air remaining at top of syringe into vial. ____ ____ ____ _____

(9) Remove needle from vial by pulling back on barrel of syringe. ____ ____ ____ _____

(10) Hold syringe at a 90-degree angle at eye level to ensure correct volume and absence of air bubbles. Remove any remaining air by tapping barrel to dislodge any air bubbles. Draw back slightly on plunger, then push plunger upward to eject air. Do not eject fluid. Recheck volume of medication. ____ ____ ____ _____

(11) If medication is to be injected into client's tissue, change needle to appropriate gauge and length according to route of medication. ____ ____ ____ _____

(12) For multidose vial, make label that includes date of mixing, concentration of drug per milliliter, and nurse's initials. ____ ____ ____ _____

C. Vial containing a powder (reconstituting medications):

(1) Remove cap covering vial of powdered medication and cap covering vial of proper diluent. Firmly swab both seals with an alcohol swab and allow to dry. ____ ____ ____ _____

(2) Draw up diluent into syringe by following steps 6B(2) through 6B(10). ____ ____ ____ _____

(3) Insert tip of needle through centre of rubber seal of powdered medication. Inject diluent into vial. Remove needle. ____ ____ ____ _____

(4) Mix medication thoroughly. Roll vial in palms. Do not shake. ____ ____ ____ _____

(5) Read label carefully to determine dose after reconstitution. ____ ____ ____ _____

(6) Prepare medication in syringe following steps 6B(2) through 6B(12). ____ ____ ____ _____

7. Dispose of soiled supplies. Place broken ampule and/or used vials and used needle in puncture-proof and leak-proof container. Clean work area and perform hand hygiene. ____ ____ ____ _____

SKILL PERFORMANCE CHECKLIST
Skill 30-8 Administering Injections

	S	U	NP	Comments
1. Review prescriber's medication order.	___	___	___	_____
2. Assess client's history of allergies.	___	___	___	_____
3. Check expiration date of medication.	___	___	___	_____
4. Observe client's verbal and non-verbal responses to receiving an injection.	___	___	___	_____
5. Assess for contraindications to subcutaneous or intramuscular injections.	___	___	___	_____
6. Perform hand hygiene. Prepare correct medication dose from ampule or vial. Check carefully. Be sure all air is expelled.	___	___	___	_____
7. Identify client.	___	___	___	_____
8. Explain steps of procedure and tell client injection will cause a slight burning or sting.	___	___	___	_____
9. Provide privacy.	___	___	___	_____
10. Perform hand hygiene. Apply disposable gloves.	___	___	___	_____
11. Keep sheet or gown draped over client's body parts not requiring exposure.	___	___	___	_____
12. Select appropriate injection site. Inspect skin surface of site for bruises, inflammation, or edema:	___	___	___	_____
A. For subcutaneous (Sub-Q) injections: Palpate sites for masses or tenderness. Avoid these areas. For daily insulin, rotate site daily. Check that needle is correct size by grasping skinfold at site with thumb and forefinger. Measure fold from top to bottom. Needle should be one-half length.	___	___	___	_____
B. For intramuscular (IM) injections: Note integrity and size of muscle and palpate for tender or hard areas. Avoid these areas. If injections are given frequently, rotate sites.	___	___	___	_____
C. For intradermal (ID) injections: Note lesions or discoloration of forearm. Select site three to four fingerwidths below antecubital space and a handwidth above wrist. If forearm cannot be used, inspect the upper back. If necessary, sites for Sub-Q injections may be used.	___	___	___	_____

Continued

	S	U	NP	Comments
13. Assist client to a comfortable position:	___	___	___	_____
A. For Sub-Q injections: Have client relax arm, leg, or abdomen, depending on site chosen.	___	___	___	_____
B. For IM injections: Have client lie flat, on side, or prone, depending on site chosen.	___	___	___	_____
C. For ID injections: Have client extend elbow and support it and forearm on flat surface.	___	___	___	_____
D. Talk with client about subject of interest.	___	___	___	_____
14. Relocate site using anatomical landmarks.	___	___	___	_____
15. Cleanse site with an antiseptic swab. Apply swab at centre of site and rotate outward in a circular direction for about 5 cm.	___	___	___	_____
16. Hold swab or gauze between third and fourth fingers of non-dominant hand.	___	___	___	_____
17. Remove needle cap or sheath from needle by pulling it straight off.	___	___	___	_____
18. Hold syringe between thumb and forefinger of dominant hand:	___	___	___	_____
A. For Sub-Q injections: Hold as dart, palm down or hold across tops of fingertips.	___	___	___	_____
B. For IM injection: Hold as dart, palm down.	___	___	___	_____
C. For ID injections: Hold bevel of needle pointing up.	___	___	___	_____
19. Administer injection:				
A. Subcutaneous injection:				
(1) For average-size client, spread skin tightly across injection site or pinch skin with non-dominant hand.	___	___	___	_____
(2) Inject needle quickly and firmly at a 45- to 90-degree angle, then release skin, if pinched.	___	___	___	_____
(3) For obese client, pinch skin at site and inject needle at 90-degree angle below tissue fold.	___	___	___	_____
(4) Inject medication slowly.	___	___	___	_____
B. Intramuscular injection:				
(1) Position non-dominant hand at proper anatomical landmarks and pull skin down to administer in a Z-track.	___ ___	___	___	_____
(2) If client's muscle mass is small, grasp body of muscle between thumb and fingers.	___	___	___	_____

Continued

	S	U	NP	Comments

(3) Inject needle quickly into muscle at a 90-degree angle. After needle enters site, grasp lower end of syringe barrel with non-dominant hand. Continue to hold skin tightly with non-dominant hand. Move dominant hand to end of plunger. Do not move syringe. ____ ____ ____ _____

(4) Pull back on plunger 5 to 10 seconds. If no blood appears, inject medicine slowly, at a rate of 10 sec/mL. ____ ____ ____ _____

(5) Wait 10 seconds, then smoothly and steadily withdraw needle and release skin. Apply gentle pressure with dry gauze if desired. ____ ____ ____ _____

C. Intradermal injection:

(1) With non-dominant hand, stretch skin across injection site with forefinger or thumb. ____ ____ ____ _____

(2) Place needle almost against client's skin and insert it slowly at a 5- to 15-degree angle until resistance is felt. Advance needle through epidermis approximately 3 mm below skin surface so that needle tip can be seen through skin. ____ ____ ____ _____

(3) Inject medication slowly. Remove needle and begin again if no resistance is felt. ____ ____ ____ _____

(4) While injecting medication, notice that a small bleb approximately 6 mm in diameter appears on skin's surface. ____ ____ ____ _____

20. Withdraw needle while applying alcohol swab or gauze gently over site. ____ ____ ____ _____

21. Apply gentle pressure. Do not massage site. Apply bandage if needed. ____ ____ ____ _____

22. Assist client to a comfortable position. ____ ____ ____ _____

23. Discard uncapped needle or needle enclosed in safety shield and attached syringe into puncture- and leak-proof receptacle. If unable to leave client's bedside, use a one-handed technique to recap needle. ____ ____ ____ _____

24. Remove and dispose of gloves. Perform hand hygiene. ____ ____ ____ _____

25. Stay with client 3 to 5 minutes and observe for any allergic reactions. ____ ____ ____ _____

Continued

	S	U	NP	Comments
26. Periodically return to client's room to ask if client feels any acute pain, burning, numbness, or tingling at injection site.	___	___	___	_____
27. Inspect site, noting any bruising or induration.	___	___	___	_____
28. Observe client's response to medication that correlates with the medication's onset, peak, and duration.	___	___	___	_____
29. Ask client to explain purpose and effects of medication.	___	___	___	_____
30. For ID injections, use skin pencil and draw circle around perimeter of injection site. Check site within 48 to 72 hours of injection.	___	___	___	_____

452

SKILL PERFORMANCE CHECKLIST
Skill 30-9 Adding Medications to Intravenous Fluid Containers

	S	U	NP	Comments
1. Check prescriber's order to determine type of intravenous (IV) solution to use medication, dosage, rout, and drug indication.	____	____	____	_____
2. Collect necessary information for safe administration of the drug.	____	____	____	_____
3. Assess for the compatibility of multiple medications in a single IV solution.	____	____	____	_____
4. Assess client's systemic fluid balance.	____	____	____	_____
5. Assess client's history of medication allergies.	____	____	____	_____
6. Assess IV insertion site for signs of infiltration or phlebitis	____	____	____	_____
7. Perform hand hygiene.	____	____	____	_____
8. Assemble supplies in medication room.	____	____	____	_____
9. Prepare prescribed medication from vial or ampule.	____	____	____	_____
10. Identify client.	____	____	____	_____
11. Assess client's understanding of medication therapy.	____	____	____	_____
12. Add medication to new container:				
A. Solutions in bags: Locate medication injection port on plastic IV solution bag. Port has small rubber stopper at end. Do not select port for the IV tubing insertion or air vent.	____	____	____	_____
B. Solutions in bottles: Locate injection site on IV solution bottle, which is often covered by a metal or plastic cap.	____	____	____	_____
C. Wipe off port or injection site with alcohol or antiseptic swab.	____	____	____	_____
D. Remove needle cap or sheath from syringe and insert needle through centre of injection port or site. Inject medication.	____	____	____	_____
E. Withdraw syringe from bag or bottle.	____	____	____	_____
F. Mix medication and IV solution by holding bag or bottle and turning it gently end to end.	____	____	____	_____
G. Complete medication label with name, dose of medication, date, time, and initials. Apply it to bottle or bag. Spike bag or bottle with IV tubing.	____	____	____	_____
13. Bring assembled items to client's bedside.	____	____	____	_____
14. Explain procedure to client and alert client to expected sensations.	____	____	____	_____

Continued

	S	U	NP	Comments
15. Regulate infusion at ordered rate.	___	___	___	_____
16. Add medication to existing container:				
A. Prepare vented IV bottle or plastic bag:				
(1) Check volume of solution remaining in bottle or bag.	___	___	___	_____
(2) Close off IV infusion clamp.	___	___	___	_____
(3) Wipe off medication port with an alcohol or antiseptic swab.	___	___	___	_____
(4) Insert syringe needle or needleless device through injection port and inject medication.	___	___	___	_____
(5) Withdraw syringe.	___	___	___	_____
(6) Lower bag or bottle from IV pole and gently mix. Re-hang bag.	___	___	___	_____
B. Complete medication label and apply it to bag or bottle.	___	___	___	_____
C. Regulate infusion to desired rate. Use IV pump if indicated.	___	___	___	_____
17. Properly dispose of equipment and supplies. Do not cap needle of syringe. Discard sheathed needles as a unit with needle covered.	___	___	___	_____
18. Perform hand hygiene.	___	___	___	_____
19. Observe client for signs and symptoms of medication reaction.	___	___	___	_____
20. Observe for signs and symptoms of fluid volume excess.	___	___	___	_____
21. Periodically return to client's room to assess IV insertion site and rate of infusion.	___	___	___	_____
22. Observe for signs or symptoms of IV infiltration.	___	___	___	_____

STUDENT: _____ DATE: _____

INSTRUCTOR: _____ DATE: _____

Skill 30-10 Administering Intravenous Medications by Intravenous Bolus

	S	U	NP	Comments
1. Check prescriber's order.	____	____	____	_____
2. Perform hand hygiene. Assess intravenous (IV) or saline (herparin) lock insertion site for infiltraticn or phlebitis.	____	____	____	_____
3. If medication is to be pushed into an IV line, assess the patency of the line by noting infusion rate.	____	____	____	_____
4. Prepare medication from vial or ampule.	____	____	____	_____
5. Perform hand hygiene. Apply gloves.	____	____	____	_____
6. Identify client.	____	____	____	_____
7. Administer medication by IV push (existing line):				
A. Select injection port of IV tubing closest to client. Whenever possible, injection port should accept a needleless syringe. Use IV filter if required.	____	____	____	_____
B. Cleanse injection port with antiseptic swab. Allow to dry.	____	____	____	_____
C. Connect syringe to IV line: Insert needleless tip or small-gauge needle of syringe containing prepared drug through centre of injection port.	____	____	____	_____
D. Occlude IV line by pinching tubing just above injection port. Aspirate for blood return.	____	____	____	_____
E. Release tubing and inject medication within recommended time. Time administration of medication. Allow IV fluids to infuse when not pushing medication.	____	____	____	_____
F. Release tubing, withdraw syringe, and recheck fluid infusion rate.	____	____	____	_____
8. Administer medication by IV push (IV lock or needleless system):				
A. Prepare flush solutions per agency policy.	____	____	____	_____
B. Administer medication.				
(1) Cleanse lock's injection port with antiseptic swab.	____	____	____	_____
(2) Insert syringe containing normal saline into injection port of IV lock.	____	____	____	_____
(3) Pull back gently on syringe plunger and look for blood return.	____	____	____	_____

Continued

	S	U	NP	Comments
(4) Flush IV lock with 1 mL saline by pushing slowly on plunger.	___	___	___	_____
(5) Remove syringe.	___	___	___	_____
(6) Cleanse lock's injection port with antiseptic swab.	___	___	___	_____
(7) Insert medication syringe into injection port.	___	___	___	_____
(8) Inject medication within recommended time. Time administration.	___	___	___	_____
(9) Withdraw syringe.	___	___	___	_____
(10) Cleanse injection port with antiseptic swab.	___	___	___	_____
(11) Attach syringe with normal saline and inject normal saline flush at the same rate that the medication was delivered.	___	___	___	_____
(12) (Heparin flush option: Insert needle of syringe containing heparin through diaphragm.)	___	___	___	_____
9. Dispose of all equipment properly.	___	___	___	_____
10. Remove and dispose of gloves. Perform hand hygiene.	___	___	___	_____
11. Observe client closely for adverse reactions during and for several minutes after administration.	___	___	___	_____

STUDENT: _____ DATE: _____

INSTRUCTOR: _____ DATE: _____

Skill 30-11 Administering Intravenous Medications by Piggyback, Intermittent Intravenous Infusion Sets, and Mini-Infusion Pumps

	S	U	NP	Comments
1. Check prescriber's order to determine type of IV solution to be used; name of medication, dose, route, time of administration, and drug indication.	____	____	____	_____
2. Collect necessary information for safe medication administration.	____	____	____	_____
3. Assess compatibility of drug with existing IV solution.	____	____	____	_____
4. Assess patency of client's existing IV infusion line by noting infusion rate of main IV line.	____	____	____	_____
5. Perform hand hygiene. Assess IV insertion site for signs of infiltration or phlebitis.	____	____	____	_____
6. Assess client's history of medication allergies.	____	____	____	_____
7. Assess client's understanding of the purpose of the drug therapy.	____	____	____	_____
8. Assemble supplies at client's bedside. Prepare client by informing him or her that medication will be given through IV equipment.	____	____	____	_____
9. Perform hand hygiene.	____	____	____	_____
10. Identify client.	____	____	____	_____
11. Explain purpose of medication and side effects to client. Encourage client to report symptoms of discomfort at site.	____	____	____	_____
12. Administer infusion:				
A. Piggyback or tandem infusion:				
(1) Connect infusion tubing to medication bag. Allow solution to fill tubing by opening regulator flow clamp. Once tubing is full, close cap and cap end of tubing.	____	____	____	_____
(2) Hang piggyback medication bag above level of primary fluid bag. Hang tandem infusion at same level as primary fluid bag.	____	____	____	_____
(3) Connect tubing of piggyback or tandem infusion to appropriate connector on primary infusion line:	____	____	____	_____
(a) Stopcock: Wipe off stopcock port with alcohol swab and connect tubing. Turn stopcock to open position.	____	____	____	_____

Continued

	S	U	NP	Comments

(b) Needleless system: Wipe off needleless port and insert tip of piggyback or tandem infusion tubing. _____ _____ _____ _____

(c) Tubing port: Connect sterile needle to end of piggyback or tandem infusion tubing, remove cap, cleanse injection port on main IV line, and insert needle through centre of port. Secure connection with tape. _____ _____ _____ _____

(4) Regulate flow rate of medication solution by adjusting regulator clamp. _____ _____ _____ _____

(5) After medication has infused, check flow regulator on primary infusion. _____ _____ _____ _____

(6) Regulate main infusion line to desired rate, if necessary. _____ _____ _____ _____

(7) Leave secondary bag and tubing in place for future drug administration or discard in appropriate containers. _____ _____ _____ _____

B. Volume-control administration set:

(1) Assemble supplies in medication room. _____ _____ _____ _____

(2) Prepare medication from vial or ampule. _____ _____ _____ _____

(3) Fill volume-control set with desired amount of fluid (50 to 100 mL) by opening clamp between volume-control set and main IV bag. _____ _____ _____ _____

(4) Close clamp and check to be sure clamp on air vent of volume-control set chamber is open. _____ _____ _____ _____

(5) Clean injection port with antiseptic swab. _____ _____ _____ _____

(6) Remove needle cap or sheath and insert syringe needle through port, then inject medication. Gently rotate volume-control set between hands. _____ _____ _____ _____

(7) Regulate IV infusion rate to allow medication to infuse in recommended time. _____ _____ _____ _____

(8) Label volume-control set with name of medication, dosage, total volume including diluent, and time of administration. _____ _____ _____ _____

(9) Dispose of uncapped needle or needle enclosed in safety shield and syringe in proper container. _____ _____ _____ _____

Continued

	S	U	NP	Comments

C. Mini-infusion administration:

(1) Connect prefilled syringe to mini-infusion tubing. ____ ____ ____ _____

(2) Carefully apply pressure to syringe plunger, allowing tubing to fill with medication. ____ ____ ____ _____

(3) Place syringe into mini-infusor pump. Be sure syringe is secure. ____ ____ ____ _____

(4) Connect mini-infusion tubing to main IV line. ____ ____ ____ _____

    (a) Stopcock: Wipe off stopcock port with alcohol swab and connect tubing. Turn stopcock to open position. ____ ____ ____ _____

    (b) Needleless system: Wipe off needleless port and insert tip of mini-infusor tubing. ____ ____ ____ _____

    (c) Tubing port: Connect sterile needle to mini-infusion tubing, remove cap, cleanse injection port on main IV line, and insert needle through centre of port. ____ ____ ____ _____

(5) Explain purpose of medication and side effects to client. Ask client to report symptoms of discomfort at site. ____ ____ ____ _____

(6) Hang infusion pump with syringe on IV pole alongside main IV bag. Set pump to deliver medication within recommended time. Press button on pump to begin infusion. Optional: set alarm. ____ ____ ____ _____

(7) After medication has infused, check flow regulator on primary infusion. Regulate main infusion line to desired rate as needed. (Note: If stopcock is used, turn off mini-infusion line.) ____ ____ ____ _____

13. Observe client for signs of adverse reactions. ____ ____ ____ _____

14. During infusion, periodically check infusion rate and condition of IV site. ____ ____ ____ _____

15. Ask client to explain purpose and side effects of medication. ____ ____ ____ _____

SKILL PERFORMANCE CHECKLIST
Skill 33-1 Applying Restraints

	S	U	NP	Comments
1. Assess client's need for restraint.	___	___	___	_____
2. Assess client's behaviour.	___	___	___	_____
3. Review agency policies regarding restraints. Determine if signed consent for use of restraint is needed.	___	___	___	_____
4. Review restraint manufacturer's instructions before entering client's room. Determine most appropriate size restraint.	___	___	___	_____
5. Perform hand hygiene and gather equipment.	___	___	___	_____
6. Introduce yourself. Explain to client and family the need for restraint. Attempt to obtain consent.	___	___	___	_____
7. Assess the area of the client's body where the restraint is to be placed.	___	___	___	_____
8. Approach client in a calm manner and explain procedure.	___	___	___	_____
9. Adjust bed to proper height and lower side rail on side of client contact.	___	___	___	_____
10. Provide privacy. Place client in proper body alignment.	___	___	___	_____
11. Pad skin and bony prominences before applying restraints.	___	___	___	_____
12. Apply restraint, making sure it is not over an IV line or other device.	___	___	___	_____
A. Jacket (vest or Posey) restraint: Apply over clothing or hospital gown. Place client's hands through armholes or sleeves, and secure according to manufacturer's directions. Place straps at client's hips.	___	___	___	_____
B. Belt restraint: Apply over clothes or gown: Remove wrinkles from front and back of restraint while placing it around client's wrist. Bring ties through slots in belt. Avoid placing belt across the chest or too tightly across the abdomen.	___	___	___	_____
C. Extremity (ankle or wrist) restraint: Limb restraint is wrapped around wrist or ankle with soft part toward skin and secured snugly in place by Velcro straps.	___	___	___	_____
D. Mitten restraint: Place hand in mitten, being sure end is brought all the way up over the wrist.	___	___	___	_____

Continued

	S	U	NP	Comments

E. Elbow restraint: Piece of fabric with slots in which tongue blades are placed so that elbow joint remains rigid.   ____ ____ ____ _____

F. Mummy restraint: Place child on blanket with shoulders at fold and feet toward opposite corner. With child's right arm straight down against body, pull right side of blanket firmly across right shoulder and chest and secure beneath left side of body. Place left arm straight against body and bring left side of blanket across shoulder and chest and beneath child's body on right side. Fold lower corner, bring over body, and tuck or fasten securely with safety pins.   ____ ____ ____ _____

13. Attach restraints to bed frame, not side rails.   ____ ____ ____ _____

14. When client is in a chair, secure jacket restraint by placing ties under armrests and securing them at the back of the chair.   ____ ____ ____ _____

15. Secure restraints with a quick-release tie.   ____ ____ ____ _____

16. Make sure two fingers will fit under secured restraint.   ____ ____ ____ _____

17. Assess proper placement of restraint and condition of client's restrained body part at least every hour or per agency policy.   ____ ____ ____ _____

18. Remove restraints at regular intervals according to agency policy. If client is violent and non-compliant, remove one restraint at a time, and/or have staff assistance while removing restraints. Client should not be left unattended at this time.   ____ ____ ____ _____

19. Secure call light or intercom within client's reach.   ____ ____ ____ _____

20. Leave client's bed or chair with wheels locked. Bed should be in lowest position.   ____ ____ ____ _____

21. Perform hand hygiene.   ____ ____ ____ _____

22. Inspect client for any injury, including all hazards of immobility, while restraints are in use.   ____ ____ ____ _____

23. Observe IV catheters, urinary catheters, and drainage tubes to determine that they are positioned correctly and that therapy remains uninterrupted.   ____ ____ ____ _____

24. Regularly reassess client's need for continued use of restraint with the intent of discontinuing restraint at the earliest possible time.   ____ ____ ____ _____

25. Provide sensory stimulation and reorient client as needed.   ____ ____ ____ _____

SKILL PERFORMANCE CHECKLIST
Skill 33-2 Seizure Precautions

	S	U	NP	Comments
1. Assess seizure history, related medical/ surgical conditions, and medication history.	___	___	___	_____
2. Inspect client's environment for safety hazards.	___	___	___	_____
3. Perform hand hygiene and prepare bed with padded side rails and headboard, bed in low position, and client positioned in side-lying position when possible.	___	___	___	_____
4. Have airway, suction equipment, clean gloves, and pillows available in room.	___	___	___	_____
5. Position client safely if seizure begins. Guide the sitting or standing client to the floor. Cradle client's head in lap or place pillow beneath it. Clear area of furniture. Lower bed and raise side rails (padded) for client in bed.	___	___	___	_____
6. Provide privacy.	___	___	___	_____
7. Turn client on side, if possible, with head flexed slightly forward.	___	___	___	_____
8. Do not restrain client. Loosen client's clothing.	___	___	___	_____
9. Do not place anything in client's mouth.	___	___	___	_____
10. Stay with client. Observe sequence and timing of seizure activity.	___	___	___	_____
11. After seizure, explain occurrence, and offer support.	___	___	___	_____
12. Following seizure, perform hand hygiene and assist client to a position of comfort; place bed in a low position with call light within reach. Provide a quiet environment.	___	___	___	_____
Status Epilepticus:				
13. For a client experiencing status epilepticus, put on disposable gloves and insert an oral airway when the jaw is relaxed between seizure activity. Hold airway and curved side up, insert downward until airway reaches back of throat, then rotate and follow natural curve of the tongue.	___	___	___	_____
14. Access oxygen/suction equipment. Prepare for IV insertion.	___	___	___	_____
15. Use pillows/pads to protect client from injuring self.	___	___	___	_____

SKILL PERFORMANCE CHECKLIST
Skill 34-1 Bathing a Client

	S	U	NP	Comments
1. Assess client's tolerance for activity, discomfort level, cognitive ability, and musculoskeletal function.	___	___	___	_____
2. Assess client's bathing preferences.	___	___	___	_____
3. Ask if client has noticed any skin problems or changes.	___	___	___	_____
4. Review orders for specific precautions concerning client's movement or positioning.	___	___	___	_____
5. Explain procedure to client and ask client about bathing preferences.	___	___	___	_____
6. Prepare room for comfort and privacy.	___	___	___	_____
7. Perform hand hygiene. Prepare equipment and supplies.	___	___	___	_____
8. Offer client bedpan or urinal. Provide towel and washcloth.	___	___	___	_____
9. Perform hand hygiene. Apply disposable gloves as needed.	___	___	___	_____
10. Bathe client:				
A. Complete or partial bed bath:				
(1) Place bed at appropriate height. Lower side rail closest to you, and assist client in assuming a comfortable position that maintains body alignment. Bring client toward side of bed closest to you.	___	___	___	_____
(2) Loosen top covers at foot of bed. Place bath blanket over top sheet. Fold and remove top sheet from under blanket.	___	___	___	_____
(3) If top sheet is to be reused, fold it for later replacement. If not, place it in linen bag.	___	___	___	_____
(4) Remove client's gown or pajamas.	___	___	___	_____
(5) Pull side rail up. Fill washbasin two-thirds full with warm water. Have client test temperature.	___	___	___	_____
(6) Remove pillow if allowed and raise head of bed 30 to 45 degrees. Place bath towel under client's head. Place second bath towel over client's chest.	___	___	___	_____
(7) Immerse washcloth in warm water and wring thoroughly. Fold washcloth around fingers of your hand to form mitt.	___	___	___	_____

Continued

	S	U	NP	Comments

(8) Inquire if client is wearing contact lenses. Wash client's eyes with plain warm water. Use different section of mitt for each eye. Move mitt from inner to outer canthus. Soak any crusts on eyelid for 2 to 3 minutes with damp cloth before attempting removal. Dry eye thoroughly but gently.

(9) Ask if client prefers to use soap on face. Wash, rinse, and thoroughly dry client's forehead, cheeks, nose, neck, and ears.

(10) Remove bath blanket from client's arm that is closest to you. Place bath towel lengthwise under arm.

(11) Bathe client's arm with soap and water using long, firm strokes from distal to proximal areas. Raise and support client's arm above head (if possible) while washing axilla.

(12) Rinse and dry arm and axilla thoroughly. Apply deodorant or talcum powder, if used.

(13) Fold bath towel in half and lay it on bed beside client. Place basin on towel. Immerse client's hand in water. Allow hand to soak for 3 to 5 minutes before washing hand and fingernails. Remove basin and dry hand well.

(14) Raise side rail and move to other side of bed. Lower side rails and repeat steps 10 through 13 for other arm.

(15) Check temperature of bath water, and change water if necessary.

(16) Cover client's chest with bath towel, and fold bath blanket down to umbilicus. Lift edge of towel away from client's chest. Bathe client's chest using long, firm strokes with mitted hand. Wash skinfolds under female clients' breasts. Keep client's chest covered between washing and rinsing. Dry well.

(17) Place bath towel(s) lengthwise over client's chest and abdomen. Fold blanket down to just above client's pubic region.

Continued

466

	S	U	NP	Comments

(18) Lift bath towel. Bathe client's abdomen with mitted hand. Stroke from side to side. Keep client's abdomen covered between washing and rinsing. Dry well.

(19) Help client put on clean gown or pajama top.

(20) Cover client's chest and abdomen with top of bath blanket. Expose client's nearer leg by folding blanket toward midline. Drape client's perineum and other leg.

(21) Bend client's leg at knee by positioning your arm under client's leg. Elevate leg from mattress slightly while grasping client's heel, and slide bath towel lengthwise under leg. Ask client to hold foot still. Place bath basin on towel on bed, and secure its position next to the foot to be washed.

(22) With one hand supporting lower leg, raise it and slide basin under lifted foot. Make sure foot is firmly placed on bottom of basin. Allow foot to soak while washing leg. If client is unable to hold leg, do not immerse; simply wash with washcloth.

(23) Use long, firm strokes in washing from client's ankle to knee and from knee to thigh, unless contraindicated. Dry well.

(24) Cleanse foot, making sure to bathe between toes. Clean and clip nails as per physician's orders. Dry well. Apply lotion to dry skin. Do not massage any reddened area on client's skin.

(25) Raise side rail and move to other side of bed. Lower side rail and repeat steps 20 through 24 for client's other leg and foot.

(26) Cover client with bath blanket, raise side rail for client's safety, and change bath water.

Continued

	S	U	NP	Comments

(27) Lower side rail. Assist client in assuming a prone or side-lying position (as applicable). Place towel lengthwise along client's side.

(28) Keep client draped by sliding bath blanket over shoulders and thighs. Wash, rinse, and dry back from neck to buttocks using long, firm strokes. Give client a back rub.

(29) Apply disposable gloves if not done previously.

(30) Assist client in assuming a side-lying or supine position. Cover chest and upper extremities with towel and lower extremities with bath blanket. Expose genitalia only. Provide perineal care, paying special attention to skin folds..

(31) Dispose of gloves in receptacle.

(32) Apply additional body lotion or oil as desired.

(33) Assist client in dressing. Comb client's hair.

(34) Make client's bed.

(35) Remove soiled linen and place it in linen bag. Clean and replace bathing equipment. Replace call light and client's personal possessions. Leave room as clean and comfortable as possible.

(36) Perform hand hygiene.

B. Tub or whirlpool bath or shower (verify if physician's order is needed):

(1) Consider client's condition, and review orders for precautions.

(2) Check tub or shower for cleanliness. Use cleaning techniques outlined in agency policy. Place rubber mat on tub or shower bottom. Place disposable bath mat or towel on floor in front of tub or shower.

(3) Collect all hygienic aids, toiletry items, and linens requested by client. Place within easy reach of tub or shower.

(4) Assist client to bathroom if necessary. Have client wear robe and slippers to bathroom.

(5) Demonstrate how to use call signal for assistance.

Continued

	S	U	NP	Comments
(6) Place "Occupied" sign on bathroom door.	___	___	___	_____
(7) Provide tub chair or shower seat if needed. Fill bathtub halfway with warm water. Ask client to test water, and adjust temperature if needed. Show client which faucet controls hot water. If client is taking a shower, turn shower on and adjust temperature before client enters shower stall.	___	___	___	_____
(8) Instruct client to use safety bars when getting in and out of tub or shower. Caution client against use of bath oil in tub water.	___	___	___	_____
(9) Instruct client not to remain in tub longer than 20 minutes. Check on client every 5 minutes. Observe client's range of motion during the bath.	___	___	___	_____
(10) Return to bathroom when client signals, and knock before entering.	___	___	___	_____
(11) Drain tub before client attempts to get out of it. Place bath towel over client's shoulders. Assist client as needed.	___	___	___	_____
(12) Observe client's skin, paying particular attention to areas that were previously soiled, reddened, or that showed early signs of breakdown.	___	___	___	_____
(13) Assist client in donning clothing, if necessary.	___	___	___	_____
(14) Assist client to room and to a comfortable position in bed or chair.	___	___	___	_____
(15) Clean tub or shower according to agency policy. Remove soiled linen and place it in linen bag. Discard disposable equipment in proper receptacle. Place "Unoccupied" sign on bathroom door. Return supplies to storage area.	___	___	___	_____
(16) Perform hand hygiene.	___	___	___	_____
11. Ask client to rate level of comfort.	___	___	___	_____

STUDENT: _____ DATE: _____

INSTRUCTOR: _____ DATE: _____

SKILL PERFORMANCE CHECKLIST
Skill 34-2 Perineal Care

	S	U	NP	Comments
1. Assess client's risk for developing infection of genitalia, urinary tract, or reproductive tract.	____	____	____	_____
2. Assess client's cognitive and musculoskeletal function.	____	____	____	_____
3. Apply disposable gloves. Assess client's genitalia for signs of inflammation, skin breakdown, or infection.	____	____	____	_____
4. Assess client's knowledge of the importance of perineal hygiene.	____	____	____	_____
5. Explain procedure and its purpose to client.	____	____	____	_____
6. Prepare necessary equipment and supplies.	____	____	____	_____
7. Provide privacy. Assemble supplies at bedside.	____	____	____	_____
8. Raise bed to comfortable working position. Lower side rail, and assist client in assuming a side-lying position. Place towel lengthwise along client's side and keep client covered with bath blanket or top sheet.	____	____	____	_____
9. Apply disposable gloves.	____	____	____	_____
10. Remove any fecal matter in a fold of underpad or toilet tissue. Cleanse buttocks and anus, washing from front to back. Clean, rinse, and dry area thoroughly. Place an absorbent pad under client's buttocks. Remove and discard underpad and replace with clean pad.	____	____	____	_____
11. Change gloves when they are soiled. Perform hand hygiene.	____	____	____	_____
12. Fold top bed linen down toward foot of bed. Raise client's gown so genital area is exposed. To protect client's privacy, "diamond" drape client.	____	____	____	_____
13. Raise side rail. Fill washbasin with warm water.	____	____	____	_____
14. Place washbasin and toilet tissue on overbed table. Place washcloths in basin.	____	____	____	_____
15. Provide perineal care:				
A. Female perineal care:				
(1) Assist client to dorsal recumbent position.	____	____	____	_____
(2) Lower side rails, and help client flex knees and spread legs. Note limitations in client's positioning.	____	____	____	_____

Continued

471

	S	U	NP	Comments

(3) Fold lower corner of bath blanket up between client's legs onto abdomen. Wash and dry client's upper thighs. _____ _____ _____ _____

(4) Wash labia majora. Use non-dominant hand to gently retract labia from thigh. With dominant hand, carefully wash in skinfolds. Wipe from perineum to rectum (front to back). Repeat on opposite side using a different section of the washcloth. Rinse and dry area thoroughly. _____ _____ _____ _____

(5) Separate labia with non-dominant hand to expose urethral meatus and vaginal orifice. With dominant hand, wash downward from pubic area toward rectum in one smooth stroke. Use separate section of cloth for each stroke. Cleanse thoroughly around labia minora, clitoris, and vaginal orifice. _____ _____ _____ _____

(6) Pour warm water over perineal area if client uses bedpan. Dry perineal area thoroughly, using front-to-back method. _____ _____ _____ _____

(7) Fold lower corner of bath blanket back between client's legs and over perineum. Ask client to lower legs and assume comfortable position. _____ _____ _____ _____

B. Male perineal care:

(1) Lower side rails, and assist client to supine position. Note any restriction in client's mobility. _____ _____ _____ _____

(2) Fold lower corner of bath blanket up between client's legs and onto abdomen. Wash and dry client's upper thighs. _____ _____ _____ _____

(3) Gently raise penis and place bath towel underneath it. Gently grasp shaft of penis. Retract foreskin if client is uncircumcised. Defer procedure until later if client has an erection. _____ _____ _____ _____

(4) Wash tip of client's penis at urethral meatus first. Using circular motion, cleanse from meatus outward. Discard washcloth and repeat with clean cloth until penis is clean. Rinse and dry area gently. _____ _____ _____ _____

Continued

	S	U	NP	Comments
(5) Return foreskin to its natural position.	___	___	___	_____
(6) Wash shaft of penis with gentle but firm downward strokes. Pay special attention to underlying surface. Rinse and dry penis thoroughly. Instruct client to spread legs apart slightly.	___	___	___	_____
(7) Gently cleanse scrotum. Lift it carefully and wash underlying skin folds. Rinse and dry.	___	___	___	_____
(8) Fold bath blanket back over client's perineum, and assist client to a side-lying position.	___	___	___	_____
16. Apply thin layer of skin barrier containing petrolatum or zinc oxide over anal and perineal skin of incontinent clients.	___	___	___	_____
17. Remove gloves and dispose of them in proper receptacle. Perform hand hygiene.	___	___	___	_____
18. Assist client in assuming a comfortable position, and cover client with sheet.	___	___	___	_____
19. Remove bath blanket and dispose of all soiled bed linen. Return unused equipment to storage area.	___	___	___	_____
20. Inspect surface of external genitalia and surrounding skin after cleansing.	___	___	___	_____
21. Ask if client feels a sense of cleanliness.				
22. Observe for abnormal drainage or discharge from client's genitalia.	___	___	___	_____

STUDENT: _____ DATE: _____

INSTRUCTOR: _____ DATE: _____

SKILL PERFORMANCE CHECKLIST
Skill 34-3 Performing Nail and Foot Care

	S	U	NP	Comments
1. Inspect all surfaces of client's fingers, toes, feet, and nails. Also inspect areas between toes, heels, and soles of feet.	____	____	____	_____
2. Assess circulation to client's toes, feet, and fingers.	____	____	____	_____
3. Observe client's walking gait.				
4. Ask female clients whether they frequently use nail polish and polish remover.	____	____	____	_____
5. Assess type of footwear worn by client.	____	____	____	_____
6. Assess client's risk for foot or nail problems.	____	____	____	_____
7. Assess types of home remedies client uses for existing foot problems.	____	____	____	_____
8. Assess client's ability to care for nails or feet.	____	____	____	_____
9. Assess client's knowledge of foot and nail care practices.	____	____	____	_____
10. Explain procedure to client.	____	____	____	_____
11. Obtain physician's order for cutting client's nails if agency policy requires it.	____	____	____	_____
12. Perform hand hygiene. Arrange equipment on overbed table.	____	____	____	_____
13. Provide privacy.	____	____	____	_____
14. Assist ambulatory client to sit in bedside chair. Help bed-bound client to supine position with head of bed elevated. Place disposable bath mat on floor under client's feet, or place towel on mattress.	____	____	____	_____
15. Fill washbasin with warm water. Test temperature.	____	____	____	_____
16. Place basin on bath mat or towel, and help client place feet in basin. Place call light within client's reach.	____	____	____	_____
17. Adjust overbed table to low position, and place it over client's lap.	____	____	____	_____
18. Fill emesis basin with warm water, and place basin on paper towels on overbed table.	____	____	____	_____
19. Instruct client to place fingers in emesis basin and to place arms in a comfortable position.	____	____	____	_____
20. Allow feet and fingernails to soak for 10 to 20 minutes unless contraindicated. Rewarm water after 10 minutes.	____	____	____	_____
21. Clean gently under fingernails with orange stick while fingers are immersed. Remove emesis basin, and dry fingers thoroughly.	____	____	____	_____

Continued

Copyright © 2006 Elsevier Canada, Inc. All rights reserved.

475

	S	U	NP	Comments
22. Clip fingernails straight across and even with tops of fingers unless contraindicated. Shape nails with emery board or file.	____	____	____	_____
23. Push client's cuticles back gently with orange stick.	____	____	____	_____
24. Move overbed table away from client.	____	____	____	_____
25. Put on disposable gloves. Scrub callused areas of feet with washcloth.	____	____	____	_____
26. Clean gently under toenails with orange stick. Remove feet from basin and dry thoroughly.	____	____	____	_____
27. Clean and trim toenails using the procedures described in steps 22 and 23. Do not file corners of toenails.	____	____	____	_____
28. Apply lotion to feet and hands, and assist client back to bed and into a comfortable position.	____	____	____	_____
29. Remove disposable gloves and place in receptacle. Clean and return equipment and supplies to proper place. Dispose of soiled linen in hamper. Perform hand hygiene.	____	____	____	_____
30. Inspect nails and surrounding skin surfaces after soaking and nail trimming.	____	____	____	_____
31. Ask client to explain or demonstrate nail care.	____	____	____	_____
32. Observe client's walk after toenail care.	____	____	____	_____

STUDENT: _____ DATE: _____

INSTRUCTOR: _____ DATE: _____

Skill 34-4 Providing Oral Hygiene

	S	U	NP	Comments
1. Perform hand hygiene. Apply disposable gloves.	____	____	____	_____
2. Inspect integrity of lips, teeth, buccal mucosa, gums, palate, and tongue.	____	____	____	_____
3. Identify presence of common oral problems.	____	____	____	_____
4. Remove gloves and perform hand hygiene.	____	____	____	_____
5. Assess risk for oral hygiene problems.	____	____	____	_____
6. Assess risk for aspiration.	____	____	____	_____
7. Determine client's oral hygiene practices.	____	____	____	_____
8. Assess client's ability to grasp and manipulate a toothbrush.	____	____	____	_____
9. Prepare equipment at bedside.	____	____	____	_____
10. Explain procedure to client and discuss preferences regarding use of hygienic aids.	____	____	____	_____
11. Place paper towels on overbed table, and arrange other equipment within easy reach.	____	____	____	_____
12. Raise bed to comfortable working position. Raise head of bed (if allowed) and lower side rail. Move client, or help client move closer. The client can also be in a side-lying position.	____	____	____	_____
13. Place towel over client's chest.	____	____	____	_____
14. Apply gloves.	____	____	____	_____
15. Apply toothpaste to toothbrush while holding brush over emesis basin. Pour small amount of water over toothpaste.	____	____	____	_____
16. Hold toothbrush bristles at a 45-degree angle to gumline. Brush inner and outer surfaces of upper and lower teeth. Clean biting surfaces of teeth, and brush sides of teeth.	____	____	____	_____
17. Have client hold brush at a 45-degree angle and lightly brush over surface and sides of tongue. Instruct client to avoid initiating gag reflex.	____	____	____	_____
18. Allow client to rinse mouth thoroughly.	____	____	____	_____
19. Allow client to gargle to rinse mouth with mouthwash as desired.	____	____	____	_____
20. Assist in wiping client's mouth.	____	____	____	_____
21. Allow client to floss.	____	____	____	_____
22. Allow client to rinse mouth thoroughly with cool water and spit into emesis basin. Assist in wiping client's mouth.	____	____	____	_____

Continued

	S	U	NP	Comments

23. Assist client to a comfortable position, remove emesis basin and bedside table, raise side rail (if used), and lower bed to original position.

24. Wipe off overbed table. Discard soiled linens and paper towels in appropriate containers. Remove and dispose of soiled gloves. Return equipment to proper place.

25. Perform hand hygiene.

26. Ask client if any area of the oral cavity feels uncomfortable or irritated.

27. Apply gloves and inspect condition of client's oral cavity.

28. Ask client to describe proper oral hygiene techniques.

29. Observe client brushing teeth.

478

STUDENT: _____ DATE: _____

INSTRUCTOR: _____ DATE: _____

SKILL PERFORMANCE CHECKLIST
Skill 34-5 Performing Mouth Care for an Unconscious or Debilitated Client

	S	U	NP	Comments
1. Perform hand hygiene. Apply disposable gloves.	____	____	____	_____
2. Assess client's risk for oral hygiene problems.	____	____	____	_____
3. Test for presence of gag reflex.	____	____	____	_____
4. Inspect condition of oral cavity.	____	____	____	_____
5. Remove gloves. Perform hand hygiene.	____	____	____	_____
6. Explain procedure to client.	____	____	____	_____
7. Apply disposable gloves.	____	____	____	_____
8. Place paper towels on overbed table and arrange equipment. If needed, prepare suction.	____	____	____	_____
9. Provide privacy.	____	____	____	_____
10. Raise bed to appropriate working height. Lower head of bed and side rail.	____	____	____	_____
11. Position client on side, close to side of bed. Turn client's head toward dependant side. Raise side rail.	____	____	____	_____
12. Place towel under head and place emesis basin under chin.	____	____	____	_____
13. Carefully separate upper and lower teeth with padded tongue blade. Insert blade when client is relaxed, if possible. Do not use force.	____	____	____	_____
14. Clean mouth using toothbrush or sponge toothettes moistened with a commercial hydrogen peroxide solution if client can tolerate; otherwise, moisten with water. Clean chewing and inner tooth surfaces first. Clean outer tooth surfaces. Swab roof of mouth, gums, and insides of cheeks. Gently swab or brush tongue, but avoid stimulating the gag reflex. Rinse client's mouth with a clean, moistened swab, toothette, or bulb syringe. Repeat rinse several times.	____	____	____	_____
15. Suction secretions as they accumulate, if necessary.	____	____	____	_____
16. Apply thin layer of water-soluble jelly to lips.	____	____	____	_____
17. Inform client that procedure is complete.	____	____	____	_____
18. Reposition client comfortably, raise side rail (if used), and return bed to original position.	____	____	____	_____
19. Clean equipment and return it to its proper place. Place soiled linen in proper receptacle.	____	____	____	_____
20. Remove and discard gloves. Perform hand hygiene.	____	____	____	_____

Continued

	S	U	NP	Comments
21. Apply clean gloves and inspect oral cavity.	____	____	____	_____
22. Ask debilitated client if mouth feels clean.	____	____	____	_____
23. Assess client's respirations on an ongoing basis.	____	____	____	_____

STUDENT: _____ DATE: _____

INSTRUCTOR: _____ DATE: _____

SKILL PERFORMANCE CHECKLIST
Skill 34-6 Making an Occupied Bed

	S	U	NP	Comments
1. Assess potential for client incontinence or for excess drainage on bed linen.	___	___	___	_____
2. Check chart concerning orders or specific precautions for movement and positioning.	___	___	___	_____
3. Explain procedure to client.	___	___	___	_____
4. Perform hand hygiene. Apply gloves if necessary.	___	___	___	_____
5. Assemble and arrange equipment on bedside chair or table.	___	___	___	_____
6. Provide privacy.	___	___	___	_____
7. Adjust bed height to comfortable working position. Lower side rail on near side of bed. Remove call light.	___	___	___	_____
8. Loosen top linen at foot of bed.	___	___	___	_____
9. Remove bedspread and blanket separately. If soiled, place in a linen bag. Do not allow linen to contact uniform. Do not fan or shake linen.	___	___	___	_____
10. Fold blanket and spread if they will be reused. Fold them into neat squares and place them over back of chair.	___	___	___	_____
11. Cover client with bath blanket in following manner: Unfold bath blanket over top sheet. Ask client to hold top edge of bath blanket, or tuck top of bath blanket under client's shoulder. Grasp top sheet under bath blanket at client's shoulders, and bring sheet down to foot of bed. Remove sheet and discard it in linen bag.	___	___	___	_____
12. With assistance, slide mattress toward head of bed.	___	___	___	_____
13. Position client on the far side of the bed, turned onto side and facing away from you. Be sure rail in front of client is up. Adjust pillow under client's head.	___	___	___	_____
14. Loosen bottom bed linens, moving from head to foot of bed. Fanfold first draw sheet and then bottom sheet toward client. Tuck edges of linen just under buttocks, back, and shoulders.	___	___	___	_____
15. Wipe off moisture on mattress with towel and appropriate disinfectant.	___	___	___	_____

Continued

	S	U	NP	Comments

16. Apply clean linen to exposed half of bed:
    A. Place clean mattress pad on bed by folding it lengthwise with centre crease in middle of bed. Fanfold top layer over mattress. ___ ___ ___ _____
    B. Unfold bottom sheet lengthwise so centre crease is situated lengthwise along centre of bed. Fanfold sheet's top layer toward centre of bed alongside client. Smooth bottom layer of sheet over mattress, and bring edge over closest side of mattress. Pull fitted sheet smoothly over mattress ends. Allow edge of flat, unfitted sheet to hang about 25 cm over mattress edge. Lower hem of bottom sheet should lie seam down and even with bottom edge of mattress. ___ ___ ___ _____

17. Mitre bottom flat sheet at head of bed:
    A. Face head of bed diagonally. Place hand away from head of bed under top corner of mattress, near mattress edge, and lift. ___ ___ ___ _____
    B. Tuck top edge of bottom sheet smoothly under mattress. ___ ___ ___ _____
    C. Face side of bed and pick up top edge of sheet at approximately 45 cm from top of mattress. ___ ___ ___ _____
    D. Lift sheet and lay it on top of mattress to form neat triangular fold, with lower base of triangle even with mattress side edge. ___ ___ ___ _____
    E. Tuck lower edge of sheet, which is hanging free below mattress, under mattress. Tuck with palms down without pulling triangular fold. ___ ___ ___ _____
    F. Hold portion of sheet covering side of mattress in place with one hand. With other hand, pick up top of triangular linen fold and bring it down over side of mattress. Tuck this portion of sheet under mattress. ___ ___ ___ _____

18. Tuck remaining portion of sheet under mattress, moving toward foot of bed. Keep linen smooth. ___ ___ ___ _____

19. (Optional): Open draw sheet so it unfolds in half. Lay centre fold along middle of bed lengthwise, and position sheet so it will be under client's buttocks and torso. Fanfold top layer toward client with edge along client's back. Smooth bottom layer out over mattress, and tuck excess edge under mattress. ___ ___ ___ _____

Continued

	S	U	NP	Comments

20. Place waterproof pad over drawsheet, with centre fold against client's side. Fanfold top layer toward client.

21. Have client roll slowly toward you, over the layers of linen. Raise side rail on working side of bed and go to other side.

22. Lower side rail. Assist client in positioning on other side, over the folds of linen. Loosen edges of soiled linen from underneath mattress.

23. Remove soiled linen by folding it into a bundle or squares, with soiled side turned in. Discard in linen bag. If necessary, wipe mattress with antiseptic solution and let mattress dry before applying new linen.

24. Spread clean, fanfolded linen smoothly over edge of mattress from head to foot of bed.

25. Assist client in rolling back into supine position. Reposition pillow.

26. Pull fitted sheet smoothly over mattress ends. Mitre top corner of bottom sheet (see step 17). When tucking corner, be sure sheet is smooth and wrinkle-free.

27. Grasp remaining edge of bottom sheet. Keep back straight and pull while tucking excess linen under mattress. Proceed from head to foot of bed.

28. Smooth fan-folded drawsheet out over bottom sheet. Grasp edge of sheet with palms down, lean back, and tuck sheet under mattress. Tuck from middle to top and then to bottom.

29. Place top sheet over client, with centre fold lengthwise down middle of bed. Open sheet from head to foot, and unfold it over client.

30. Ask client to hold clean top sheet, or tuck sheet around client's shoulders. Remove bath blanket and discard in linen bag.

31. Place blanket on bed, unfolding it so that crease runs lengthwise along middle of bed. Unfold blanket to cover client. Top edge of blanket should be parallel with edge of top sheet and 15 to 20 cm down from top sheet's edge.

32. Place spread over bed according to step 31. Be sure top edge of spread extends about 2.5 cm above blanket's edge. Tuck top edge of spread over and under top edge of blanket.

33. Make cuff by turning edge of top sheet down over edge of blanket and spread.

Continued

	S	U	NP	Comments

34. Standing at foot of bed, lift mattress corner slightly with one hand and tuck top linens under mattress. Top sheet and blanket are tucked under together. Allow for movement of client's feet. (Making a horizontal toe pleat is an option.) ____ ____ ____ _____

35. Make modified mitred corner with top sheet, blanket, and spread: ____ ____ ____ _____
    A. Pick up side edge of top sheet, blanket, and spread approximately 45 cm from foot of mattress. Lift linens to form triangular fold, and lay it on bed. ____ ____ ____ _____
    B. Tuck lower edge of sheet, which is hanging free below mattress, under mattress. Do not pull triangular fold. ____ ____ ____ _____
    C. Pick up triangular fold, and bring it down over mattress while holding linen in place along side of mattress. Do not tuck tip of triangle. ____ ____ ____ _____

36. Raise side rail. Make other side of bed. Spread sheet, blanket, and bedspread out evenly. Fold top edge of spread over blanket, and make cuff with top sheet (see step 33). Make modified mitred corner at foot of bed (see step 35). ____ ____ ____ _____

37. Change pillowcase:
    A. Have client raise head. Remove pillow while supporting client's neck. ____ ____ ____ _____
    B. Remove soiled pillowcase and discard in linen bag. ____ ____ ____ _____
    C. Grasp clean pillowcase at centre of closed end. Gather case, turning it inside out over hand holding it. With the same hand, pick up middle of one end of pillow. Pull pillowcase down over pillow with other hand. ____ ____ ____ _____
    D. Fit pillow corners evenly in corners of pillowcase. ____ ____ ____ _____

38. Place call light within client's reach. Return bed to comfortable position. ____ ____ ____ _____

39. Open room curtains. Rearrange furniture. Place personal items easily within client's reach on overbed table or bedside stand. Return bed to comfortable height. ____ ____ ____ _____

40. Discard dirty linen and perform hand hygiene. ____ ____ ____ _____
41. Ask if client feels comfortable. ____ ____ ____ _____
42. Inspect skin for irritation. ____ ____ ____ _____
43. Observe for signs of fatigue, dyspnea, pain, or discomfort. ____ ____ ____ _____

SKILL PERFORMANCE CHECKLIST
Skill 35-1 Suctioning

	S	U	NP	Comments
1. Assess signs and symptoms of upper and lower airway obstruction requiring nasotracheal or orotracheal suctioning.	____	____	____	_____
2. Assess signs and symptoms associated with hypoxia and hypercapnia.	____	____	____	_____
3. Determine factors that normally influence upper or lower airway functioning.	____	____	____	_____
4. Assess client's understanding of procedure.	____	____	____	_____
5. Obtain physician's order if indicated by agency policy.	____	____	____	_____
6. Explain to client purpose of procedure and expected sensations. Encourage client to cough out secretions. Splint surgical incisions, if necessary.	____	____	____	_____
7. Explain importance of and encourage coughing during procedure.	____	____	____	_____
8. Help client to assume comfortable position.	____	____	____	_____
9. Place pulse oximeter on client's finger. Take reading and leave pulse oximeter in place.	____	____	____	_____
10. Place towel across client's chest.	____	____	____	_____
11. Perform hand hygiene.	____	____	____	_____
12. Preparation for all types of suctioning:				
A. Open suction kit or catheter with use of aseptic technique. Place sterile drape (if available) across client's chest or on the overbed table.	____	____	____	_____
B. Unwrap or open sterile basin and place on bedside table. Fill with about 100 mL of sterile normal saline solution or water.	____	____	____	_____
C. Connect one end of connecting tubing to suction machine. Place other end in convenient location near client. Check that equipment is functioning properly by suctioning a small amount of water from basin.	____	____	____	_____
D. Turn on suction device. Set regulator to appropriate negative pressure.	____	____	____	_____
13. Suction airway.				
A. Oropharyngeal suctioning:				
(1) Apply disposable glove to dominant hand.	____	____	____	_____
(2) Consider applying mask or face shield.	____	____	____	_____

Continued

	S	U	NP	Comments

(3) Attach suction catheter to connecting tubing. Remove oxygen mask if present.

(4) Insert catheter into client's mouth along gumline to pharynx. With suction applied, move catheter around mouth until secretions are cleared.

(5) Encourage client to cough, and repeat suctioning if needed. Replace oxygen mask if used.

(6) Suction water from basin through catheter until catheter is cleared of secretions.

(7) Place catheter in a clean, dry area with suction turned off or within client's reach, with suction on.

B. Nasopharyngeal and nasotracheal suctioning

(1) Increase supplemental oxygen therapy to 100% as indicated or as ordered. Encourage client to deep breathe.

(2) Open lubricant. Squeeze small amount onto open sterile catheter package.

(3) Apply sterile glove to each hand, or apply non-sterile glove to non-dominant hand and sterile glove to dominant hand.

(4) Pick up suction catheter with dominant hand without touching non-sterile surfaces. Pick up connecting tubing with non-dominant hand. Secure catheter to tubing.

(5) Suctioning small amount of normal saline solution from basin.

(6) Coat distal 6 to 8 cm of catheter with water-soluble lubricant.

(7) Remove oxygen delivery device, if applicable, with non-dominant hand. Without applying suction, gently insert catheter into naris during inhalation.

(8) *Nasopharyngeal:* Follow natural course of naris; slightly slant catheter downward and advance to back of pharynx. Insert catheter appropriate distance for child or adult.

Continued

486

	S	U	NP	Comments

(a) Apply intermittent suction for up to 10 to 15 seconds by placing and releasing non-dominant thumb over catheter vent. Slowly withdraw catheter while rotating it back and forth between thumb and forefinger.

(9) *Nasotracheal:* Follow natural course of naris and advance catheter slightly slanted and downward to just above entrance into trachea. Allow client to take a breath. Insert catheter appropriate distance for child or adult.

(a) Positioning option for nasotracheal suctioning: Turning client's head to right helps to suction left mainstem bronchus; turning head to left helps to suction right mainstem bronchus. If resistance is felt after insertion of catheter for maximum recommended distance, pull catheter back 1 cm before applying suction.

(b) Apply intermittent suction for up to 10 to 15 seconds by placing and releasing non-dominant thumb over vent of catheter and slowly withdrawing catheter while rotating it back and forth between dominant thumb and forefinger. Encourage client to cough. Replace oxygen device, if applicable.

(10) Rinse catheter and connecting tubing with normal saline or water until cleared.

(11) Assess for need to repeat suctioning procedure. Allow adequate time between suction passes. Ask client to deep breathe and cough.

C. Artificial airway suctioning
(1) Apply face shield.
(2) Prepare proper suction catheter.
(3) Apply one sterile glove to each hand, or apply non-sterile glove to non-dominant hand and sterile glove to dominant hand.

Continued

	S	U	NP	Comments

(4) Pick up suction catheter with dominant hand without touching non-sterile surfaces. Pick up connecting tubing with non-dominant hand. Secure catheter to tubing.

(5) Check that equipment is functioning properly by suctioning small amount of saline from basin.

(6) Hyperinflate and/or hyperoxygenate client before suctioning.

(7) Open swivel adapter or remove oxygen or humidity delivery device with non-dominant hand.

(8) Without applying suction, insert catheter into artificial airway using dominant thumb and forefinger until resistance is met or client coughs; then pull back 1 cm.

(9) Apply intermittent suction, and slowly withdraw catheter while rotating it back and forth between dominant thumb and forefinger. Encourage client to cough. Watch for respiratory distress.

(10) Close swivel adapter or replace oxygen delivery device.

(11) Encourage client to deep breathe, if able.

(12) Rinse catheter and connecting tubing with normal saline until clear. Use continuous suction.

(13) Assess client's cardiopulmonary status. Repeat steps 13C(6) through 13C(12) once or twice more to clear secretions. Allow adequate time between suction passes. Perform oropharyngeal and nasopharyngeal suctioning. Do not reinsert into endotracheal or tracheostomy tube.

14. Complete procedure:

A. Disconnect catheter. Roll catheter around fingers of dominant hand. Pull glove off inside out so that catheter remains in glove. Pull off other glove over first glove. Discard into appropriate receptacle. Turn off suction device.

Continued

488

	S	U	NP	Comments
B. Remove towel or drape and discard in appropriate receptacle.	___	___	___	_____
C. Reposition client as indicated by condition. Reapply clean gloves for client's personal care.	___	___	___	_____
D. If indicated, readjust oxygen to original level.	___	___	___	_____
E. Discard remainder of normal saline into appropriate receptacle. Discard or clean and replace basin.	___	___	___	_____
F. Remove and discard face shield, and perform hand hygiene.	___	___	___	_____
G. Place unopened suction kit on suction machine table or at head of bed according to institution preference.	___	___	___	_____
15. Compare client's vital signs and O_2 saturation before and after suctioning.	___	___	___	_____
16. Ask client if breathing is easier and if congestion is decreased.	___	___	___	_____
17. Observe airway secretions.	___	___	___	_____

SKILL PERFORMANCE CHECKLIST
Skill 35-2 Care of an Artificial Airway

	S	U	NP	Comments
1. Perform cardiopulmonary assessment.	___	___	___	_____
2. Explain procedure to client.	___	___	___	_____
3. Position client.	___	___	___	_____
4. Place towel across client's chest.	___	___	___	_____
5. Perform hand hygiene.	___	___	___	_____
6. Perform airway care:				
A. Endotracheal (ET) tube care:				
(1) Observe for signs and symptoms indicating the need to perform care of the artificial airway.	___	___	___	_____
(2) Identify factors that increase risk of complications from ET tubes.	___	___	___	_____
(3) Suction ET tube:	___	___	___	_____
(a) Instruct client not to bite or move ET tube.	___	___	___	_____
(b) Leave Yankauer suction catheter connected to suction source.	___	___	___	_____
(4) Prepare tape. Cut piece of tape long enough to go completely around client's head from naris to naris plus 15 cm—about 30 to 60 cm (for adult). Lay adhesive side up on bedside table. Cut and lay 8 to 16 cm of tape, adhesive side down, in centre of long strip to prevent tape from sticking to hair.	___	___	___	_____
(5) Have an assistant apply a pair of gloves and hold ET tube firmly so that tube does not move.	___	___	___	_____
(a) Carefully remove tape from ET tube and client's face. If tape is difficult to remove, moisten with water or adhesive tape remover. Discard tape in appropriate receptacle if nearby. If not, place soiled tape on bedside table or on distant end of towel.	___	___	___	_____
(b) Use adhesive remover swab to remove excess adhesive left on face after tape removal.	___	___	___	_____
(c) Remove oral airway or bite block if present.	___	___	___	_____

Continued

	S	U	NP	Comments

(d) Clean mouth, gums, and teeth opposite ET tube with mouthwash solution and 4 × 4 gauze, sponge-tipped applicators, or saline swabs. Brush teeth as indicated. If necessary, administer oropharyngeal suctioning with Yankauer catheter.

(e) Note "cm" ET tube marking at lips or gums. With help of assistant, move ET tube to opposite side or centre of mouth. Do not change tube depth.

(f) Repeat oral cleaning on opposite side of mouth.

(g) Clean face and neck with soapy washcloth; rinse and dry. Shave male client as necessary.

(h) Use tincture of benzoin swab or pour small amount of tincture of benzoin on clean 2 × 2 gauze and dot on upper lip (oral ET tube) or across nose (nasal ET tube) and cheeks to ear. Allow to dry completely.

(i) Slip tape under client's head and neck, adhesive side up. Take care not to twist tape or catch hair. Do not allow tape to stick to itself. It helps to stick tape gently to tongue blade, which serves as a guide as tape is passed behind client's head. Centre tape so that double-faced tape extends around back of neck from ear to ear.

(j) On one side of face, secure tape from ear to naris (nasal ET tube) or edge of mouth (oral ET tube). Tear remaining tape in half lengthwise, forming two pieces that are 1- to 2-cm wide. Secure bottom half of tape across upper lip (oral ET tube) or across top of nose (nasal ET tube). Wrap top half of tape around tube.

Continued

492

	S	U	NP	Comments

(k) Gently pull other side of tape firmly to pick up slack and secure to remaining side of face. Assistant can release hold when tube is secure. Nurse may want assistant to help reinsert oral airway.
    ____ ____ ____ _____

(l) Clean oral airway in warm soapy water and rinse well. Hydrogen peroxide can aid in removal of crusted secretions. Shake excess water from oral airway.
    ____ ____ ____ _____

(m) For unconscious client, reinsert oral airway without pushing tongue into oropharynx.
    ____ ____ ____ _____

B. Tracheostomy care:

(1) Observe for signs and symptoms of need to perform tracheostomy care.
    ____ ____ ____ _____

(2) Suction tracheostomy. Before removing gloves, remove soiled tracheostomy dressing and discard in glove with coiled catheter.
    ____ ____ ____ _____

(3) While client is replenishing oxygen stores, prepare equipment on bedside table. Open sterile tracheostomy kit. Open three 4 × 4 gauze packages using aseptic technique and pour normal saline (NS) on one package and hydrogen peroxide on another. Leave third package dry. Prepare equipment:
    ____ ____ ____ _____

(a) Open two packages of cotton-tipped swabs and pour NS on one package and hydrogen peroxide on the other.
    ____ ____ ____ _____

(b) Open sterile tracheostomy package.
    ____ ____ ____ _____

(c) Unwrap sterile basin and pour about 2 cm of hydrogen peroxide into it.
    ____ ____ ____ _____

(d) Open small sterile brush package and place aseptically into sterile basin.
    ____ ____ ____ _____

(e) If using large roll of twill tape, cut appropriate length of tape and lay aside in dry area. Do not recap hydrogen peroxide and NS.
    ____ ____ ____ _____

Continued

	S	U	NP	Comments

(4) Apply gloves. Keep dominate hand sterile throughout procedure. ____ ____ ____ _____

(5) Remove oxygen source. ____ ____ ____ _____

(6) If a non-disposable inner cannula is used:

    (a) Remove cannula with non-dominant hand. Drop cannula into hydrogen peroxide basin. ____ ____ ____ _____

    (b) Place tracheostomy collar or T tube and ventilator oxygen source over or near outer cannula. ____ ____ ____ _____

    (c) To prevent oxygen desaturation in affected clients, quickly pick up inner cannula and use small brush to remove secretions from inside and outside. ____ ____ ____ _____

    (d) Hold inner cannula over basin and rinse with NS, using non-dominant hand to pour. ____ ____ ____ _____

    (e) Replace inner cannula and secure "locking" mechanism. Reapply ventilator or oxygen sources. ____ ____ ____ _____

(7) If a disposable inner cannula is used:

    (a) Remove cannula from manufacturer's packaging. ____ ____ ____ _____

    (b) Withdraw inner cannula and replace with new cannula. Lock into position. ____ ____ ____ _____

    (c) Dispose of contaminated cannula in appropriate receptacle and apply oxygen source. ____ ____ ____ _____

(8) Using hydrogen peroxide-prepared cotton-tipped swabs and 4×4 gauze, clean exposed outer cannula surfaces and stoma under faceplate, extending 5 to 10 cm in all directions from stoma. Clean in circular motion from stoma site outward, using dominant hand to handle sterile supplies. ____ ____ ____ _____

(9) Using NS-prepared cotton-tipped swabs and 4×4 gauze, rinse hydrogen peroxide from tracheostomy tube and skin surfaces. ____ ____ ____ _____

(10) Using dry 4×4 gauze, pat lightly at skin and exposed outer cannula surfaces. ____ ____ ____ _____

(11) Instruct assistant, if available, to hold tracheostomy tube securely in place while ties are cut. ____ ____ ____ _____

Continued

	S	U	NP	Comments
(a) Cut length of twill tape long enough to go around client's neck two times, about 60 to 75 cm for an adult. Cut ends on a diagonal.	___	___	___	_____
(b) Insert one end of tie through faceplate eyelet and pull ends even.	___	___	___	_____
(c) Slide both ends of tie behind head and around neck to other eyelet, and insert one tie through second eyelet.	___	___	___	_____
(d) Pull snugly.	___	___	___	_____
(e) Tie ends securely in double square knot, allowing space for only one finger in tie.	___	___	___	_____
(f) Insert fresh tracheostomy dressing under clean ties and faceplate.	___	___	___	_____
(g) Position client comfortably and assess respiratory status.	___	___	___	_____
7. Replace any oxygen delivery devices.	___	___	___	_____
8. Remove and discard gloves. Perform hand hygiene.	___	___	___	_____
9. Compare respiratory assessments made before and after artificial airway care.	___	___	___	_____
10. Observe depth and position of tubes.	___	___	___	_____
11. Assess security of tape or commercial ET or ET tube holder by tugging at tube.	___	___	___	_____
12. Assess skin around mouth and oral mucosa (ET tube) and tracheostomy stoma for drainage, pressure, and signs of irritation.	___	___	___	_____

STUDENT: _____ DATE: _____

INSTRUCTOR: _____ DATE: _____

Skill 35-3 Care of Clients With Chest Tubes

	S	U	NP	Comments
1. Perform hand hygiene and assess client for respiratory distress and chest pain, breath sounds over affected lung area, and vital signs.	___	___	___	_____
2. Observe the following:				
A. Chest tube dressing and site surrounding insertion.	___	___	___	_____
B. Tubing, for kinks, dependent loops, or clots	___	___	___	_____
C. Chest drainage system	___	___	___	_____
3. Provide two shodded hemostats or approved clamps for each chest tube, and attach them to top of client's bed with adhesive tape.	___	___	___	_____
4. Position client in one of the following ways:				
A. Semi-Fowler's position to evacuate air (pneumothorax)	___	___	___	_____
B. High-Fowler's position to drain fluid (hemothorax), effusion.	___	___	___	_____
5. Maintain tube connection between chest and drainage tubes intact.	___	___	___	_____
6. Ensure tubing is laying horizontally across the client bed or chair before dropping vertically into the drainage bottle. If the client is in a chair and the tubing is coiled, lift the tubing every 15 minutes to promote drainage.	___	___	___	_____
7. Adjust tubing to hang in straight line from top of mattress to drainage chamber. Indicate time that drainage began.	___	___	___	_____
8. Strip or milk chest tube only if indicated.	___	___	___	_____
9. Perform hand hygiene.	___	___	___	_____
10. Evaluate:				
A. Chest tube dressing.	___	___	___	_____
B. Tubing should be free of kinks and dependent loops.	___	___	___	_____
C. Chest drainage system: should be upright and below level of tube insertion. Note presence of clots or debris in tubing.	___	___	___	_____
D. Water seal.	___	___	___	_____
(1) Waterless system: diagnostic indicator for fluctuations with client's inspirations and expirations	___	___	___	_____
(2) Water-seal system: bubbling in the water-seal chamber	___	___	___	_____

Continued

	S	U	NP	Comments
E. Waterless system: Bubbling is diagnostic indicator.	___	___	___	_____
F. Type and amount of fluid drainage: Note colour and amount of drainage, client's vital signs, and skin colour.	___	___	___	_____
G. Water-sealed system: bubbling in the suction control chamber (when suction is being used)	___	___	___	_____
H. Waterless system: The suction control (float ball) indicates the amount of suction that the client's intrapleural space is receiving.	___	___	___	_____
I. Lungs: auscultate and observe for symmetry.	___	___	___	_____
J. Pain: ask client to evaluate pain on a level of 0 to 10.	___	___	___	_____

STUDENT: _____ DATE: _____

INSTRUCTOR: _____ DATE: _____

SKILL PERFORMANCE CHECKLIST
Skill 35-4 Applying a Nasal Cannula or Oxygen Mask

	S	U	NP	Comments
1. Inspect client for signs and symptoms associated with hypoxia and presence of airway secretions.	____	____	____	_____
2. Explain procedure and purpose to client and family.	____	____	____	_____
3. Perform hand hygiene.	____	____	____	_____
4. Attach nasal cannula to oxygen tubing and attach to humidified oxygen source, adjusted to prescribed flow rate.	____	____	____	_____
5. Place tips of cannula into nares. Adjust band until cannula fits snugly and comfortably.	____	____	____	_____
6. Secure oxygen tubing to clothes, maintaining sufficient slack.	____	____	____	_____
7. Check cannula every 8 hours. Keep humidification jar filled at all times.	____	____	____	_____
8. Observe client's nares and superior surface of both ears for skin breakdown.	____	____	____	_____
9. Check oxygen flow rate and physician's orders every 8 hours.	____	____	____	_____
10. Perform hand hygiene.	____	____	____	_____
11. Inspect client for relief of symptoms.	____	____	____	_____

STUDENT: _____ DATE: _____

INSTRUCTOR: _____ DATE: _____

Skill 35-5 Using Home Liquid Oxygen Equipment

	S	U	NP	Comments
1. Assess:				
A. Client's need for home oxygen therapy.	____	____	____	_____
B. Client's or family's ability to use oxygen equipment properly, or for appropriate use of oxygen equipment in home setting.	____	____	____	_____
C. Client's and family's ability to observe for signs and symptoms of hypoxia.	____	____	____	_____
2. Explain procedure to client and family.	____	____	____	_____
3. Perform hand hygiene.	____	____	____	_____
4. Demonstrate steps for oxygen therapy.	____	____	____	_____
5. Prepare primary and portable oxygen:	____	____	____	_____
A. Place primary oxygen source in clutter-free environment.	____	____	____	_____
B. Check oxygen levels of both sources by reading gauge on top.	____	____	____	_____
C. Refill portable source by placing on top of primary source and pressing down firmly. Check oxygen gauge to determine fullness of portable source.	____	____	____	_____
D. Select prescribed rate.	____	____	____	_____
E. Connect nasal cannula and oxygen tubing to oxygen source.	____	____	____	_____
F. Perform hand hygiene.	____	____	____	_____
6. Have client or family perform each step with guidance.	____	____	____	_____

STUDENT: _____ DATE: _____

INSTRUCTOR: _____ DATE: _____

Skill 36-1 Initiating a Peripheral Intravenous Infusion

	S	U	NP	Comments
1. Review physician's order. Follow six rights for administration of medication.	___	___	___	_____
2. Observe client for signs and symptoms indicating fluid or electrolyte imbalances.	___	___	___	_____
3. Assess client's prior experience with intravenous (IV) therapy and client's arm placement preference.	___	___	___	_____
4. Determine if client is to have surgery or blood transfusion.	___	___	___	_____
5. Assess laboratory data and client's allergies.	___	___	___	_____
6. Assess client for risk factors.	___	___	___	_____
7. Explain procedure to client.	___	___	___	_____
8. Perform hand hygiene.	___	___	___	_____
9. Assist client to a comfortable sitting or lying position.	___	___	___	_____
10. Organize equipment on bedside stand or overbed table.	___	___	___	_____
11. Change client's gown to a more easily removable gown with snaps at shoulder, if available.	___	___	___	_____
12. Open sterile packages using sterile technique.	___	___	___	_____
13. Check IV solution. Make sure prescribed additives (e.g., potassium, vitamins) have been added. Check solution for colour, clarity, and expiration date. Check bag for leaks.	___	___	___	_____
14. Open infusion set.	___	___	___	_____
15. Place roller clamp about 2 to 5 cm below drip chamber and move roller clamp to "off" position.	___	___	___	_____
16. Remove protective sheath over IV tubing port.	___	___	___	_____
17. Insert infusion set into fluid bag or bottle by removing protector cap from tubing insertion spike (keeping spike sterile), and insert spike into opening of IV bag. Cleanse rubber stopper on bottled solution with antiseptic, and insert spike into black rubber stopper of IV bottle. Hang solution container on IV pole at minimum height of 90 cm above planned insertion site.	___	___	___	_____
18. Compress drip chamber and release, allowing it to fill one-third to one-half full. Open clamp and prime infusion by filling with IV solution.	___	___	___	_____

Continued

	S	U	NP	Comments

19. Remove tubing protector cap and slowly release roller clamp to allow fluid to travel from drip chamber through tubing to needle adapter. Return roller clamp to "off" position after tubing is primed.

20. Clear tubing of air bubbles. Firmly tap IV tubing where air bubbles are located. Check entire length of tubing to ensure that all air bubbles are removed.

21. Replace tubing cap protector on end of tubing.

22. Optional: Prepare heparin or normal saline lock for infusion. Use a sterile technique to connect the IV plug to the loop or short extension tubing. Inject 1 to 3 mL normal saline through the plug and through the loop or short extension tubing.

23. Apply disposable gloves. Eye protection and mask may be applied, if indicated.

24. Identify site for IV replacement. Place tourniquet 10 to 15 cm above insertion site. Position tourniquet so that the ends are away from the site. Check presence of radial pulse. OPTION: Apply blood pressure (BP) cuff instead of tourniquet. Inflate to a level just below client's normal diastolic pressure. Maintain inflation at that pressure until venipuncture is completed.

25. Select the vein.
    A. Use the most distal site in the non-dominant arm, if possible.
    B. Avoid areas that are painful to palpation.
    C. Select a vein large enough for catheter placement.
    D. Choose a site that will not interfere with client's activities of daily or planned procedures.
    E. Use the fingertips to palpate the vein by pressing downward and noting the resilient, soft, bouncy feeling as the pressure is released.
    F. Promote venous distension by instructing the client to open and close the fist several times, lowering the client's arm in a dependent position, applying warmth to the arm for several minutes, and/or rubbing or stroking the client's arm from distal to proximal below proposed site.

Continued

504

	S	U	NP	Comments

G. Avoid sites distal to previous venipuncture site, sclerosed or hardened cordlike veins, infiltrated site or phlebotic vessels, bruised areas, and areas of venous valves or bifurcation. Avoid veins in antecubital fossa and ventral surface of the wrist.   ____ ____ ____ _____

H. Avoid fragile dorsal veins in older adults and vessels in an extremity with compromised circulation.   ____ ____ ____ _____

26. Release tourniquet temporarily. Clip excess hair at site, if necessary.   ____ ____ ____ _____

27. (If area of insertion appears to need cleansing, use soap and water first.) Cleanse insertion site using firm, circular motion (centre to outward) from insertion site. Use antiseptic prep as a single agent or in combination, according to agency policy. Avoid touching the cleansed site. Allow the site to dry for at least 2 minutes. If skin is touched after cleansing, repeat cleansing procedure.   ____ ____ ____ _____

28. Reapply tourniquet or BP cuff.   ____ ____ ____ _____

29. Perform venipuncture. Anchor vein by placing thumb over vein and stretching skin against the direction of insertion 5 to 7.5 cm distal to the site. Puncture skin and vein, holding catheter at 10- to 30-degree angle with bevel pointed upward.   ____ ____ ____ _____

A. Butterfly needle: Hold needle at 10- to 30-degree angle with bevel up slightly distal to actual site of venipuncture.   ____ ____ ____ _____

B. Needleless over-the-needle catheter (ONC) safety device: Insert ONC with bevel up at 10- to 30-degree angle slightly distal to actual site of venipuncture in the direction of the vein.   ____ ____ ____ _____

30. Look for blood return through tubing of butterfly needle or flashback chamber of ONC. Lower catheter/needle until almost flush with skin. Advance butterfly needle until hub rests at venipuncture site. Advance ONC 0.5 cm into vein and then loosen stylet. Advance catheter into vein until hub rests at venipuncture site. Do not reinsert the stylet once it is loosened.   ____ ____ ____ _____

Continued

	S	U	NP	Comments

31. Stabilize the catheter. Apply gentle, firm pressure with index finger of non-dominant hand 3 cm above insertion site. Release tourniquet or BP cuff with dominant hand and retract stylet from ONC. Do not recap the stylet. Slide the catheter off the stylet while gliding the protective guard over the stylet.

32. Connect needle adapter of primed fluid administration set or heparin lock to hub of ONC or butterfly tubing. Do not touch point of entry of adapter.

33. Release roller clamp slowly to begin infusion at a rate to maintain patency of IV line.
   A. Intermittent infusion: Continue to stabilize catheter with non-dominant hand and attach injection cap of adapter. Insert pre-filled flush solution into injection cap. Flush slowly. Maintain thumb pressure on syringe during withdrawal or close clamp on extension tubing of injection cap while still flushing last 0.2 to 0.4 mL of flush solution.

34. Tape or secure catheter.
   A. If applying transparent dressing, secure catheter with non-dominant hand while preparing to apply dressing.
   B. If applying a gauze dressing:
     (1) Tape the IV catheter. Place narrow piece (1-cm wide) of sterile tape under hub of catheter with adhesive side up and criss-cross tape over hub to form a chevron.
     (2) Place tape only on the catheter, *never* over the insertion site. Secure the site to allow easy visual inspection. Avoid applying tape around the extremity.

35. Apply sterile dressing over site.
   A. Transparent dressing:
     (1) Carefully remove adherent backing. Apply one edge of dressing and then gently smooth remaining dressing over site, leaving end of catheter hub uncovered.
     (2) Take 2.5-cm piece of tape and place from end of catheter hub to insertion site over dressing.
     (3) Apply chevron and place only over tape, not dressing.

Continued

	S	U	NP	Comments

B. Sterile gauze dressing:
    (1) Fold 2 × 2 gauze in half and cover with 1-inch tape. Place under tubing/catheter hub junction.   _____ _____ _____ _____
    (2) Place a 2 × 2 gauze pad over venipuncture site and catheter hub. Secure edges with tape.   _____ _____ _____ _____
    (3) Curl loop of tubing alongside arm and secure with tape.   _____ _____ _____ _____

36. For IV fluid administration, adjust flow rate to correct drops per minute or connect to electronic infusion device (EID):   _____ _____ _____ _____
    A. For heparin lock, flush with 1 to 3 mL of heparin (10 to 100 units/ml).   _____ _____ _____ _____
    B. For saline lock, flush with 1 to 3 mL of sterile normal saline.   _____ _____ _____ _____

37. Label dressing with date, time, gauge size and length of catheter, placement of IV line and dressing, and your initials.   _____ _____ _____ _____

38. Dispose of used needles in appropriate sharps container. Discard supplies. Remove gloves and perform hand hygiene.   _____ _____ _____ _____

39. Observe client every hour to determine if fluid is infusing correctly.   _____ _____ _____ _____
    A. Check if correct amount of solution is infused and prescribed by looking at time tape.   _____ _____ _____ _____
    B. Count flow or check rate on infusion pump.   _____ _____ _____ _____
    C. Check patency of IV catheter or needle.   _____ _____ _____ _____
    D. Observe client for signs of discomfort.   _____ _____ _____ _____
    E. Inspect insertion site for absence of phlebitis, infiltration, or inflammation.   _____ _____ _____ _____

40. Observe client every hour to determine response to therapy.   _____ _____ _____ _____

STUDENT: _____ DATE: _____

INSTRUCTOR: _____ DATE: _____

SKILL PERFORMANCE CHECKLIST
Skill 36-2 Regulating Intravenous Flow Rate

	S	U	NP	Comments
1. Check client's medical record for correct solution, additives, and time of infusion.	____	____	____	_____
2. Perform hand hygiene. Observe for patency of intravenous (IV) line and needle or catheter.	____	____	____	_____
3. Check client's knowledge of how positioning of IV site affects flow rate.	____	____	____	_____
4. Verify with client how venipuncture site feels.	____	____	____	_____
5. Calculate flow rate.	____	____	____	_____
6. Check calibration (drop factor) in drops per milliliter (gtt/ml) of infusion set.	____	____	____	_____
7. Calculate flow rate (hourly volume) of prescribed infusion.	____	____	____	_____
8. Read prescriber's orders and follow six rights for correct solution and proper additives.	____	____	____	_____
9. Determine how long each litre of fluid should run.	____	____	____	_____
10. Place adhesive or fluid indicator tape on IV bottle or bag next to volume markings.	____	____	____	_____
11. Calculate minute rate based on drop factor of 60 gtt/mL.	____	____	____	_____
12. Establish rate by counting drops in drip chamber for 1 minute, then adjust roller clamp to increase or decrease rate of infusion.	____	____	____	_____
13. Follow this procedure for infusion controller or pump:				
A. Place electronic eye on drip chamber below origin of drop and above fluid level in chamber or consult manufacturer's directions for setup of the infusion. If controller is used, ensure that IV bag is 1 m above the IV site.	____	____	____	_____
B. Place IV infusion tubing within ridges of control box in direction of flow or consult manufacturer's directions for use of pump. Close door to control chamber. Turn on pump. Select drops per minute or volume per hour. Open rate control clamp and press start button.	____	____	____	_____
C. Monitor infusion rates and IV site for infiltration according to agency policy.	____	____	____	_____
D. Assess patency and integrity of system when alarm sounds.	____	____	____	_____

Continued

	S	U	NP	Comments

14. Follow this procedure for volume control device:

    A. Place volume control device between IV bag and insertion spike of infusion set using sterile technique.   ____ ____ ____ _____

    B. Place 2 hours' allotment of fluid into chamber device.   ____ ____ ____ _____

    C. Assess system at least hourly. Add fluid to volume control device as needed. Regulate flow rate.   ____ ____ ____ _____

15. Observe client for signs of over-hydration or dehydration.   ____ ____ ____ _____

16. Evaluate infusion site for signs of infiltration, inflammation, clot in catheter, or kink or knot in infusion tubing.   ____ ____ ____ _____

SKILL PERFORMANCE CHECKLIST
Skill 36-3 Maintenance of an IV System

	S	U	NP	Comments

Changing intravenous (IV) solution:

1. Check physician's order. _____ _____ _____ _____

2. Clarify rate, if necessary. Note date and time solution was last changed. _____ _____ _____ _____

3. Determine compatibility of IV fluids and additives. _____ _____ _____ _____

4. Determine client's understanding of need for continued IV therapy. _____ _____ _____ _____

5. Assess patency of current IV access site. _____ _____ _____ _____

6. Have next solution prepared at least 1 hour before needed. Check that solution is correct and properly labelled. Check solution expiration date and for the presence of precipitate and discolouration. _____ _____ _____ _____

7. Prepare to change solution when less than 50 mL of fluid remains in bottle or bag or when new type of solution is ordered. _____ _____ _____ _____

8. Explain procedure to client. _____ _____ _____ _____

9. Ensure drip chamber at least half full. _____ _____ _____ _____

10. Perform hand hygiene. _____ _____ _____ _____

11. Prepare new solution for changing. If using plastic bag, remove protective cover from IV tubing port. If using glass bottle, remove metal cap and metal and rubber disks. _____ _____ _____ _____

12. Move roller clamp to stop flow rate. _____ _____ _____ _____

13. Remove old IV fluid container from IV pole. _____ _____ _____ _____

14. Remove spike from old solution bag or bottle and, without touching tip, insert spike into new bag or bottle. _____ _____ _____ _____

15. Hang new bag or bottle of solution on IV pole. _____ _____ _____ _____

16. Check for air in tubing. Remove bubbles by closing the roller clamp, stretching the tubing downward, and tapping the tubing with the finger. For larger amounts of air, swab injection port below the air with alcohol and allow to dry. Connect a syringe to this port and aspirate the air into the syringe. Reduce air in tubing by priming slowly instead of allowing a wide open flow. _____ _____ _____ _____

17. Ensure drip chamber one-third to one-half full. If the drip chamber is too full, pinch off tubing below the drip chamber, invert the container, squeeze the drip chamber, hang up the bottle, and release the tubing. _____ _____ _____ _____

Continued

	S	U	NP	Comments

18. Regulate flow to prescribed rate.
19. Mark the date and time on label and tape it on bag.
20. Observe client for signs of overhydration or dehydration.
21. Observe IV system for patency and development of complications.

Changing IV tubing:

22. Determine when new infusion set is needed. Observe for occlusions in tubing.
23. Explain procedure to client.
24. Perform hand hygiene.
25. Open new infusion set, keeping protective coverings over infusion spike and distal adapter. Secure all junctions with Luer-loks, clasping devices, or threaded devices.
26. Apply non-sterile, disposable gloves.
27. If needle or catheter hub is not visible, remove IV dressing while maintaining stability of catheter. If transparent dressing must be removed, place small piece of sterile tape across hub temporarily to anchor catheter during disconnection. Do not remove tape securing needle or catheter to skin with gauze dressing.
28. For IV continuous infusion:
    A. Move roller clamp on new IV tubing to "off" position.
    B. Slow rate of infusion by regulating drip rate on old tubing. Maintain keep vein open (KVO) rate.
    C. Compress and fill drip chamber.
    D. Remove IV container from pole, invert container and remove old tubing from container. Carefully hold container while hanging or taping drip chamber on IV pole 1m above IV site.
    E. Place insertion spike of new tubing into old solution bag opening and hang solution bag on IV pole.
    F. Compress and release drip chamber on new tubing. Slowly fill drip chamber one-third to one-half full.
    G. Slowly open roller clamp, remove protective cap from needle adapter (if necessary), and flush new tubing with solution. Replace cap.
    H. Turn roller clamp on old tubing to "off" position.

Continued

	S	U	NP	Comments

29. For heparin lock:
 A. Use sterile technique to connect the new injection cap to the loop or tubing. ___ ___ ___ _____
 B. Swab injection cap with antiseptic. Insert syringe with 1 to 3 mL saline and inject through the injection cap into the loop or short extension tubing. ___ ___ ___ _____
30. Stabilize hub of catheter and apply pressure over vein just above catheter tip, at least 3 cm above insertion site. Gently disconnect old tubing. Maintain stability of hub and quickly insert needle adapter of new tubing or saline/heparin lock into hub. ___ ___ ___ _____
31. Open roller clamp on new tubing. Allow solution to run rapidly for 30 to 60 seconds. ___ ___ ___ _____
32. Regulate IV drip according to orders and monitor rate hourly. ___ ___ ___ _____
33. Apply new dressing if necessary. ___ ___ ___ _____
34. Discard old tubing in proper container. ___ ___ ___ _____
35. Remove and dispose of gloves. Perform hand hygiene. ___ ___ ___ _____
36. Evaluate flow rate and observe connection site for leakage. ___ ___ ___ _____
37. Check physicians order for discontinuing IV. ___ ___ ___ _____
38. Explain procedure to client. ___ ___ ___ _____
39. Perform hand hygiene and apply disposable gloves. ___ ___ ___ _____
40. Turn IV tubing roller clamp to "off" position. Remove tape securing tubing. ___ ___ ___ _____
41. Remove IV site dressing and tape while stabilizing catheter. ___ ___ ___ _____
42. With dry gauze or alcohol swab held over site, apply light pressure and withdraw the catheter, using a slow steady movement, keeping the hub parallel to the skin. ___ ___ ___ _____
43. Apply pressure to the site for 2 or 3 minutes, using the dry, sterile gauze pad. Secure with tape. ___ ___ ___ _____
44. Inspect the catheter for intactness, noting tip integrity and length. ___ ___ ___ _____
45. Discard used supplies. ___ ___ ___ _____
46. Remove and discard gloves, and perform hand hygiene. ___ ___ ___ _____
47. Instruct client to report any redness, pain, drainage, or swelling that may occur after catheter removal. ___ ___ ___ _____

STUDENT: _____ DATE: _____

INSTRUCTOR: _____ DATE: _____

SKILL PERFORMANCE CHECKLIST
Skill 36-4 Changing a Peripheral Intravenous Dressing

	S	U	NP	Comments
1. Determine when dressing was last changed.	____	____	____	_____
2. Perform hand hygiene. Observe present dressing for moisture and intactness.	____	____	____	_____
3. Observe intravenous (IV) system for proper functioning. Palpate the catheter site through the intact dressing for inflammation or discomfort.	____	____	____	_____
4. Inspect exposed catheter site for swelling or blanching.	____	____	____	_____
5. Assess client's understanding of need for continued IV infusion.	____	____	____	_____
6. Explain procedure to client and family.	____	____	____	_____
7. Perform hand hygiene. Apply disposable gloves.	____	____	____	_____
8. Remove tape, gauze, and/or transparent dressing from old dressing one layer at a time, leaving tape (if present) that secures the IV needle in place. When removing transparent dressing, hold catheter hub and tubing with non-dominant hand.	____	____	____	_____
9. Observe insertion site for signs and/or symptoms of infection. If present, remove catheter and insert a new IV in another site.	____	____	____	_____
10. If infiltration, phlebitis, or clot occurs or if ordered by physician, stop infusion and discontinue IV. Restart new IV if continued therapy is necessary. Place moist warm compress over area of phlebitis.	____	____	____	_____
11. If IV is infusing properly, gently remove tape securing catheter. Stabilize needle or catheter with one hand. Use adhesive remover to cleanse skin and remove adhesive residue, if needed.	____	____	____	_____
12. Keep one finger over catheter at all times until tape or dressing is replaced.	____	____	____	_____
13. Cleanse peripheral IV insertion site with antiseptic swab, starting at insertion site and working outward, creating concentric circles. Allow swab to air-dry completely.	____	____	____	_____
14. Apply new transparent or gauze dressing.	____	____	____	_____
15. Remove and discard gloves.	____	____	____	_____

Continued

	S	U	NP	Comments
16. Anchor IV tubing with additional pieces of tape. Minimize tape placed over transparent polyurethane dressing.	____	____	____	_____
17. Write insertion date (if known), date and time of dressing change, size and gauge of catheter, and your initials, directly on dressing.	____	____	____	_____
18. Discard equipment and perform hand hygiene.	____	____	____	_____
19. Observe functioning and patency of IV system in response to changing dressing.	____	____	____	_____
20. Monitor client's body temperature.	____	____	____	_____

SKILL PERFORMANCE CHECKLIST
Skill 39-1 Inserting a Small-Bore Nasoenteral Tube for Enteral Feedings

	S	U	NP	Comments
1. Assess client for the need for enteral tube feeding.	____	____	____	_____
2. Perform hand hygiene. Assess patency of nares. Examine each naris for skin breakdown.	____	____	____	_____
3. Assess the gag reflex.	____	____	____	_____
4. Review client's medical history for nasal problems.	____	____	____	_____
5. Review physician's order for type of tube and enteral feeding schedule.	____	____	____	_____
6. Auscultate abdomen for bowel sounds.	____	____	____	_____
7. Perform hand hygiene.	____	____	____	_____
8. Explain procedure to client and how to communicate during intubation by raising index finger to indicate gagging or discomfort.	____	____	____	_____
9. Stand on same side of bed as nares for insertion. Assist client to high-Fowler's position unless contraindicated. Place pillow behind client's head and shoulders.	____	____	____	_____
10. Place bath towel over client's chest. Keep facial tissues within reach.	____	____	____	_____
11. Determine length of tube to be inserted and mark with tape: Measure distance from tip of client's nose to earlobe to xiphoid process of sternum.	____	____	____	_____
12. Prepare nasogastric or nasointestinal tube for intubation:	____	____	____	_____
A. Do not ice plastic tubes.	____	____	____	_____
B. Inject 10 mL of water from 30 mL or larger Luer-Lok or catheter-tip syringe into the tube.	____	____	____	_____
C. Make certain that guidewire is securely positioned against weighted tip and that both Luer-Lok connections are snugly fitted together.	____	____	____	_____
13. Cut tape 10 cm long or prepare tube fixation device.	____	____	____	_____
14. Apply disposable gloves.	____	____	____	_____
15. Dip tube with surface lubricant into glass of water.	____	____	____	_____
16. Insert tube through client's nostril to back of throat. Aim back and down toward ear.	____	____	____	_____
17. Have client flex head toward chest after tube has passed through nasopharynx.	____	____	____	_____

Continued

	S	U	NP	Comments

18. Emphasize client's need to breathe through mouth and swallow during procedure. ____ ____ ____ _____

19. When tip of tube reaches carina (about 25 cm in an adult), stop, hold end of twice near ear and listen for air exchange from the distal portion of the tube. ____ ____ ____ _____

20. Advance tube each time client swallows until desired length has been passed. ____ ____ ____ _____

21. Check for position of tube in back of throat with penlight and tongue blade. ____ ____ ____ _____

22. Perform measures to verify placement of tube. ____ ____ ____ _____

23. Anchor tube to nose, avoiding pressure on nares. Mark exit site with indelible ink. Select one of the following: ____ ____ ____ _____

   A. Apply tape. ____ ____ ____ _____

     (1) Apply tincture of benzoin or other skin adhesive on tip of client's nose and tube. Allow to become "tacky." ____ ____ ____ _____

     (2) Remove gloves and split one end of tape lengthwise 5 cm. ____ ____ ____ _____

     (3) Place the intact end of tape over bridge of client's nose. Wrap each of the 5 cm strips around tube as it exits client's nose. ____ ____ ____ _____

   B. Apply tube fixation device using shaped adhesive patch. ____ ____ ____ _____

     (1) Apply wide end of adhesive patch to nose. ____ ____ ____ _____

     (2) Slip connector around tube as it exits nose. ____ ____ ____ _____

24. Fasten end of nasogastric tube to client's gown by looping rubber band around tube in slip knot. Pin rubber band to gown. ____ ____ ____ _____

25. For intestinal placement, position client on right side if possible until confirmation of placement. Otherwise, assist client to a comfortable position. Remove gloves. Perform hand hygiene. ____ ____ ____ _____

26. Obtain x-ray film of client's abdomen. ____ ____ ____ _____

27. Apply clean gloves and administer oral hygiene. Cleanse tubing at nostril. ____ ____ ____ _____

28. Remove gloves. Dispose of equipment and perform hand hygiene. ____ ____ ____ _____

29. Inspect client's nares and oropharynx for any irritation after insertion. ____ ____ ____ _____

30. Ask if client feels comfortable.

31. Observe client for difficulty breathing, coughing, or gagging. ____ ____ ____ _____

32. Auscultate lung sounds. ____ ____ ____ _____

SKILL PERFORMANCE CHECKLIST
Skill 39-2 Administering Enteral Tube Feedings via Nasoenteral Tubes

	S	U	NP	Comments
1. Assess client's need for enteral tube feedings.	____	____	____	_____
2. Evaluate client's nutritional status. Obtain client's baseline weight and laboratory values. Assess client for fluid volume excess or deficit, and electrolyte and metabolic abnormalities.	____	____	____	_____
3. Verify physician's order for formula, rate, route, and frequency of feeding.	____	____	____	_____
4. Explain procedure to client.	____	____	____	_____
5. Perform hand hygiene.	____	____	____	_____
6. Auscultate for bowel sounds before feeding.	____	____	____	_____
7. Prepare feeding container to administer formula:	____	____	____	_____
A. Check expiration date of formula and integrity of container.	____	____	____	_____
B. Have formula at room temperature.	____	____	____	_____
C. Connect tubing to container as needed or prepare ready-to-hang container.	____	____	____	_____
D. Shake formula container well and fill container and tubing with formula. Open stopcock on tubing and fill with formula to remove air. Hang on intravenous (IV) pole.	____	____	____	_____
8. Have syringe ready and be sure formula is at room temperature for intermittent feeding.	____	____	____	_____
9. Place client in high-Fowler's position or elevate head of bed 30 degrees.	____	____	____	_____
10. Determine tube placement.	____	____	____	_____
11. Check for gastric residual.	____	____	____	_____
12. Flush tubing with 30 mL water.	____	____	____	_____
13. Initiate feeding:				
A. Syringe or intermittent feeding:				
(1) Pinch proximal end of feeding tube.	____	____	____	_____
(2) Remove plunger from syringe and attach barrel of syringe to end of tube.	____	____	____	_____
(3) Fill syringe with measured amount of formula. Release tube and hold syringe high enough to allow it to be emptied gradually by gravity. Refill. Repeat until prescribed amount has been delivered to the client.	____	____	____	_____

Continued

	S	U	NP	Comments
(4) If feeding bag is used, hang feeding bag on IV pole. Fill bag with prescribed amount of formula and allow bag to empty gradually over at least 30 minutes.	___	___	___	_____
B. Continuous-drip method:				
(1) Hang feeding bag and tubing on IV pole.	___	___	___	_____
(2) Connect distal end of tubing to the proximal end of the feeding tube.	___	___	___	_____
(3) Connect tubing through infusion pump and set rate.	___	___	___	_____
14. Advance tube feeding gradually.	___	___	___	_____
15. Following intermittent infusion or at end of continuous infusion, flush nasoenteral tubing with 30 mL of water. Repeat every 4 to 6 hours. Remove gloves and/or perform hand hygiene.	___	___	___	_____
16. When tube feedings are not being administered, cap or clamp the proximal end of the feeding tube.	___	___	___	_____
17. Rinse bag and tubing with warm water whenever feedings are interrupted.	___	___	___	_____
18. Change bag and tubing every 24 hours.	___	___	___	_____
19. Measure amount of aspirate every 8 to 12 hours.	___	___	___	_____
20. Monitor finger-stick blood glucose every 6 hours until maximum administration is reached and maintained for 24 hours.	___	___	___	_____
21. Monitor intake and output every 8 hours and do 24-hour totals.	___	___	___	_____
22. Weigh client daily until maximum administration rate is reached and maintained for 24 hours, then weigh client three times per week.	___	___	___	_____
23. Observe return of normal laboratory values.	___	___	___	_____

STUDENT: _____ DATE: _____

INSTRUCTOR: _____ DATE: _____

Skill Performance Checklist
Skill 39-3 Administering Enteral Feedings via Gastrostomy or Jejunostomy Tube

	S	U	NP	Comments
1. Assess client's need for enteral tube feedings.	___	___	___	_____
2. Auscultate for bowel sounds before feeding. Consult physician if bowel sounds are absent.	___	___	___	_____
3. Obtain baseline weight and laboratory values.	___	___	___	_____
4. Verify physician's order for formula, rate, route, and frequency.	___	___	___	_____
5. Perform hand hygiene.	___	___	___	_____
6. Assess gastronomy/jejunostomy site for breakdown, irritation, or drainage.	___	___	___	_____
7. Explain procedure to client.	___	___	___	_____
8. Prepare feeding container to administer formula:				
A. Have tube feeding at room temperature.	___	___	___	_____
B. Connect tubing to container as needed or prepare ready-to-hang bag.	___	___	___	_____
C. Shake formula well. Fill container and tubing with formula.	___	___	___	_____
9. For intermittent feeding, have syringe ready and be sure formula is at room temperature.	___	___	___	_____
10. Elevate head of bed 30 to 45 degrees.	___	___	___	_____
11. Apply gloves and verify tube placement:	___	___	___	_____
A. Gastrostomy tube: Attach syringe and aspirate client's gastric secretions, observe their appearance and check pH. Return aspirated contents unless the volume exceeds 100 mL. If the volume is greater than 100 mL on several consecutive occasions, hold feeding and notify physician.	___	___	___	_____
B. Jejunostomy tube: Aspirate intestinal secretions, observe their appearance, and check pH.	___	___	___	_____
12. Flush tube with 30 mL of water.	___	___	___	_____
13. Initiate feedings:				
A. Syringe feedings:				
(1) Pinch proximal end of gastrostomy/jejunostomy tube.	___	___	___	_____
(2) Remove plunger and attach barrel of syringe to end of tube, then fill syringe with formula.	___	___	___	_____

Continued

(3) Release tube and elevate syringe. Allow syringe to empty gradually by gravity. Refill until prescribed amount of formula has been delivered to client.

B. Continuous-drip feedings:

   (1) Verify that volume in container is sufficient or length of feeding.

   (2) Hang container on IV pole and clear tubing of air.

   (3) Thread tubing into pump according to manufacturer's directions.

   (4) Connect tubing to end of feeding tube.

   (5) Begin infusion at prescribed rate.

14. Administer water via tube as ordered.

15. Flush tube with 30 mL of water every 4 to 6 hours and before and after administering medications via feeding tube.

16. Cap or clamp proximal end of tube between feedings.

17. Rinse container and tubing with warm water after intermittent feedings.

18. Assess skin around tube exit site. Cleanse skin daily with warm water and mild soap. Tubing exit site is left open to air. If a dressing is needed because of drainage, assess drainage and change dressing as needed.

19. Dispose of supplies and perform hand hygiene.

20. Evaluate client's tolerance to tube feeding. Measure the amount of aspirate (residual) every 8 to 12 hours.

21. Monitor finger-stick blood glucose every 6 hours until maximum administration rate is reached and maintained for 24 hours.

22. Monitor intake and output every 24 hours.

23. Weigh client daily until maximum administration rate is reached and maintained for 24 hours, then weigh client three times per week.

24. Observe return of normal laboratory values.

25. Inspect stoma site for skin integrity.

STUDENT: _____ DATE: _____

INSTRUCTOR: _____ DATE: _____

Skill 40-1 Collecting a Midstream (Clean-Voided) Urine Specimen

	S	U	NP	Comments
1. Assess client's voiding status.	___	___	___	_____
2. Assess client's understanding of procedure.	___	___	___	_____
3. Explain procedure to client.	___	___	___	_____
4. Provide fluids a half-hour before collecting specimen, unless contraindicated.	___	___	___	_____
5. Provide privacy.	___	___	___	_____
6. Have client cleanse perineal area, or assist client with this process.	___	___	___	_____
7. Perform hand hygiene and apply non-sterile gloves. Assist female client onto bedpan if non-ambulatory.	___	___	___	_____
8. Change gloves if necessary.	___	___	___	_____
9. Using surgical asepsis, open sterile kit and prepare sterile supplies. Apply sterile gloves after opening sterile specimen cup, placing cap with sterile inside surface up; do not touch inside of container or cap.	___	___	___	_____
10. Pour antiseptic over cotton balls or gauze.	___	___	___	_____
11. Assist or allow client to cleanse perineal area and collect specimen:	___	___	___	_____
A. Female client:				
(1) Cleanse client's perineal area. Rinse and dry per agency policy.	___	___	___	_____
(2) After client begins urinating, pass container into stream and collect 30 to 60 mL of urine.	___	___	___	_____
B. Male client:				
(1) Cleanse client's penis. Rinse and dry per agency policy.	___	___	___	_____
(2) After client begins urinating, pass container into stream and collect 30 to 60 mL of urine.	___	___	___	_____
12. Remove container before urine flow stops.	___	___	___	_____
13. Place cap on container.	___	___	___	_____
14. Cleanse urine from outside of container. Place container in plastic specimen bag.	___	___	___	_____
15. Remove bedpan (if applicable) and assist client to a comfortable position. Provide hand-washing basin, if needed.	___	___	___	_____
16. Label specimen and attach laboratory requisition slip.	___	___	___	_____

Continued

	S	U	NP	Comments
17. Remove and dispose of gloves and perform hand hygiene.	___	___	___	_____
18. Take specimen to laboratory within 15 minutes or refrigerate.	___	___	___	_____

STUDENT: _____ DATE: _____

INSTRUCTOR: _____ DATE: _____

SKILL PERFORMANCE CHECKLIST
Skill 40-2 Inserting a Straight or In-Dwelling Catheter

	S	U	NP	Comments
1. Assess client's urinary status.	____	____	____	_____
2. Review client's medical record.	____	____	____	_____
3. Assess client's knowledge of the purpose of catheterization.	____	____	____	_____
4. Explain procedure to client.	____	____	____	_____
5. Arrange for assistance if necessary.	____	____	____	_____
6. Perform hand hygiene.	____	____	____	_____
7. Provide privacy.	____	____	____	_____
8. Raise bed to appropriate working height.	____	____	____	_____
9. Stand on left side of bed if right-handed (or vice versa). Clear bedside table and arrange equipment.	____	____	____	_____
10. Raise side rail on opposite side of bed, and put side rail down on working side.	____	____		_____
11. Place waterproof pad under client.	____	____	____	_____
12. Position client:				
A. Female client:				
(1) Assist client to dorsal recumbent position. Ask client to relax thighs so hip joints can be externally rotated.	____	____	____	_____
(2) Position client in side-lying position with upper leg flexed at hip if client cannot be in dorsal recumbent position. If this position is used, drape rectal area to reduce chance of cross-contamination.	____	____	____	_____
B. Male client: Assist client to supine position with thighs slightly abducted.	____	____	____	_____
13. Drape client:				
A. Female client: Diamond-drape client.	____	____	____	_____
B. Male client: Drape client's upper trunk with bath blanket and cover lower extremities with bed sheets so only genitalia are exposed.	____	____	____	_____
14. Apply disposable gloves. Wash client's perineal area with soap and water as needed. Dry area thoroughly. Remove gloves and discard. Perform hand hygiene.	____	____	____	_____
15. Position light to illuminate perineal area.	____	____	____	_____
16. Open package containing drainage system. Place drainage bag over edge of bottom bed frame, and bring drainage tube up between side rail and mattress.	____	____	____	_____

Continued

	S	U	NP	Comments

17. Open catheterization kit according to directions, keeping bottom of container sterile.   ____ ____ ____ _____

18. Place plastic bag that contained kit to use for waste disposal.   ____ ____ ____ _____

19. Apply sterile gloves.   ____ ____ ____ _____

20. Organize supplies on sterile field. Open inner sterile package containing catheter. Pour sterile antiseptic solution into correct compartment containing sterile cotton balls. Open packet containing lubricant. Remove specimen container (lid should be loosely placed on top) and prefilled syringe from collection compartment of tray, and set them aside on sterile field.   ____ ____ ____ _____

21. Test balloon by injecting fluid from prefilled syringe into balloon port.   ____ ____ ____ _____

22. Lubricate 2.5 to 5 cm of catheter for female clients and 12.5 to 17.5 cm for male clients.   ____ ____ ____ _____

23. Apply sterile drape:
    A. Female client:
       (1) Allow top edge of drape to form cuff over both gloved hands. Place drape down on bed between client's thighs. Slip cuffed edge just under client's buttocks, taking care not to touch contaminated surface with gloves.   ____ ____ ____ _____
       (2) Pick up fenestrated sterile drape and allow it to unfold without touching an unsterile object. Apply drape over client's perineum, exposing labia, taking care not to touch contaminated surface with gloves.   ____ ____ ____ _____
    B. Male client:
       (1) First method: Apply drape over thighs and under penis without completely opening fenestrated drape.   ____ ____ ____ _____
       (2) Second method: Apply drape over thighs just below penis. Pick up fenestrated sterile drape, allow it to unfold, and drape it over penis with fenestrated slit resting over penis.   ____ ____ ____ _____

24. Place sterile tray and contents on sterile drape. Open specimen container.   ____ ____ ____ _____

25. Cleanse urethral meatus:
    A. Female client:
       (1) Retract labia with non-dominant hand to fully expose urethral meatus. Maintain position of non-dominant hand throughout procedure.   ____ ____ ____ _____

Continued

526

	S	U	NP	Comments

(2) Using forceps in sterile dominant hand, pick up cotton ball saturated with antiseptic solution and clean perineal area, wiping front to back from clitoris toward anus. Using a new cotton ball for each area, wipe along the far labial fold, near labial fold, and directly over centre of urethral meatus.

B. Male client:

(1) If client is not circumcised, retract foreskin with non-dominant hand. Grasp penis at shaft just below glans. Retract urethral meatus between thumb and forefinger. Maintain non-dominant hand in this position throughout procedure.

(2) With forceps, pick up cotton ball saturated with antiseptic solution and clean penis. Move cotton ball in circular motion from urethral meatus down to base of glans. Repeat cleansing three more times, using clean cotton ball each time.

26. Pick up catheter with gloved dominant hand 7.5 to 10 cm from catheter tip. Hold end of catheter loosely coiled in palm of dominant hand.

27. Insert catheter:

A. Female client:

(1) Ask client to bear down gently as if to void, and slowly insert catheter through urethral meatus.

(2) Advance catheter a total of 5 to 7.5 cm in adult or until urine flows out catheter's end. Advance catheter another 2.5 to 5 cm when urine appears. Do not use force against resistance. Place end of catheter in urine tray receptacle.

(3) Release labia and hold catheter securely with non-dominant hand. Slowly inflate balloon of in-dwelling catheter.

B. Male client:

(1) Lift client's penis to position perpendicular to client's body and apply light traction.

Continued

	S	U	NP	Comments

(2) Ask client to bear down as if to void urine, and slowly insert catheter through urethral meatus.

(3) Advance catheter 17 to 22.5 cm (7-9 inches) in adult or until urine flows out catheter's end. Withdraw catheter if resistance is felt. Advance catheter another 2.5 to 5 cm when urine appears. Do not force to insert catheter.

(4) Lower client's penis and hold catheter securely in non-dominant hand. Place end of catheter in urine tray. Inflate balloon of in-dwelling catheter.

(5) Reposition the foreskin.

28. Collect urine specimen as needed. Fill specimen cup or jar to desired level by holding end of catheter in dominant hand over cup.

29. Allow bladder to empty fully if institution policy permits.

30. Inflate balloon fully per manufacturer's recommendation and then release catheter with non-dominant hand and pull gently.

31. Attach end of in-dwelling catheter to collecting tube of drainage system. Drainage bag must be below level of bladder; attach bag to bed frame, do not place bag on side rails of bed.

32. Anchor catheter.

    A. Female client: Secure catheter tubing to client's inner thigh with strip of non-allergenic tape or tube holder. Allow for slack for client movement.

    B. Male client: Secure catheter tubing to top of thigh or lower abdomen (with penis directed toward chest). Allow for slack for client movement.

33. Assist client to a comfortable position. Wash and dry perineal area as needed.

34. Dispose of equipment, drapes, and urine in proper receptacles.

35. Perform hand hygiene.

36. Palpate bladder.

37. Ask if client is comfortable.

38. Observe character and amount of urine in drainage system.

39. Determine that no urine is leaking from catheter or tubing connections.

Continued

528

	S	U	NP	Comments
40. Record and report catheterization, characteristics and amount of urine, specimen collection (if performed), and client's response to procedure and teaching concepts.	____	____	____	_____
41. Initiate intake and output records.	____	____	____	_____

STUDENT: _____ DATE: _____

INSTRUCTOR: _____ DATE: _____

SKILL PERFORMANCE CHECKLIST
Skill 40-3 In-Dwelling Catheter Care

	S	U	NP	Comments
1. Assess client for bowel incontinence or discomfort or provide care as per agency routine.	____	____	____	_____
2. Explain procedure to client.	____	____	____	_____
3. Provide privacy.	____	____	____	_____
4. Perform hand hygiene.	____	____	____	_____
5. Position client properly.	____	____	____	_____
6. Place waterproof pad under client.	____	____	____	_____
7. Drape client.	____	____	____	_____
8. Apply disposable gloves.	____	____	____	_____
9. Remove anchor device to free catheter tubing.	____	____	____	_____
10. With non-dominant hand:				
A. Female				
(1) Gently retract labia to fully expose urethral meatus and catheter insertion site, maintaining position of hand throughout procedure.	____	____	____	_____
B. Male				
(1) Retract foreskin if not circumcised, and hold penis at shaft just below glans, maintaining position throughout procedure.	____	____	____	_____
11. Assess urethral meatus and surrounding tissue for inflammation, swelling, and discharge. Note amount, colour, odour, and consistency of discharge. Ask client if any burning or discomfort is felt.	____	____	____	_____
12. Cleanse perineal tissue:				
A. Female				
(1) Use clean cloth, soap, and water. Cleanse around urethral meatus and catheter. Cleaning from pubis toward anus, clean labia minora. Use a clean side of cloth for each wipe. Clean around anus. Dry each area well.	____	____	____	_____
B. Male				
(1) While spreading urethral meatus, cleanse around catheter first, and then wipe in circular motion around meatus and glans.	____	____	____	_____

Continued

	S	U	NP	Comments
14. With soap and water, wipe in a circular motion approximately 10 cm down the length of the catheter.	____	____	____	_____
15. Apply antibiotic ointment (if ordered) at meatus and along 2.5 cm of catheter.	____	____	____	_____
16. Reposition male client's foreskin.	____	____	____	_____
17. Assist client to a comfortable position.	____	____	____	_____
18. Dispose of supplies and gloves. Perform hand hygiene.	____	____	____	_____

STUDENT: _____ DATE: _____

INSTRUCTOR: _____ DATE: _____

Skill 40-4 Closed and Open Catheter Irrigation

	S	U	NP	Comments
1. Assess physician's order.	____	____	____	_____
2. Assess colour of urine and presence of mucus or sediment.	____	____	____	_____
3. Determine type of catheter in place, triple or double lumen.	____	____	____	_____
4. Determine patency of drainage tubing.	____	____	____	_____
5. Measure urine in drainage bag.	____	____	____	_____
6. Explain procedure and purpose to client.	____	____	____	_____
7. Perform hand hygiene and apply clean gloves for closed methods.	____	____	____	_____
8. Provide privacy. Expose catheter. Drape client.	____	____	____	_____
9. Assess lower abdomen for bladder distension.	____	____	____	_____
10. Position client in dorsal recumbent or supine position.	____	____	____	_____
11. Closed intermittent irrigation:				
A. Prepare solution in sterile graduated cup.	____	____	____	_____
B. Draw solution into syringe.	____	____	____	_____
C. Clamp in-dwelling catheter below injection port.	____	____	____	_____
D. Cleanse injection port with swab.	____	____	____	_____
E. Insert syringe at 30-degree angle toward bladder.	____	____	____	_____
F. Slowly inject fluid into catheter and bladder.	____	____	____	_____
G. Withdraw syringe, remove clamp, and allow solution to drain into bag. If ordered, keep clamped to allow solution to remain in bladder for 20 to 30 minutes.	____	____	____	_____
12. Closed continuous irrigation:				
A. Using aseptic technique, insert tip of irrigation tubing into bag containing solution.	____	____	____	_____
B. Close clamp on tubing and hang bag of solution on IV pole.	____	____	____	_____
C. Open clamp and allow solution to flow through tubing, keeping end of tubing sterile. Close clamp.	____	____	____	_____
D. Wipe off irrigation port of triple lumen catheter or attach sterile Y connector to double lumen catheter and then attach to irrigation tubing.	____	____	____	_____

Continued

	S	U	NP	Comments

E. Be sure that drainage bag and tubing are securely connected to drainage port of triple lumen catheter or other arm of Y connector.

F. For intermittent flow, clamp tubing on drainage system, open clamp on irrigation tubing, and allow prescribed amount of fluid to enter bladder. Close irrigation clamp, open drainage tubing clamp. (Optional: Leave clamp closed for 20 to 30 minutes if ordered.)

G. For continuous drainage, calculate drip rate and adjust clamp on irrigation tubing accordingly. Ensure clamp on drainage tubing is open, and check volume of drainage in drainage bag. Ensure drainage tubing is patent, and avoid kinks.

13. Open irrigation (when double lumen catheter is in place):

A. Prepare sterile supplies.

B. Apply sterile gloves.

C. Position waterproof drape under catheter.

D. Aspirate 30 mL of solution into sterile irrigating syringe.

E. Move sterile collection close to client's thighs.

F. Disconnect catheter from drainage tubing, allowing urine from catheter to flow into basin. Allow urine in tubing to flow into drainage bag. Cover end of tubing with sterile cap. Position tubing in a safe place.

G. Insert syringe into lumen, and gently instill solution.

H. Withdraw syringe, lower catheter, and allow solution to drain into basin. Repeat until solution has been used or until drainage is clear, depending on purpose of irrigation.

I. If solution does not return, have client turn onto side facing you or gently aspirate solution.

J. After irrigation is complete, remove protector cap from tubing, cleanse end, and re-establish drainage system.

14. Re-anchor catheter to client with tape or elastic tube holder.

15. Assist client to comfortable position.

16. Lower bed to lowest position. Put side rails up if appropriate.

Continued

	S	U	NP	Comments
17. Dispose of contaminated supplies, remove gloves, and perform hand hygiene.	____	____	____	_____
18. Calculate fluid used and subtract from total output.	____	____	____	_____
19. Assess characteristics of output: viscosity, colour, and presence of matter (e.g., sediment, clots, blood).	____	____	____	_____

STUDENT: _____ DATE: _____

INSTRUCTOR: _____ DATE: _____

Skill 41-1 Administering a Cleansing Enema

	S	U	NP	Comments
1. Assess status of client.	____	____	____	_____
2. Assess client for presence of increased intracranial pressure, glaucoma, or recent rectal or prostate surgery.	____	____	____	_____
3. Check client's medical record.	____	____	____	_____
4. Review physician's order for enema.	____	____	____	_____
5. Determine client's understanding of purpose of enema.	____	____	____	_____
6. Perform hand hygiene. Collect appropriate equipment.	____	____	____	_____
7. Identify client and explain procedure.	____	____	____	_____
8. Assemble enema bag with appropriate solution and rectal tube.	____	____	____	_____
9. Perform hand hygiene and apply gloves.	____	____	____	_____
10. Provide privacy.	____	____	____	_____
11. Raise bed to appropriate working height and raise side rail on client's left side.	____	____	____	_____
12. Assist client to left side-lying position with right knee flexed.	____	____	____	_____
13. Place waterproof pad under client's hips and buttocks.	____	____	____	_____
14. Cover client with bath blanket so that only rectal area is exposed and anus is clearly visible.	____	____	____	_____
15. Place bedpan or commode in easily accessible position.	____	____	____	_____
16. Administer enema:				
A. Enema bag:				
(1) Add warmed solution to enema bag. Warm tap water as it flows from faucet, place saline container in basin of hot water before adding saline to enema bag, and check temperature of solution.	____	____	____	_____
(2) Raise container, release clamp, and allow solution to flow long enough to fill tubing.	____	____	____	_____
(3) Reclamp tubing.	____	____	____	_____
(4) Lubricate 6 to 8 cm of rectal tube with lubricating jelly.	____	____	____	_____
(5) Gently separate buttocks and locate anus. Instruct client to relax by breathing out slowly through mouth.	____	____	____	_____

Continued

	S	U	NP	Comments
(6) Insert tip of rectal tube slowly by pointing tip in direction of client's umbilicus (7.5 to 10 cm in adult, 5 to 7.5 cm in child, 2.5 to 3.75 cm in infant).	___	___	___	_____
(7) Hold tubing in rectum constantly until end of fluid instillation.	___	___	___	_____
(8) Open regulating clamp, and allow solution to enter slowly, with container at client's hip level.	___	___	___	_____
(9) Raise enema container slowly to appropriate level above client's anus.	___	___	___	_____
(10) Lower container or clamp tubing if client complains of cramping or if fluid escapes around rectal tube.	___	___	___	_____
(11) Clamp tubing after all solution is instilled.	___	___	___	_____

B. Prepackaged disposable container:

	S	U	NP	Comments
(1) Remove plastic cap from rectal tip.	___	___	___	_____
(2) Gently separate buttocks and locate rectum. Instruct client to relax by breathing out slowly through mouth.	___	___	___	_____
(3) Insert tip of bottle gently into rectum (7.5 to 10 cm in adult, 5 to 7.5 cm in child, 2.5 to 3.75 cm in infant).	___	___	___	_____
(4) Squeeze bottle until all of solution has entered rectum and colon. Instruct client to retain solution until the urge to defecate occurs, usually 2 to 5 minutes.	___	___	___	_____
17. Place layers of toilet tissue around tube at anus and gently withdraw rectal tube.	___	___	___	_____
18. Explain to client that feeling of distention is normal. Ask client to retain solution as long as possible while lying quietly in bed. For infant or young child, gently hold buttocks together for a few minutes.	___	___	___	_____
19. Discard enema container and tubing in receptacle, or rinse container thoroughly with soap and warm water if it is to be reused.	___	___	___	_____
20. Assist client to bathroom or help position client on bedpan.	___	___	___	_____
21. Observe character of client's feces and solution (caution client against flushing toilet before inspection).	___	___	___	_____
22. Assist client as needed to wash anal area with warm soap and water.	___	___	___	_____
23. Remove and discard gloves. Perform hand hygiene.	___	___	___	_____

Continued

538

	S	U	NP	Comments
24. Inspect colour, consistency, and amount of stool and fluid passed.	____	____	____	_____
25. Assess condition of client's abdomen. Cramping, rigidity, or distension can indicate a serious problem.	____	____	____	_____

STUDENT: _____ DATE: _____

INSTRUCTOR: _____ DATE: _____

Skill 41-2 Inserting and Maintaining a Nasogastric Tube

	S	U	NP	Comments
1. Perform hand hygiene. Inspect condition of client's nasal and oral cavities.	____	____	____	_____
2. Ask if client has history of nasal surgery and note if deviated nasal septum is present.	____	____	____	_____
3. Palpate client's abdomen for distention, pain, and rigidity. Auscultate for bowel sounds.	____	____	____	_____
4. Assess client's level of consciousness and ability to follow instructions.	____	____	____	_____
5. Check medical record for physician's order, type of nasogastric (NG) tube to be placed, and whether tube is to be attached to suction or drainage bag.	____	____	____	_____
6. Perform hand hygiene. Prepare equipment at bedside.	____	____	____	_____
7. Identify the client and explain procedure to client.	____	____	____	_____
8. Apply disposable gloves.	____	____	____	_____
9. Position client in high-Fowler's position with pillow behind client's head and shoulders. Raise bed to a comfortable working level.	____	____	____	_____
10. Place bath towel over client's chest. Give facial tissues to client. Place emesis basin within reach.	____	____	____	_____
11. Provide privacy.	____	____	____	_____
12. Stand on client's right side if you are right-handed and on left side if left-handed.	____	____	____	_____
13. Instruct client to relax and breathe normally while occluding one naris. Repeat for other naris. Select nostril with greater air flow.	____	____	____	_____
14. Measure distance to insert tube:	____	____	____	_____
A. Measure distance from tip of nose to earlobe to xiphoid process.	____	____	____	_____
B. First mark 50-cm point on tube, then do traditional measurement. Tube insertion should be midway point between 50 cm and traditional mark.	____	____	____	_____
15. Mark length of tube to be inserted with small piece of tape placed so it can easily be removed.	____	____	____	_____
16. Curve 10 to 15 cm of end of tube tightly around index finger, then release.	____	____	____	_____
17. Lubricate 7.5 to 10 cm of end of tube with water-soluble lubricating jelly.	____	____	____	_____

Continued

	S	U	NP	Comments

18. Alert client that procedure is to begin.

19. Instruct client to extend neck back against pillow. Insert tube slowly through naris, with curved end pointing downward.

20. Continue to pass tube along floor of nasal passage, aiming down toward ear. If resistance is felt, apply gentle downward pressure to advance tube (do not force past resistance).

21. If resistance is met, try to rotate the tube and see if it advances. If there is still resistance, withdraw tube, allow client to rest, relubricate tube, and insert into client's other naris.

22. Continue insertion of tube until just past nasopharynx by gently rotating tube toward opposite naris.
   A. Stop tube advancement, allow client to relax, and provide tissues.
   B. Explain to client that next step requires that client swallow. Give client glass of water, unless contraindicated.

23. With tube just above client's oropharynx, instruct client to flex head forward, take a small sip of water, and swallow. Advance tube 2.5 to 5 cm with each swallow of water. If client is not allowed fluids, instruct client to dry swallow or suck air through straw.

24. If client begins to cough, gag, or choke, withdraw tube slightly (do not remove) and stop advancement. Instruct client to breathe easily and take sips of water.

25. If client continues to gag and cough, or complains that tube feels as though it is coiling in the back of throat, check back of oropharynx using tongue blade. If tube is coiled, withdraw it until the tip is back in the oropharynx. Then reinsert with client swallowing.

26. Continue to advance tube with swallowing until tape or mark is reached. Temporarily anchor tube to client's cheek with a piece of tape until tube placement is checked.

27. Verify tube placement (check agency policy for preferred method):
   A. Ask client to talk.
   B. Inspect posterior pharynx for presence of coiled tube.
   C. Aspirate gently back on syringe to obtain gastric contents. Observe colour.

Continued

542

	S	U	NP	Comments
D. Measure pH of aspirate with colour-coded pH paper that has range of whole numbers from 1 to 11.	___	___	___	_____
E. Measure pH of aspirate with colour-coded pH paper with range of whole numbers 1 to 11.	___	___	___	_____
F. Have ordered x-ray examination performed of chest/abdomen.	___	___	___	_____

28. Anchor the tube:

	S	U	NP	Comments
A. Clamp end of tube or connect it to drainage bag or suction machine after insertion.	___	___	___	_____
B. Tape tube to nose; avoid putting pressure on nares:	___	___	___	_____
(1) Before taping tube to nose, apply small amount of tincture of benzoin to lower end of nose and allow to dry (optional). Be sure that top end of tape over nose is secure.	___	___	___	_____
(2) Carefully wrap two split ends of tape around tube.	___	___	___	_____
(3) Alternatively, apply tube fixation device using shaped adhesive patch.	___	___	___	_____
C. Fasten end of NG tube to client's gown by looping rubber band around tube in slip knot. Pin rubber band to gown.	___	___	___	_____
D. Elevate head of bed 30 degrees, unless contraindicated.	___	___	___	_____
E. Explain to client that sensation of tube should decrease somewhat with time.	___	___	___	_____
F. Remove and dispose of gloves and perform hand hygiene.	___	___	___	_____

29. Identify tube placement in nose with mark or tape or measure length from nares to connector.

	S	U	NP	Comments
	___	___	___	_____

30. Irrigate tube:

	S	U	NP	Comments
A. Wash hands and apply disposable gloves.	___	___	___	_____
B. Check for tube placement. Reconnect NG tube to connecting tube.	___	___	___	_____
C. Draw up 30 mL of normal saline into Asepto or catheter-tipped syringe.	___	___	___	_____
D. Clamp NG tube. Disconnect it from connection tubing and lay end of connection tubing on towel.	___	___	___	_____
E. Insert tip of irrigating syringe into end of NG tube. Remove clamp. Hold syringe with tip pointed at floor and inject saline slowly and evenly. Do not force solution.	___	___	___	_____

Continued

543

	S	U	NP	Comments
F. If resistance occurs, check for kinks in tubing. Turn client onto left side. Report repeated resistance to physician.	___	___	___	_____
G. After instilling saline, immediately aspirate or pull back slowly on syringe to withdraw fluid. If amount aspirated is greater than amount instilled, record the difference as output. If amount aspirated is less than amount instilled, record the difference as intake.	___	___	___	_____
H. Reconnect NG tube to drainage or suction. (If solution does not return, repeat irrigation).	___	___	___	_____
I. Remove and dispose of gloves and perform hand hygiene.	___	___	___	_____
31. Observe amount and character of contents drainage from NG tube. Ask if client feels nauseated.	___	___	___	_____
32. Palpate client's abdomen periodically, noting any distension, pain, and rigidity and auscultate for the presence of bowel sounds. Turn off suction while auscultating.	___	___	___	_____
33. Inspect condition of nares and nose.	___	___	___	_____
34. Observe position of tubing.	___	___	___	_____
35. Ask if client feels sore throat or irritation in pharynx.	___	___	___	_____
36. Discontinuation of NG tube:				
A. Verify order to discontinue NG tube.	___	___	___	_____
B. Explain procedure to client and reassure client that removal is less distressing than insertion.	___	___	___	_____
C. Perform hand hygiene and apply disposable gloves.	___	___	___	_____
D. Turn off suction and disconnect NG tube from drainage bag or suction. Remove tape from bridge of nose and unpin tube from gown.	___	___	___	_____
E. Stand on client's right side if you are right-handed and left side if you are left-handed.	___	___	___	_____
F. Hand the client facial tissue. Place clean towel across client's chest. Instruct client to take and hold a deep breath.	___	___	___	_____
G. Clamp or kink tubing securely and then pull tube out steadily and smoothly into towel held in other hand while client holds breath.	___	___	___	_____

Continued

544

	S	U	NP	Comments
H. Measure amount of drainage and note character of content. Dispose of tube and drainage equipment.	____	____	____	_____
I. Clean nares and provide mouth care.	____	____	____	_____
J. Assist client to a comfortable position and explain procedure for drinking fluids, if not contraindicated.	____	____	____	_____
37. Clean equipment and return to proper place. Place soiled linen in proper receptacle.	____	____	____	_____
38. Remove and dispose of gloves and perform hand hygiene.	____	____	____	_____
39. Inspect condition of nares and nose.	____	____	____	_____
40. Ask if client feels sore throat or irritation in the pharynx.	____	____	____	_____

SKILL PERFORMANCE CHECKLIST
Skill 41-3 Pouching an Ostomy

	S	U	NP	Comments
1. Perform hand hygiene and auscultate for bowel sounds.	___	___	___	_____
2. Observe client's skin barrier and pouch for leakage and length of time in place.	___	___	___	_____
3. Observe stoma for colour, swelling, trauma, and healing.	___	___	___	_____
4. Measure the stoma with each pouching change.	___	___	___	_____
5. Observe abdominal incision (if present).	___	___	___	_____
6. Observe effluent from stoma and keep a record of intake and output. Ask client about skin tenderness. Remove gloves and perform hand hygiene.	___	___	___	_____
7. Assess client's abdomen for best type of pouching system to use.	___	___	___	_____
8. Assess client's self-care ability.	___	___	___	_____
9. After skin barrier and pouch removal, assess client's skin around stoma. Keep pouch loosely attached to stoma to collect any drainage while the system is being changed.	___	___	___	_____
10. Determine client's emotional response and knowledge and understanding of an ostomy and its care.	___	___	___	_____
11. Explain procedure to client. Encourage client's interaction and questions.	___	___	___	_____
12. Assemble equipment. Provide privacy.	___	___	___	_____
13. Position client either standing or supine and drape. If seated, position either on or in front of the toilet.	___	___	___	_____
14. Perform hand hygiene. Apply disposable gloves.	___	___	___	_____
15. Place towel or disposable waterproof barrier under client.	___	___	___	_____
16. Remove used pouch and skin barrier gently by pushing the skin away from the barrier.	___	___	___	_____
17. Cleanse peristomal skin gently with warm tap water using gauze pads or clean washcloth. Do not scrub the skin. Dry area completely by patting the skin with gauze or towel.	___	___	___	_____
18. Measure the stoma for correct size of pouching system needed.	___	___	___	_____

Continued

	S	U	NP	Comments

19. Select appropriate pouch for client based on assessment. With a custom cut-to-fit pouch, use an ostomy guide to cut opening on the pouch 2 mm larger than stoma before removing backing. Prepare pouch by removing backing from barrier and adhesive. With ileostomy, apply thin circle of barrier paste around opening in pouch. Allow to dry.

20. Apply skin barrier and pouch. If creases occur next to stoma, use barrier paste to fill in; let dry 1 to 2 minutes.

   A. For one-piece pouching system:

   (1) Use skin sealant wipes on skin directly under adhesive skin barrier or pouch; allow to dry. Press the adhesive backing of the pouch and/or skin barrier smoothly against the skin, starting from the bottom and working up and around the sides.

   (2) Hold pouch by barrier, centre over stoma, and press down gently on barrier. Bottom of pouch should point toward client's knees.

   (3) Maintain gentle finger pressure around barrier for 1 to 2 minutes.

   B. For two-piece pouching system: Apply flange as in steps above for one-piece system, then snap on pouch and maintain finger pressure.

   C. For both pouching systems, gently tug on the pouch in a downward direction.

21. Apply non-allergenic paper tape around pectin skin barrier using "picture frame" method. A belt may be attached for extra security, rather than tape.

22. A small amount of ostomy deodorant may be put in pouch.

23. Fold bottom of drainable open-ended pouches up once and close with closure device.

24. Properly dispose of old pouch and soiled equipment. Spray room deodorant if necessary.

25. Remove gloves and perform hand hygiene.

26. Change pouch every 3 to 7 days unless leaking.

27. Ask if client feels discomfort around stoma.

Continued

	S	U	NP	Comments
28. Note appearance of stoma around skin and existing incision (if present) while pouch is removed and skin is cleansed. Reinspect condition of skin barrier and adhesive.	___	___	___	_____
29. Auscultate bowel sounds and observe characteristics of stool.	___	___	___	_____
30. Observe client's non-verbal behaviours as pouch is applied. Ask if client has any questions about pouching.	___	___	___	_____

SKILL PERFORMANCE CHECKLIST
Skill 42-1 Moving and Positioning Clients in Bed

	S	U	NP	Comments
1. Assess client's body alignment and comfort level while client is lying down.	___	___	___	_____
2. Assess for risk factors that may contribute to complications of immobility.	___	___	___	_____
3. Assess client's physical ability to help with moving and positioning.	___	___	___	_____
4. Check physician's order.	___	___	___	_____
5. Perform hand hygiene.	___	___	___	_____
6. Assess for presence of tubes, incisions, and equipment.	___	___	___	_____
7. Assess ability and motivation of client, family members, and primary caregiver to participate in moving and positioning client in bed in anticipation of discharge to home.	___	___	___	_____
8. Raise bed to comfortable working height. Get extra help if needed.	___	___	___	_____
9. Perform hand hygiene.	___	___	___	_____
10. Explain procedure to client.	___	___	___	_____
11. Position client flat, if tolerated.	___	___	___	_____
12. Position client in bed:				
A. Assist client to move up in bed (one or two nurses). NOTE: Only a young child or a lightweight client requiring minimal assistance can be safely moved by one nurse:				
(1) Remove pillow from under head and shoulders, and place pillow at head of bed. Ask client to cross arms across the chest.	___	___	___	_____
(2) Face head of bed.				
(a) Each nurse should have one arm under client's shoulders and one arm under client's thighs.	___	___	___	_____

Continued

	S	U	NP	Comments

(b) Alternative position: Position one nurse at client's upper body. Nurse's arm nearest head of bed should be under client's head and opposite shoulder, other arm should be under client's closest arm and shoulder. Position other nurse at client's lower torso. The nurse's arms should be under client's lower back and torso.

(3) Place feet apart, with foot nearest head of bed behind other foot. ____ ____ ____ _____

(4) Ask client to flex knees with feet on bed surface. ____ ____ ____ _____

(5) Instruct client to flex neck, tilting chin toward chest. ____ ____ ____ _____

(6) Instruct client to push with feet on bed surface. ____ ____ ____ _____

(7) Flex knees and hips, bringing forearms closer to level of bed. ____ ____ ____ _____

(8) Instruct client to push with heels and elevate trunk while breathing out, thus moving toward head of bed on count of three. ____ ____ ____ _____

(9) On count of three, rock and shift weight from front to back leg. At the same time, client pushes with heels and elevates trunk. ____ ____ ____ _____

B. Move immobile client up in bed with drawsheet or pull sheet (two nurses):

(1) Place drawsheet or pull sheet under client by turning client side to side. Drawsheet extends from shoulders to thighs. Return to supine position. ____ ____ ____ _____

(2) Position one nurse at each side of client. ____ ____ ____ _____

(3) Grasp drawsheet or pull sheet firmly near the client. ____ ____ ____ _____

(4) Place feet apart with forward-backward stance. Flex knees and hips. Shift weight from front to back leg, and move client and drawsheet or pull sheet to desired position in bed. ____ ____ ____ _____

(5) Realign client in correct body alignment. ____ ____ ____ _____

Continued

552

	S	U	NP	Comments

C. Position client in supported Fowler's position:

(1) Elevate head of bed 45 to 60 degrees. ____ ____ ____ _____

(2) Rest client's head against mattress or on small pillow. ____ ____ ____ _____

(3) Use pillows to support client's arms and hands if client does not have control of use of them. ____ ____ ____ _____

(4) Position pillow at lower back. ____ ____ ____ _____

(5) Place small pillow or roll under thigh. ____ ____ ____ _____

(6) Place small pillow or roll under ankles. ____ ____ ____ _____

D. Position hemiplegic client in supported Fowler's position:

(1) Elevate head of bed 45 to 60 degrees. ____ ____ ____ _____

(2) Position client in sitting position as straight as possible. ____ ____ ____ _____

(3) Position head on small pillow with chin slightly forward. Hyperextension of the neck must be avoided. ____ ____ ____ _____

(4) Flex client's knees and hips by using pillow or folded blanket under knees. ____ ____ ____ _____

(5) Support feet in dorsiflexion with firm pillow or footboard. ____ ____ ____ _____

E. Position client in supine position:

(1) Place client on back, with head of bed flat. ____ ____ ____ _____

(2) Place small rolled towel under lumbar area of back. ____ ____ ____ _____

(3) Place pillow under upper shoulders, neck, or head. ____ ____ ____ _____

(4) Place trochanter rolls or sandbags parallel to lateral surface of thighs. ____ ____ ____ _____

(5) Place small pillow or roll under ankles to elevate heels. ____ ____ ____ _____

(6) Place foot board or firm pillows against bottom of feet. ____ ____ ____ _____

(7) Place high-top sneakers or foot splints on feet. ____ ____ ____ _____

(8) Place pillows under client's pronated forearms, and keep client's upper arms parallel to client's body. ____ ____ ____ _____

(9) Place hand rolls in client's hands. ____ ____ ____ _____

F. Position hemiplegic client in supine position:

(1) Place client on back, with head of bed flat. ____ ____ ____ _____

Continued

	S	U	NP	Comments

    (2) Place folded towel or small pillow under client's shoulder or affected side.

    (3) Keep affected arm away from client's body, with elbow extended and palm up.

    (4) Place folded towel under client's hip on involved side.

    (5) Flex client's affected knee 30 degrees by supporting it on a pillow or folded blanket.

    (6) Support client's feet with soft pillows at right angle to leg.

G. Position client in prone position:

    (1) With client supine, roll client over arm positioned close to body, with elbow straight, and hand under hip. Position on abdomen in centre of bed.

    (2) Turn client's head to one side and support head with small pillow.

    (3) Place small pillow under client's abdomen, below level of diaphragm.

    (4) Support arms in flexed position level at shoulders.

    (5) Support lower legs with pillows to elevate toes.

H. Position hemiplegic client in prone position:

    (1) Move client toward unaffected side.

    (2) Roll client onto side.

    (3) Place pillow on client's abdomen.

    (4) Roll client onto abdomen by positioning involved arm close to client's body, with elbow straight and hand under hip. Roll client carefully over arm.

    (5) Turn client's head toward involved side.

    (6) Position client's involved arm out to side with elbow bent, hand toward head of bed, and fingers extended (if possible).

    (7) Flex knees slightly by placing pillow under legs from knees to ankles.

    (8) Keep feet at right angles by using pillow high enough to keep toes off mattress.

Continued

554

	S	U	NP	Comments

I. Position client in lateral position:
    (1) Lower head of bed completely or as low as client can tolerate. ____ ____ ____ _____
    (2) Position client to side of bed. ____ ____ ____ _____
    (3) Prepare to turn client onto side. Flex client's knee that will not be next to mattress. Place one hand on client's hip and one hand on client's shoulder. ____ ____ ____ _____
    (4) Roll client onto side, toward you. ____ ____ ____ _____
    (5) Place pillow under client's head and neck. ____ ____ ____ _____
    (6) Bring shoulder blade forward. ____ ____ ____ _____
    (7) Position both arms in slightly flexed position. Upper arm is supported by pillow level with shoulder, other arm, by mattress. ____ ____ ____ _____
    (8) Place tuck-back pillow behind client's back. ____ ____ ____ _____
    (9) Place pillow under semiflexed upper leg for support. ____ ____ ____ _____
    (10) Place sandbag parallel to plantar surface of dependent foot. ____ ____ ____ _____

J. Position client in Sims' position:
    (1) Lower head of bed completely. ____ ____ ____ _____
    (2) Place client in supine position. ____ ____ ____ _____
    (3) Position client in lateral position, with dependent arm straight along client's body and with client lying partially on abdomen.
    (4) Carefully lift client's dependent shoulder and bring arm back behind client. ____ ____ ____ _____
    (5) Place small pillow under client's head. ____ ____ ____ _____
    (6) Place pillow under flexed upper arm, supporting arm level with shoulder. ____ ____ ____ _____
    (7) Place pillow under flexed upper legs, supporting leg level with hip. ____ ____ ____ _____
    (8) Place sandbags or pillows parallel to plantar surface of foot. ____ ____ ____ _____

K. Logrolling the client (three nurses):
    (1) Place pillow between client's knees. ____ ____ ____ _____
    (2) Cross client's arms over chest. ____ ____ ____ _____
    (3) Position two nurses on side of bed to which the client will be turned. Position third nurse on the other side of bed. ____ ____ ____ _____

Continued

	S	U	NP	Comments
(4) Fanfold or roll the drawsheet or pull sheet.	___	___	___	_____
(5) Move the client as one unit in a smooth, continuous motion on the count of three.	___	___	___	_____
(6) Nurse on the opposite side of the bed places pillows along the length of the client.	___	___	___	_____
(7) Gently lean the client as a unit back toward the pillows.	___	___	___	_____
13. Perform hand hygiene.	___	___	___	_____
14. Evaluate client's comfort level and ability to assist in position change.	___	___	___	_____
15. Evaluate client's body alignment and presence of any pressure areas.	___	___	___	_____

STUDENT: _____ DATE: _____

INSTRUCTOR: _____ DATE: _____

SKILL PERFORMANCE CHECKLIST
Skill 42-2 Using Safe and Effective Transfer Techniques

	S	U	NP	Comments
1. Assess the client for the following:				
A. Muscle strength (legs and upper arms)	___	___	___	_____
B. Joint mobility and contracture formation	___	___	___	_____
C. Paralysis or paresis (spastic or flaccid)	___	___	___	_____
D. Orthostatic hypotension	___	___	___	_____
E. Activity tolerance	___	___	___	_____
F. Presence of pain	___	___	___	_____
G. Vital signs	___	___	___	_____
2. Assess client's sensory status.	___	___	___	_____
3. Assess client's cognitive status.	___	___	___	_____
4. Assess client's level of motivation.	___	___	___	_____
5. Assess previous mode of transfer (if applicable).	___	___	___	_____
6. Assess client's specific risk of falling when transferred.	___	___	___	_____
7. Assess special transfer equipment needed for home setting. Assess home environment for hazards	___	___		_____
8. Perform hand hygiene.	___	___	___	_____
9. Explain procedure to client.	___	___	___	_____
10. Transfer client:				
A. Assist client to sitting position (bed at waist level):				
(1) Place client in supine position.	___	___	___	_____
(2) Face head of bed at a 45-degree angle and remove pillows.	___	___	___	_____
(3) Place feet apart, with foot nearer bed behind other foot, continuing at a 45-degree angle to head of bed.	___	___	___	_____
(4) Place hand farther from client under shoulders, supporting client's head and neck.	___	___	___	_____
(5) Place other hand on bed surface.	___	___	___	_____
(6) Raise client to sitting position by shifting weight from front to back leg. Pivot feet as weight is shifted.	___	___	___	_____
(7) Push against bed using arm that is placed on bed surface.	___	___	___	_____
B. Assist client to sitting position on side of bed with bed in low position:				
(1) Turn client to side, facing you on side of bed on which client will be sitting.	___	___	___	_____

Continued

	S	U	NP	Comments

(2) With client supine, raise head of bed 30 degrees.

(3) Stand opposite client's hips. Turn diagonally so you face client and far corner of foot of bed.

(4) Place feet apart, with foot closer to head of bed in front of other foot.

(5) Place arm nearer head of bed under client's shoulder, supporting client's head and neck.

(6) Place other arm over client's thighs.

(7) Move client's lower legs and feet over side of bed. Pivot toward rear leg, allowing client's upper legs to swing downward.

(8) At same time, shift weight to rear leg and elevate client. Pivot feet in the direction of movement to avoid twisting of upper body.

C. Transfer client from bed to chair with bed in low position:

(1) Assist client to sitting position on side of bed. Position chair at 45-degree angle to bed.

(2) Apply transfer belt of other transfer aid.

(3) Ensure that client has stable, non-skid shoes. Client's strong leg is forward and weak leg is back.

(4) Spread feet apart.

(5) Flex hips and knees, and align knees with client's knees.

(6) Grasp transfer belt from underneath.

(7) Rock client up to standing position on count of three while straightening hips and legs and keeping knees slightly flexed. Instruct client to use hands to push up, unless contraindicated.

(8) Maintain stability of client's weak or paralyzed leg with knee.

(9) Pivot on foot farther from chair. Instruct client to stand straight. Pivot body in direction of chair, instructing client to take small steps toward chair. Ask client to tell you when the chair touches the back of his or her knees.

Continued

558

	S	U	NP	Comments

(10) Instruct client to use armrests on chair for support, and ease client into chair.

(11) Flex hips and knees while lowering client into chair.

(12) Assess client for proper alignment for sitting position. Provide support for paralyzed extremities. Use lap board or sling to support flaccid arm. Stabilize legs with bath blanket or pillow.

(13) Praise client's progress, effort, and performance.

D. Perform three-person carry from bed to stretcher (bed at stretcher level):

(1) Stand side by side with two other nurses, facing side of client's bed.

(2) Assume responsibility for one of three areas: head and shoulders, hips and thighs, or ankles.

(3) Assume wide base of support with foot closer to stretcher in front and knees slightly flexed.

(4) Lifters will place arms under client's head and shoulders, hips and thighs, and ankles, with fingers securely around other side of client's body.

(5) Lifters will roll client toward their chests. On count of three, lift client and hold against chest.

(6) On second count of three, all lifters step back and pivot toward stretcher, moving forward if needed.

(7) Gently lower client onto centre of stretcher by flexing knees and hips until elbows are level with edge of stretcher.

(8) Assess body alignment, place safety straps across client's body, and raise side rails.

E. Use mechanical/hydraulic lift to transfer client from bed to chair:

(1) Bring lift to bedside.

(2) Position chair near bed and allow adequate space to manoeuvre lift.

(3) Raise bed to high position, with mattress flat. Lower side rail.

(4) Keep bed side rail up on side opposite nurse.

Continued

	S	U	NP	Comments
(5) Roll client away from you.	___	___	___	_____
(6) Place hammock or canvas strips under client to form sling; fit lower edge under client's knees and upper edge under client's shoulders.	___	___	___	_____
(7) Raise side rail of bed.	___	___	___	_____
(8) Go to opposite side of bed and lower side rail.	___	___	___	_____
(9) Roll client to opposite side and pull hammock or canvas strips through.	___	___	___	_____
(10) Roll client supine onto canvas seat.	___	___	___	_____
(11) Remove client's glasses, if appropriate.	___	___	___	_____
(12) Place lift's horseshoe bar under side of bed (on side with chair).	___	___	___	_____
(13) Lower horizontal bar to sling level by releasing hydraulic valve. Lock valve.	___	___	___	_____
(14) Attach hooks on strap (chain) to holes in sling. Hook short chains or straps to top holes of sling, and hook longer chains to bottom of sling.	___	___	___	_____
(15) Elevate head of bed.	___	___	___	_____
(16) Fold client's arms over chest.	___	___	___	_____
(17) Pump hydraulic handle using long, slow, even strokes until client is raised off bed.	___	___	___	_____
(18) Use steering handle to pull lift from bed and manoeuvre to chair.	___	___	___	_____
(19) Roll base around chair.	___	___	___	_____
(20) Release check valve slowly and lower client into chair.	___	___	___	_____
(21) Close check valve as soon as client is down and straps can be released.	___	___	___	_____
(22) Remove straps and mechanical/ hydraulic lift.	___	___	___	_____
(23) Check client's sitting alignment.	___	___	___	_____
11. Perform hand hygiene.	___	___	___	_____
12. Assess client's tolerance and level of fatigue and comfort with each transfer.	___	___	___	_____
13. Following each transfer, evaluate client's body alignment.	___	___	___	_____

STUDENT: _____ DATE: _____

INSTRUCTOR: _____ DATE: _____

SKILL PERFORMANCE CHECKLIST
Skill 43-1 Assessment for Risk of Pressure Ulcer Development

	S	U	NP	Comments
1. Identify at-risk individuals needing prevention and the factors placing them at risk.	____	____	____	_____
A. Use a validated risk assessment tool such as the Braden Scale.	____	____	____	_____
B. Assess the client upon admission.	____	____	____	_____
C. Inspect the condition of the client's skin at least once a day and examine all bony prominences, noting skin integrity. If redness or discolouration is noted, use thumb to gently palpate area of redness. The discolouration may vary from pink to deep red.	____	____	____	_____
D. Observe all assistive devices for pressure points.	____	____	____	_____
2. Determine client's ability to communicate discomfort.	____	____	____	_____
3. Assess extent that skin is exposed to moisture.	____	____	____	_____
4. Evaluate client's activity level.	____	____	____	_____
5. Assess food intake pattern.	____	____	____	_____
6. Evaluate presence of friction and/or shear.	____	____	____	_____
7. Document the risk assessment.	____	____	____	_____
8. Provide education to client and family regarding pressure ulcer risk and prevention.	____	____	____	_____
9. Evaluate measures to reduce pressure ulcer development:				
A. Observe client's skin for areas at risk.	____	____	____	_____
B. Observe tolerance of client for positioning.	____	____	____	_____
C. Monitor success of toileting program.	____	____	____	_____
D. Evaluate nutrition and laboratory values.	____	____	____	_____

SKILL PERFORMANCE CHECKLIST
Skill 43-2 Treating Pressure Ulcers

	S	U	NP	Comments
1. Assess client's level of comfort and need for pain medication.	___	___	___	_____
2. Determine if client has allergies to topical agents.	___	___	___	_____
3. Review order for topical agent or dressing. Position client to allow dressing removal.	___	___	___	_____
4. Provide privacy.	___	___	___	_____
5. Perform hand hygiene. Apply disposable gloves. Remove dressing.	___	___	___	_____
6. Assess pressure ulcer(s):				
A. Note colour, type, and percentage of tissue present in the wound base.	___	___	___	_____
B. Measure width and length of the ulcer(s). Width is determined by measuring the dimension from left to right, and the length is from top to bottom.	___	___	___	_____
C. Measure depth of pressure ulcer using sterile cotton-tipped applicator or other device.	___	___	___	_____
D. Measure depth of undermining skin using a cotton-tipped applicator and gently probing under skin edges.	___	___	___	_____
7. Assess the periwound skin; check for maceration, redness, denuded areas.	___	___	___	_____
8. Change to sterile gloves (check agency policy).	___	___	___	_____
9. Cleanse ulcer thoroughly with normal saline or cleansing agent: Use irrigating syringe for deep ulcers.	___	___	___	_____
10. Apply topical agents as prescribed:				
A. Enzymes:				
(1) Apply thin, even layer of ointment over necrotic areas of ulcer only.	___	___	___	_____
(2) Apply gauze dressing directly over ulcer.	___	___	___	_____
(3) Tape dressing securely in place.	___	___	___	_____
B. Hydrogel:				
(1) Cover surface of ulcer with hydrogel using applicator or gloved hand.	___	___	___	_____
(2) Apply dry gauze, hydrocolloid, or transparent dressing over wound and adhere to intact skin.	___	___	___	_____
C. Calcium alginate:				
(1) Pack wound with alginate using applicator or gloved hand.	___	___	___	_____

Continued

	S	U	NP	Comments

(2) Apply dry gauze, foam, or
    hydrocolloid over alginate.
    Tape in place.

11. Remove gloves and dispose of soiled
    supplies. Perform hand hygiene.

12. Complete ulcer information required for one
    of the wound-healing scales per agency's
    protocol.

13. Compare subsequent ulcer measurements.

14. Do *not* use the pressure ulcer staging system
    to measure pressure ulcer healing.

STUDENT: _____ DATE: _____

INSTRUCTOR: _____ DATE: _____

Skill 43-3 Performing Wound Irrigation

	S	U	NP	Comments
1. Assess client's level of pain. Administer prescribed analgesic 30 to 45 minutes before starting wound irrigation procedure.	____	____	____	_____
2. Review medical record for prescription for irrigation of open wound and type of solution to be used.	____	____	____	_____
3. Assess signs and symptoms related to client's open wound.	____	____	____	_____
4. Explain procedure to client.	____	____	____	_____
5. Perform hand hygiene.	____	____	____	_____
6. Assist client to a comfortable position that will permit gravitational flow of irrigating solution through wound and into collection receptacle. Position client so that wound is vertical to collection basin.	____	____	____	_____
7. Warm irrigation solution to approximate body temperature.	____	____	____	_____
8. Form cuff on waterproof bag and place it near bed.	____	____	____	_____
9. Provide privacy.	____	____	____	_____
10. Apply gown and goggles, if needed.	____	____	____	_____
11. Apply disposable gloves. Remove soiled dressing and discard in waterproof bag. Remove and dispose of gloves.	____	____	____	_____
12. Prepare equipment and open sterile supplies.	____	____	____	_____
13. Apply sterile gloves.	____	____	____	_____
14. To irrigate wound with wide opening:				
A. Fill 35-mL syringe with irrigation solution.	____	____	____	_____
B. Attach 19-gauge needle or angiocatheter.	____	____	____	_____
C. Hold syringe tip 2.5 cm above upper end of wound and over area being cleansed.	____	____	____	_____
D. Flush wound with continuous pressure. Repeat steps 14 a, b, and c until solution draining into basin is clear.	____	____	____	_____
15. To irrigate deep wound with very small opening:				
A. Attach soft angiocatheter to filled irrigating syringe.	____	____	____	_____
B. Lubricate tip of catheter with irrigating solution, then gently insert tip of catheter and pull out about 1 cm.	____	____	____	_____
C. Flush wound with slow continuous pressure.	____	____	____	_____

Continued

	S	U	NP	Comments
D. Pinch off catheter just below syringe while keeping catheter in place.	___	___	___	_____
E. Remove and refill syringe. Reconnect to catheter and repeat until solution draining into basin is clear.	___	___	___	_____

16. To cleanse wound with hand-held shower:
  A. With client seated comfortably in shower chair, adjust spray to gentle flow; water temperature should be warm.
  B. Cover shower head with clean washcloth, if needed.
  C. Shower wound for 5 to 10 minutes with showerhead 30 cm from wound.
17. Obtain cultures, if needed, after cleansing wound with non-bacteriostatic saline.
18. Dry wound edges with gauze; dry client if shower or whirlpool is used.
19. Apply appropriate dressing.
20. Remove gloves and, if worn, mask, goggles, and gown.
21. Dispose of equipment and soiled supplies. Perform hand hygiene.
22. Assist client to comfortable position.
23. Assess type of tissue in the wound bed.
24. Inspect dressing periodically.
25. Evaluate skin integrity.
26. Observe client for signs of discomfort.
27. Observe for presence of retained irrigant.

STUDENT: _____ DATE: _____

INSTRUCTOR: _____ DATE: _____

Skill 43-4 Applying Dry and Wet-to-Dry Dressings

	S	U	NP	Comments
1. Perform hand hygiene. Obtain information about size and location of wound to be dressed.	____	____	____	_____
2. Assess client's level of comfort.	____	____	____	_____
3. Review orders for dressing change procedure.	____	____	____	_____
4. Explain procedure to client and instruct client not to touch wound area or sterile supplies.	____	____	____	_____
5. Provide privacy.	____	____	____	_____
6. Assist client to a comfortable position. Drape client with bath blanket to expose only wound site.	____	____	____	_____
7. Place disposable bag within reach of work area. Fold top of bag to make cuff.	____	____	____	_____
8. Apply face mask and protective eyewear, if required. Perform hand hygiene.	____	____	____	_____
9. Apply disposable gloves and remove tape, bandage, or ties from wound site.	____	____	____	_____
10. Remove tape: Pull parallel to skin, toward dressing, and remove remaining adhesive from client's skin.	____	____	____	_____
11. With gloved hand, carefully remove gauze dressings one layer at a time, taking care not to dislodge drains or tubes. If dressing sticks on a wet-to-dry dressing, alert client of potential discomfort and gently free dressing (do not moisten it).	____	____	____	_____
12. Observe character and amount of drainage on dressing and appearance of wound.	____	____	____	_____
13. Fold dressings with drainage contained inside, and remove gloves inside out. With small dressings, remove gloves inside out over dressing. Dispose of gloves and soiled dressings. Perform hand hygiene.	____	____	____	_____
14. Open sterile dressing tray or individually wrapped sterile supplies. Place on bedside table.	____	____	____	_____
15. Cleanse wound:				
A. Pour ordered solution into sterile irrigation container.	____	____	____	_____
B. Using syringe, gently allow solution to flow over wound.	____	____	____	_____

Continued

	S	U	NP	Comments

C. Continue until the irrigation flow is clear. _____ _____ _____ _____

D. Dry surrounding skin. _____ _____ _____ _____

16. Apply dressing:

   A. Dry dressing:

      (1) Apply sterile gloves. _____ _____ _____ _____

      (2) Inspect wound for appearance, drains, drainage, and integrity. _____ _____ _____ _____

      (3) Cleanse wound with solution. _____ _____ _____ _____

      (4) Dry area. _____ _____ _____ _____

      (5) Apply sterile dry dressing covering wound. _____ _____ _____ _____

      (6) Apply topper dressing if indicated. _____ _____ _____ _____

   B. Wet-to-dry dressing:

      (1) Apply disposable gloves. _____ _____ _____ _____

      (2) Remove old dressings; discard. _____ _____ _____ _____

      (3) Assess surrounding skin. Discard gloves. _____ _____ _____ _____

      (4) Apply sterile gloves. _____ _____ _____ _____

      (5) Cleanse wound base with normal saline. Assess wound base. _____ _____ _____ _____

      (6) Moisten gauze with prescribed solution. Wring gauze out. Unfold. _____ _____ _____ _____

      (7) Apply moist, fine-mesh, open-weave gauze as a single layer directly onto the wound surface. If wound is deep, gently pack dressing into wound base with sterile gloves or forceps until all wound surfaces are in contact with the gauze. If tunnelling is present, use a cotton-tipped applicator to place gauze into tunnelled area. _____ _____ _____ _____

      (8) Cover with sterile dry gauze and topper dressing. _____ _____ _____ _____

17. Secure dressing.

   A. Tape: Apply non-allergenic tape to dressing. _____ _____ _____ _____

   B. Montgomery ties:

      (1) Expose adhesive surface of tape on end of each tie. _____ _____ _____ _____

      (2) Place ties on opposites of dressing. _____ _____ _____ _____

      (3) Place adhesive directly on skin or use skin barrier. _____ _____ _____ _____

      (4) Secure dressing by lacing ties across it. _____ _____ _____ _____

   C. For dressings on an extremity, secure dressing with roller gauze or Surgiflex elastic net. _____ _____ _____ _____

19. Dispose of supplies and perform hand hygiene. _____ _____ _____ _____

20. Assist client to a comfortable position. _____ _____ _____ _____

Skill 43-5 Implementation of Vacuum-Assisted Closure

	S	U	NP	Comments
1. Perform hand hygiene. Assemble supplies.	____	____	____	_____
2. Position client comfortably and drape to expose only wound site. Instruct client not to touch wound or sterile supplies.	____	____	____	_____
3. Place disposable waterproof bag within reach of work area with top folded to make a cuff.	____	____	____	_____
4. Push therapy on/off button.	____	____	____	_____
A. Keeping tube connectors with V.A.C. unit, disconnect tubes from each other to drain fluids into canister.	____	____	____	_____
B. Before lowering, tighten clamp on canister tube.	____	____	____	_____
5. With dressing tube unclamped, introduce 10 to 30 mL of normal saline, if ordered, into tubing to soak underneath foam.	____	____	____	_____
6. Gently stretch transparent film horizontally and slowly pull up from the skin.	____	____	____	_____
7. Remove old V.A.C. dressing, observing appearance and drainage on dressing. Avoid tension on any drains that are present. Discard dressing and remove gloves.	____	____	____	_____
8. Apply sterile or disposable gloves. Irrigate the wound with normal saline or other solution as ordered. Gently blot to dry.	____	____	____	_____
9. Measure wound as ordered. Remove and discard gloves.	____	____	____	_____
10. Depending on the type of wound, apply sterile gloves or new disposable gloves.	____	____	____	_____
11. Prepare V.A.C. foam.	____	____	____	_____
A. Select appropriate foam.	____	____	____	_____
B. Using sterile scissors, cut foam to wound size.	____	____	____	_____
12. Gently place foam in wound; be sure that the foam is in contact with entire wound base, margins, and tunnelled and undermined areas.	____	____	____	_____
13. Apply wrinkle-free transparent dressing over foam and secure tubing to the unit.	____	____	____	_____
14. Apply skin protectant to skin around the wound.	____	____	____	_____
15. Apply Wound V.A.C. dressing. Secure tubing to transparent film, aligning drainage holes to ensure an occlusive seal. Do not apply tension to drape and tubing.	____	____	____	_____

Continued

	S	U	NP	Comments

16. Secure tubing several centimetres away from the dressing.

17. Connect the tubing from the dressing to the tubing from the canister and V.A.C. unit.

    A. Remove canister from sterile packaging and push into V.A.C. unit until a click is heard. An alarm will sound if the canister is not properly engaged.

    B. Connect the dressing tubing to the canister tubing. Make sure both clamps are open.

    C. Place V.A.C. unit on a level surface or hang from the foot of the bed. The unit will alarm and deactivate therapy if the unit is tilted beyond 45 degrees.

    D. Press in green-lit power button and set pressure as ordered.

18. Discard old dressing materials; remove gloves and perform hand hygiene.

19. Inspect Wound V.A.C. system to verify that negative pressure is achieved.

    A. Verify that display screen reads THERAPY ON.

    B. Be sure clamps are open and tubing is patent.

    C. Identify air leaks by listening with stethoscope or by moving hand around edges of wound while applying light pressure.

    D. If a leak is present, use strips of transparent film to patch areas.

20. Compare wound with baseline wound assessment.

21. Verify airtight dressing seal and proper negative pressure.

STUDENT: _____ DATE: _____

INSTRUCTOR: _____ DATE: _____

SKILL PERFORMANCE CHECKLIST
Skill 43-6 Applying an Abdominal or Breast Binder

	S	U	NP	Comments
1. Observe client with need for support of thorax or abdomen. Observe client's ability to breathe deeply and cough effectively.	____	____	____	_____
2. Review medical record if medical prescription for particular binder is required and reasons for application.	____	____	____	_____
3. Inspect skin for actual or potential alterations in integrity.	____	____	____	_____
4. Inspect any surgical dressings.	____	____	____	_____
5. Assess client's comfort level.	____	____	____	_____
6. Gather necessary data regarding size of client and appropriate binder.	____	____	____	_____
7. Explain procedure to client.	____	____	____	_____
8. Teach procedure to client or caregiver.	____	____	____	_____
9. Perform hand hygiene. Apply disposable gloves if likely to contact wound drainage.	____	____	____	_____
10. Provide privacy.	____	____	____	_____
11. Apply binder:				
A. Abdominal binder:				
(1) Position client in supine position with head slightly elevated and knees slightly flexed.	____ ____	____ ____	____ ____	_____ _____
(2) Fanfold far side of binder toward midline of binder.	____	____	____	_____
(3) Instruct and assist client in rolling away from you and toward raised side rail while firmly supporting abdominal incision and dressing with hands.	____	____	____	_____
(4) Place fanfolded ends of binder under client.	____	____	____	_____
(5) Instruct or assist client to roll over onto folded ends.	____	____	____	_____
(6) Unfold and stretch ends out smoothly on far side of bed.	____	____	____	_____
(7) Instruct client to roll back into supine position.	____	____	____	_____
(8) Adjust binder so that supine client is centred over binder using symphysis pubis and costal margins as lower and upper landmarks.	____	____	____	_____

Continued

	S	U	NP	Comments

(9) Close binder. Pull one end over centre of client's abdomen. While maintaining tension on that end of binder, pull opposite end over centre and secure with Velcro closure tabs, metal fasteners, or horizontally placed safety pins. _____ _____ _____ _____

B. Breast binder:

  (1) Assist client in placing arms through binder's armholes. _____ _____ _____ _____

  (2) Assist client to supine position in bed. _____ _____ _____ _____

  (3) Pad area under breasts, if necessary. _____ _____ _____ _____

  (4) Using Velcro closure tabs or horizontally placed safety pins, secure binder at nipple level first. Continue closure process above and then below nipple line until entire binder is closed. _____ _____ _____ _____

  (5) Make appropriate adjustments, including individualizing fit of shoulder straps and pinning waistline darts to reduce binder size. _____ _____ _____ _____

  (6) Instruct and observe client reapplying breast binder. _____ _____ _____ _____

12. Remove gloves and perform hand hygiene. _____ _____ _____ _____

13. Assess client's comfort level, using analogue scale of 0 to 10 and noting any objective signs and symptoms. _____ _____ _____ _____

14. Adjust binder as necessary. _____ _____ _____ _____

15. Observe site for skin integrity, circulation, and characteristics of the wound. _____ _____ _____ _____

16. Assess client's ability to ventilate properly. _____ _____ _____ _____

17. Identify client's need for assistance with daily activities. _____ _____ _____ _____

SKILL PERFORMANCE CHECKLIST
Skill 43-7 Applying an Elastic Bandage

	S	U	NP	Comments
1. Perform hand hygiene and apply gloves, if necessary. Inspect skin for alterations in integrity.	____	____	____	_____
2. Inspect surgical dressing. Remove gloves and perform hand hygiene.	____	____	____	_____
3. Observe distal circulation by noting temperature, colour, and sensation of body part to be wrapped.	____	____	____	_____
4. Review medical record.	____	____	____	_____
5. Identify and primary caregiver's present knowledge level and skill if bandaging will be continued when at home.	____	____	____	_____
6. Explain procedure to client.	____	____	____	_____
7. Teach bandaging skill to client or caregiver.	____	____	____	_____
8. Perform hand hygiene. Apply disposable gloves if drainage is present.	____	____	____	_____
9. Provide privacy.	____	____	____	_____
10. Assist client to a comfortable position.	____	____	____	_____
11. Hold roll of elastic bandage in dominant hand and use other hand to lightly hold beginning of bandage at distal body part. Continue transferring roll to dominant hand as bandage is wrapped.	____	____	____	_____
12. Apply bandage from distal point toward proximal boundary using a variety of turns to cover various shapes of body parts.	____	____	____	_____
13. Unroll and very slightly stretch bandage.	____	____	____	_____
14. Overlap turns by one-half to two-thirds width of bandage roll.	____	____	____	_____
15. Secure first bandage with clip or tape before applying additional rolls. Apply additional rolls without leaving any uncovered skin surface. Secure final bandage applied.	____	____	____	_____
16. Remove gloves if worn and perform hand hygiene.	____	____	____	_____
17. Assess distal circulation when bandage application is complete and at least twice during each 8-hour period.				
A. Observe skin colour.	____	____	____	_____
B. Palpate skin for warmth.	____	____	____	_____
C. Palpate pulses and compare bilaterally.	____	____	____	_____

Continued

	S	U	NP	Comments
D. Ask if client is aware of pain, numbness, tingling, or other discomfort.	____	____	____	_____
E. Observe mobility of extremity.	____	____	____	_____
18. Have client or caregiver demonstrate bandage application.	____	____	____	_____

SKILL PERFORMANCE CHECKLIST
Skill 43-8 Applying a Warm, Moist Compress to an Open Wound

	S	U	NP	Comments
1. Refer to physician's order for type of compress, location and duration of application, desired temperature, and agency policies regarding temperature of compress.	___	___	___	_____
2. Refer to medical record to identify any systemic contraindications to heat application.	___	___	___	_____
3. Perform hand hygiene.	___	___	___	_____
4. Inspect condition of exposed skin and wound on which compress is to be applied.	___	___	___	_____
5. Assess client's extremities for sensitivity to temperature and pain.	___	___	___	_____
6. Assemble equipment and supplies.	___	___	___	_____
7. Explain steps of procedure and purpose to client. Describe sensations to be felt. Explain precautions to prevent burning.	___	___	___	_____
8. Provide privacy.	___	___	___	_____
9. Assist client to a comfortable position and place waterproof pad under area to be treated.	___	___	___	_____
10. Expose body part to be covered with compress and drape client with bath blanket.	___	___	___	_____
11. Prepare compress:				
A. Pour solution into sterile container.	___	___	___	_____
B. If using portable heating source, warm solution. Commercially prepared compresses may remain under infrared lamp until just before use. Open sterile packages and drop gauze into container to become immersed in solution.	___	___	___	_____
12. Apply disposable gloves. Remove any dressing covering wound. Dispose of gloves and dressings.	___	___	___	_____
13. Assess condition of wound and surrounding skin.	___	___	___	_____
14. Apply sterile gloves.	___	___	___	_____
15. Pick up one layer of immersed gauze, wring out any excess solution, and apply it lightly to open wound.	___	___	___	_____
16. In a few seconds, lift edge of gauze to assess for redness.	___	___	___	_____

Continued

	S	U	NP	Comments

17. If client tolerates compress, pack gauze snugly against the wound. Be sure all wound surfaces are covered by the warm compress. ____ ____ ____ _____

18. Cover moist compress with dry sterile dressing and bath towel. If necessary, pin or tie in place. Remove sterile gloves. ____ ____ ____ _____

19. Apply waterproof heating pad over towel (optional). Keep it in place for desired duration of application. ____ ____ ____ _____

20. Change warm compress using sterile technique every 5 minutes or as ordered during duration of therapy. ____ ____ ____ _____

21. Inspect affected area covered by compress and heating pad every 5 to 10 minutes. ____ ____ ____ _____

22. Ask every 5 to 10 minutes if client notices any unusual burning sensation not felt before application. ____ ____ ____ _____

23. After prescribed time, apply disposable gloves and remove pad, towel, and compress. Reassess wound and condition of skin, and replace dry sterile dressing as ordered. ____ ____ ____ _____

24. Assist client to preferred comfortable position. ____ ____ ____ _____

25. Dispose of equipment and soiled compress. Perform hand hygiene. ____ ____ ____ _____

26. Have client explain and demonstrate application. ____ ____ ____ _____

576

STUDENT: _____ DATE: _____

INSTRUCTOR: _____ DATE: _____

Skill 45-1 Demonstrating Post-operative Exercises

	S	U	NP	Comments
1. Assess client for risk of post-operative respiratory complications.	____	____	____	_____
2. Assess client's ability to cough and deep breathe.	____	____	____	_____
3. Assess risk for post-operative thrombus formation.	____	____	____	_____
4. Assess client's ability to move independently while in bed.	____	____	____	_____
5. Explain purpose and importance of exercises.	____	____	____	_____
6. Demonstrate exercises:				
A. Diaphragmatic breathing				
(1) Assist client to comfortable sitting position on side of bed or in chair or standing position.	____	____	____	_____
(2) Stand or sit facing client.	____	____	____	_____
(3) Instruct client to place palms of hands across from each other, down and along lower borders of anterior rib cage. Place tips of third fingers lightly together. Demonstrate for client.	____	____	____	_____
(4) Have client take slow, deep breaths, inhaling through nose and pushing abdomen against hands. Tell client to feel middle fingers separate during inhalation. Demonstrate.	____	____	____	_____
(5) Explain that client will feel normal downward movement of diaphragm during inspiration. Explain that abdominal organs descend and chest wall expands.	____	____	____	_____
(6) Avoid using chest and shoulders while inhaling and instruct client in same manner.	____	____	____	_____
(7) Have client hold slow, deep breath for count of three and then slowly exhale through mouth as if blowing out a candle (pursed lips). Tell client middle fingertips will touch as chest wall contracts.	____	____	____	_____
(8) Repeat breathing exercise 3 to 5 times.	____	____	____	_____

Continued

	S	U	NP	Comments
(9) Have client practice exercise. Instruct client to take 10 slow, deep breaths every hour while awake during post-operative period until mobile.	___	___	___	_____
B. Incentive spirometry:				
(1) Perform hand hygiene.	___	___	___	_____
(2) Position client in semi- or high-Fowler's position.	___	___	___	_____
(3) Set the spirometer to the volume level to be attained.	___	___	___	_____
(4) Demonstrate correct use of spirometer mouthpiece.	___	___	___	_____
(5) Instruct client to inhale slowly and maintain constant flow through unit, attempting to reach goal volume. When maximal inspiration is reached, client should hold breath for 2 to 3 seconds and then exhale slowly. Number of breaths should not exceed 10 to 12/min each session.	___	___	___	_____
(6) Instruct client to breathe normally for short period.	___	___	___	_____
(7) Instruct client to repeat manoeuvre until goals are achieved.	___	___	___	_____
(8) Perform hand hygiene.	___	___	___	_____
C. Positive expiratory pressure (PEP) therapy and "huff" coughing:				
(1) Perform hand hygiene.	___	___	___	_____
(2) Set PEP device for the setting ordered.	___	___	___	_____
(3) Instruct client to assume semi-Fowler's or high-Fowler's position and place nose clip on client's nose.	___	___	___	_____
(4) Have client place lips around mouthpiece. Client should take a full breath and then exhale two to three times longer than inhalation. Pattern should be repeated for 10 to 20 breaths.	___	___	___	_____
(5) Remove device from client's mouth and have client take a slow, deep breath and hold for 3 seconds.	___	___	___	_____
(6) Instruct client to exhale in quick, short, forced inhalations, or "huffs".	___	___	___	_____
D. Controlled coughing:				
(1) Explain importance of maintaining upright position.	___	___	___	_____
(2) Demonstrate coughing. Take two slow, deep breaths, inhaling through nose and exhaling through mouth.	___	___	___	_____

Continued

578

	S	U	NP	Comments

(3) Inhale deeply third time and hold breath to count of three. Cough fully for two or three consecutive coughs without inhaling between coughs. (Tell client to push all air out of lungs.)

(4) Caution client against just clearing throat instead of coughing. Explain that coughing will not cause injury to incision when done correctly.

(5) If surgical incision will be abdominal or thoracic, teach client to place one hand over incisional area and other hand on top of first. Client presses gently against incisional area to splint or support it. Pillow over incision is optional.

(6) Client continues to practise coughing exercises, splinting imaginary incision. Instruct client to cough two to three times every 2 hours while awake.

(7) Instruct client to examine sputum for consistency, odour, amount, and colour changes.

E. Turning

(1) Instruct client to assume supine position and move to side of bed if permitted by surgery. Have bend knees and press heels against the mattress to raise and move buttocks. Top side rails on both sides of bed are up.

(2) Instruct client to place right hand over incisional area to splint it.

(3) Instruct client to keep right leg straight and flex left knee up. If back or vascular surgery was performed, client will need to logroll or will require assistance with turning.

(4) Have client grab right side rail with left hand, pull toward right, and roll onto right side.

(5) Instruct client to turn every 2 hours while awake.

Continued

	S	U	NP	Comments

F. Leg exercises

(1) Have client assume supine position in bed. Demonstrate leg exercises by performing passive range-of-motion exercises and simultaneously explaining exercise.

(2) Rotate each ankle in complete circle. Instruct client to draw imaginary circles with big toe. Repeat five times.

(3) Alternate dorsiflexion and plantar flexion of both feet. Direct client to feel calf muscles contract and relax alternately. Repeat five times.

(4) Perform quadriceps setting by tightening thigh and bringing knee down toward mattress, then relaxing. Repeat five times.

(5) Have client alternately raise each leg straight up from bed surface, keeping legs straight, and then have client bend leg at hip and knee. Repeat five times.

7. Have client practise exercises at least every 2 hours while awake. Instruct client to coordinate turning and leg exercises with diaphragmatic breathing, incentive spirometry, and coughing exercises.

8. Observe client's ability to perform all exercises. sencentive spirometry, and coughing exercises

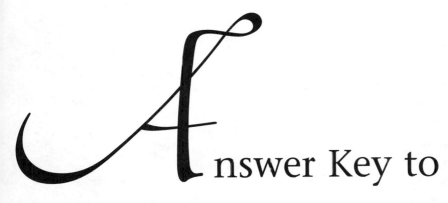

Answer Key to Review Questions

CHAPTER 1

1. d
2. a
3. a
4. b
5. c
6. b
7. c
8. b
9. d

CHAPTER 2

1. a
2. b
3. a
4. b
5. b

CHAPTER 3

1. a
2. d
3. b
4. b
5. d

CHAPTER 4

1. c
2. a
3. a
4. d
5. c

CHAPTER 5

1. a
2. a
3. d
4. c
5. c

CHAPTER 6

1. c
2. d
3. c
4. b
5. c

CHAPTER 7

1. d
2. d
3. a
4. b
5. a

CHAPTER 8

1. a
2. d
3. b
4. d
5. d
6. d
7. a
8. b
9. b
10. d

CHAPTER 9

1. b
2. b
3. a
4. b
5. c

CHAPTER 10

1. c
2. c
3. d
4. c
5. c

CHAPTER 11

1. b
2. c
3. a
4. b

CHAPTER 12

1. c
2. c
3. c
4. b
5. d
6. c
7. a
8. d

CHAPTER 13

1. b
2. c
3. c
4. c
5. d

CHAPTER 14

1. a
2. b
3. b
4. b
5. a

CHAPTER 15

1. c
2. c
3. d
4. a
5. c

CHAPTER 16

1. a
2. c
3. a
4. c
5. d
6. c

CHAPTER 17

1. b
2. c
3. d
4. c
5. b

CHAPTER 18

1. B
2. C
3. A
4. C
5. D

CHAPTER 19

1. c
2. d
3. d
4. d
5. c
6. d

CHAPTER 20

1. a
2. b
3. c
4. a
5. a

CHAPTER 21

1. b
2. a
3. b
4. c
5. b

CHAPTER 22

1. c
2. c
3. d
4. c
5. d

CHAPTER 23

1. b
2. d
3. c
4. a
5. d

CHAPTER 24

1. a
2. a
3. a
4. a
5. c

CHAPTER 25

1. c
2. c
3. b
4. c
5. d

CHAPTER 26

1. d
2. a
3. a
4. a
5. c
6. d

CHAPTER 27

1. d
2. d
3. b
4. c
5. c

CHAPTER 28

1. d
2. a
3. c
4. c
5. c
6. d

CHAPTER 29

1. d
2. b
3. d
4. a
5. b
6. b

CHAPTER 30

1. b
2. a
3. a
4. a
5. b
6. a

CHAPTER 31

1. c
2. b
3. d
4. a

CHAPTER 32

1. c
2. b
3. a
4. b
5. d

CHAPTER 33

1. d
2. d
3. c
4. d
5. a

CHAPTER 34

1. b
2. a
3. c
4. b
5. c

CHAPTER 35

1. a
2. c
3. b
4. b
5. d
6. b

CHAPTER 36

1. b
2. c
3. a
4. c
5. b

CHAPTER 37

1. a
2. a
3. c
4. d
5. b

CHAPTER 38

1. b
2. d
3. a
4. b
5. c

CHAPTER 39

1. c
2. d
3. c
4. c
5. b
6. a

CHAPTER 40

1. a
2. b
3. b
4. a
5. d

CHAPTER 41

1. b
2. a
3. c
4. b
5. c

CHAPTER 42

1. a
2. d
3. d
4. a
5. d

CHAPTER 43

1. b
2. b
3. a
4. c
5. b
6. d

CHAPTER 44

1. c
2. a
3. b
4. c
5. a

CHAPTER 45

1. d
2. c
3. b
4. a
5. b

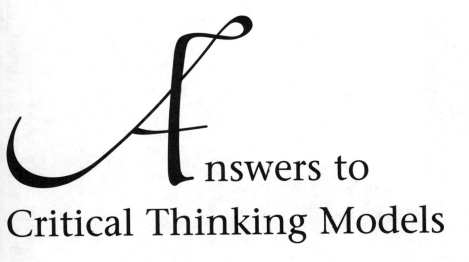

Answers to
Critical Thinking Models

KNOWLEDGE

- Components of self-concept (identity, body image, self-esteem, role performance)
- Self-concept stressors related to identity, body image, self-esteem, role
- Therapeutic communication principles, non-verbal indicators of distress
- Cultural factors that influence self-concept
- Growth and development (middle-age adult)
- Pharmacologic effects of medicine (pain medication)

EXPERIENCE

- Caring for a client who had an alteration in body image, self-esteem, role, or identity
- Personal experience of threat to self-concept

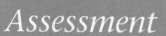

Assessment

- Observe the Mrs. Johnson's behaviours that suggest an alteration in self-concept
- Assess Mrs. Johnson's cultural background
- Assess Mrs. Johnson's coping skills and resources
- Converse with Mrs. Johnson to determine her feelings, perceptions about changes in body image, self-esteem, or role
- Assess the quality of Mrs. Johnson's relationships

STANDARDS

- Support Mrs. Johnson's autonomy to make choices and express values that support positive self-concept
- Apply intellectual standards of relevance and plausibility for care to be acceptable to Mrs. Johnson
- Safeguard Mrs. Johnson's right to privacy by judiciously protecting information of a confidential nature

ATTITUDES

- Display curiosity in considering why Mrs. Johnson might be behaving or responding in this manner
- Display integrity when beliefs and values differ from Mrs. Johnson's; admit to any inconsistencies in own values or in the client's
- Risk taking may be necessary in developing a trusting relationship with Mrs. Johnson

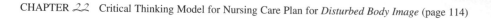

CHAPTER 22   Critical Thinking Model for Nursing Care Plan for *Disturbed Body Image* (page 114)

KNOWLEDGE

- A basic understanding of sexual development, sexual orientation, socio-cultural dimensions, the impact of self-concept, STDs, safe sex practices
- Ways to phrase questions regarding sexuality and functioning
- Disease conditions that affect sexual functioning
- How interpersonal relationship factors may affect sexual functioning

EXPERIENCE

- Jack needs to explore his discomfort with discussing topics related to sexuality and develop a plan for addressing these discomforts
- Jack needs to reflect on his personal sexual experiences and how he has responded

Assessment

- Assess Mr. Clement's developmental stage in regard to sexuality
- Consider self-concept as a factor that will influence sexual satisfaction and functioning
- Physical assessment of urogenital area
- Determine Mr. Clement's sexual concerns
- Assess safer sex practices and the use of contraception
- Assess the medical conditions and medications which may be affecting his sexual functioning
- Assess the impact of high-risk behaviours on sexual health

STANDARDS

- Jack needs to apply intellectual standards of relevance and plausibility for care to be acceptable to Mr. Clement
- Jack needs to safeguard Mr. Clement's right to privacy by judiciously protecting information of a confidential nature
- Jack needs to apply the principles of ethic of care

ATTITUDES

- Jack needs to display curiosity, consider why Mr. Clement might behave or respond in a particular manner
- Jack needs to display integrity; his beliefs and values may differ from Mr. Clement's
- Jack needs to admit to any inconsistencies in his and Mr. Clement's values
- Risk taking: Jack needs to be willing to explore both personal and Mr. Clement's sexual issues and concerns

CHAPTER 23   Critical Thinking Model for Nursing Care Plan for *Sexual Dysfunction* (page 121)

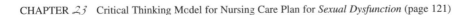

KNOWLEDGE

- The concepts of faith, hope, spiritual well-being, and religion
- Caring practices in the individual approach to a client
- Available services in the community (health care providers and agencies)

EXPERIENCE

- Leah's past experience in selecting interventions that support client's spiritual well-being

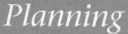

Planning

- Leah needs to collaborate with James and his family on choice of interventions
- Consult with pastoral care, or other clergy or spiritual leaders as appropriate
- Incorporate religious rituals specific to James
- Ask if the client's expectations have been met

STANDARDS

- Standards of autonomy and self determination to support Jame's decisions about the plan

ATTITUDES

- Leah will exhibit confidence in her skills and know to develop a trusting relationship with James
- Be open to any possible conflict between the client's opinion and Leah's; decide how to reach mutually beneficial outcomes

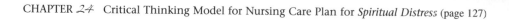

CHAPTER 24 Critical Thinking Model for Nursing Care Plan for *Spiritual Distress* (page 127)

KNOWLEDGE

- Characteristics of a resolution of grief

EXPERIENCE

- Previous client responses to planned nursing interventions for symptom management or the loss of a significant other

Evaluation

- Evaluate signs and symptoms of Mrs. Miller's grief
- Evaluate extended family members' ability to provide supportive care

STANDARDS

- Use established expected outcomes to evaluate Mrs. Miller's response to care (eg., ability to discuss loss)
- Evaluate Mrs. Miller's role in the grieving process

ATTITUDES

- Persevere in seeking successful comfort measures for Mrs. Miller

CHAPTER 25 Critical Thinking Model for Nursing Care Plan for *Ineffective Coping* (page 133)

KNOWLEDGE

- Characteristics of adaptive behaviours
- Characteristics of continuing stress response
- Differentiation of stress and trauma

EXPERIENCE

- Previous client responses to planned nursing interventions

Evaluation

- Reassess Carl for the presence of new or recurring stress-related problems or symptoms (fatigue, changes in energy level, weight, or eating habits)
- Determine if change in care promoted Carl's adaptation to stress
- Evaluate if Carl's expectations have been achieved

STANDARDS

- Use of established expected outcomes to evaluate Carl's plan of care (rest and relaxation, stable weight, positive feelings about wife and their relationship)
- Apply the intellectual standard of relevance; be sure that Carl achieves goals relevant to his needs

ATTITUDES

- Maya needs to demonstrate perseverance in redesigning interventions to promote Carl's adaptation to stress
- Maya needs to display integrity in accurately evaluating nursing interventions

CHAPTER 26 Critical Thinking Model for Nursing Care Plan for *Caregiver Role Strain* (page 139)

KNOWLEDGE

- The role of physiotherapists and exercise trainers in improving Mrs. Smith's activity and exercise program
- Determine Mrs. Smith's ability to increase her level of activity
- Impact of medication on Mrs. Smith's activity tolerance

EXPERIENCE

- Erich needs to consider previous client and personal experiences to therapies designed to improve exercise and activity tolerance
- Erich's personal experience with exercise regimens

Planning

- Erich needs to consult and collaborate with members of the health team to increase Mrs. Smith' activity
- Involve Mrs. Smith and her family in designing her activity and exercise plan
- Erich needs to consider Mrs. Smith' ability to increase her activity level and follow an exercise program

STANDARDS

- Therapies need to be individualized to Mrs. Smith's activity tolerance
- Erich needs to apply the goals of the Health Canada Physical Activity Unit in the application

ATTITUDES

- Erich needs to be responsible and creative in designing interventions to improve Mrs. Smith's activity tolerance

CHAPTER 32 Critical Thinking Model for Nursing Care Plan for *Activity Intolerance* (page 199)

KNOWLEDGE

- Basic human needs
- The potential risks to a client's safety from physical and environmental hazards
- The influence of developmental stage on safety needs (older adult)
- The influence of illness and medications on Ms. Cohen's safety (immobilization and visual impairment)

EXPERIENCE

- Past experiences of Mr. Key in caring for clients with mobility or sensory impairments that threaten safety
- Personal experiences in caring for the older adult

Assessment

- Identification of actual and potential threats to Ms. Cohen's safety
- Determine the impact of Ms. Cohen's underlying disease on her safety
- The presence of risks for Ms. Cohen's developmental stage

STANDARDS

- Mr. Key needs to apply intellectual standards of accuracy, significance, completeness, and fairness when assessing for threats to Ms. Cohen's safety
- Fall prevention or restraint protocols

ATTITUDES

- Perseverance is needed when identifying all threats to Ms. Cohen's safety
- Responsibility for collecting unbiased accurate data regarding Ms. Cohen's threat to safety
- Fairness is appropriate to objectively evaluate the risk to Ms. Cohen's safety within the home and the community

CHAPTER *33* Critical Thinking Model for Nursing Care Plan for *Risk for Injury* (page 205)

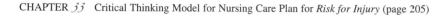

KNOWLEDGE

- Principles of comfort and safety
- Adult learning principles to apply when educating the client and family
- Services available through community agencies

EXPERIENCE

- Care of previous clients that required adaptation of hygiene approaches

Planning

- Involve Mrs. Wyatt and her family in planning and adapting approaches as well as in hygiene instruction
- Know community resources applicable to Mrs. Wyatt's needs
- Consider the timing of other care activities when choosing the best time for hygienic care

STANDARDS

- Individualize the hygiene care to meet Mrs. Wyatt's preferences
- Apply standards of safety and promotion of client dignity

ATTITUDES

- Jeannette needs to be creative when adapting approaches to any self-care limitations that Mrs. Wyatt might have
- Jeannette needs to take responsibility for following standards of good hygiene practice

CHAPTER 34   Critical Thinking Model for Nursing Care Plan for *Ineffective Tissue Perfusion, Improper Foot Care/Hygiene* (page 213)

KNOWLEDGE

- Cardiac and respiratory anatomy and physiology
- Cardiopulmonary pathophysiology
- Clinical signs and symptoms of altered oxygenation
- Developmental factors affecting oxygenation
- Impact on lifestyle
- Environmental impact

EXPERIENCE

- Caring for clients with impaired oxygenation, activity intolerance, and respiratory infections
- Observations of changes in client respiratory patterns made during poor air quality days
- Personal experience with how a change in altitudes or physical conditioning affects respiratory patterns
- Personal experience with respiratory infections or cardiopulmonary alterations

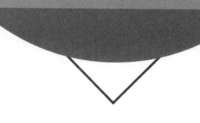

Assessment

- Identify recurring and present signs and symptoms associated with Mr. Edwards' impaired oxygenation
- Determine the presence of risk factors that apply to Mr. Edwards
- Ask Mr. Edwards about the use of medication
- Determine Mr. Edwards' activity status
- Determine Mr. Edwards' tolerance to activity

STANDARDS

- Apply intellectual standards of clarity, precision, specificity, and accuracy when obtaining a health history from Mr. Edwards

ATTITUDES

- Carry out the responsibility of obtaining correct information about Mr. Edwards
- Display confidence while assessing the extent of Mr. Edwards' respiratory alterations

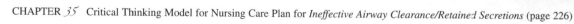

CHAPTER *35* Critical Thinking Model for Nursing Care Plan for *Ineffective Airway Clearance/Retained Secretions* (page 226)

KNOWLEDGE

- Consider the other health care professionals caring for Mrs. Bottomley
- The impact of specific fluid regimens on the Mrs. Bottomley's fluid balance
- The impact of new medications on Mrs. Bottomley's fluid balance

EXPERIENCE

- Consider the previous clinical assignments you have had and how those clients responded to nursing therapies (what worked and what didn't)

Planning

- Select nursing interventions to promote fluid, electrolyte, and acid-base balance
- Consult with pharmacists and nutritionists
- Involve Mrs. Bottomley and her family in designing the interventions

STANDARDS

- Therapies need to be individualized to Mrs. Bottomley's fluid balance and acid-base requirements
- Apply agency and professional standards for prevention of intravascular infections

ATTITUDES

- Use creativity to plan interventions that will achieve an effective airway and integrate those into Mrs. Bottomley's activities of daily living
- Be responsible in planning nursing interventions consistent with the client's fluid balance and acid-base requirements and with standards of practice

CHAPTER 36 Critical Thinking Model for Nursing Care Plan for *Fluid and Electrolyte Alterations* (page 239)

KNOWLEDGE

- The characteristics of a desirable sleep pattern
- Behaviours reflecting adequate sleep

EXPERIENCE

- Previous clients' responses to planned nursing interventions for promoting sleep
- Previous experience in adapting sleep therapies to personal needs

Evaluation

- Evaluate signs and symptoms of Julie's sleep disturbance
- Review Julie's sleep pattern
- Ask Julie's sleep partner to report response to therapies
- Ask if expectations of care are being met

STANDARDS

- Use of established expected outcomes to evaluate Julie's responses to care (eg., improved duration of sleep, fewer awakenings)

ATTITUDES

- Humility may apply if an intervention is unsuccessful; rethink the approach
- In the case of chronic sleep problems, perseverance is needed in staying with the plan of care or in trying new approaches

CHAPTER *37* Critical Thinking Model for Nursing Care Plan for *Disturbed Sleep Pattern* (page 248)

KNOWLEDGE

- Physiology of pain
- Factors that potentially increase or decrease responses to pain
- Pathophysiology of conditions causing pain
- Awareness of biases affecting pain assessment and treatment
- Cultural variations in how pain is expressed
- Knowledge of nonverbal communication

EXPERIENCE

- Caring for clients with acute, chronic, and cancer pain
- Caring for clients who experienced pain as a result of a health care therapy
- Personal experience with pain

Assessment

- Determine Mrs. Mays' perspective of pain including history of pain, its meaning, and physical emotional and social effects
- Objectively measure the characteristics of Mrs. Mays' pain
- Review potential factors affecting Mrs. Mays' pain

STANDARDS

- Refer to AHCPR and RNAO guidelines for acute pain assessment and management
- Apply intellectual standards (clarity, specificity, accuracy, and completeness) when gathering assessment

ATTITUDES

- Display confidence when assessing pain to relieve Mrs. Mays' anxiety
- Display integrity and fairness to prevent prejudice from affecting assessment

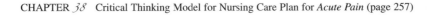

CHAPTER *38* Critical Thinking Model for Nursing Care Plan for *Acute Pain* (page 257)

KNOWLEDGE

- Roles of dietitians and nutritionists in caring for clients with altered nutrition
- Impact of community support groups and other resources in assisting clients to manage nutrition
- Impact of bad diets on client's overall nutritional status

EXPERIENCE

- Previous client responses to nursing interventions for altered nutrition
- Personal experiences with dietary change strategies (what worked and what did not)

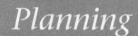

Planning

- Select nursing interventions to promote optimal nutrition
- Select nursing interventions consistent with therapeutic diets
- Consult with other health care professinonals (dietitians, nutritionists, physicians, pharmacists, and physiotherapists and occupational therapists) to adopt interventions that reflect Mrs. Cooper's needs
- Involve Mrs. Cooper's family when designing interventions

STANDARDS

- Individualize therapy according to client needs
- Select therapies consistent with established standards of normal nutrition
- Select therapies consistent with established standards for therapeutic diets

ATTITUDES

- Display confidence in selecting interventions
- Creatively adapt interventions for the client's physical limitations, culture, personal preferences, budget, and home care needs

CHAPTER *39* Critical Thinking Model for Nursing Care Plan for *Imbalanced Nutrition: Less Than Body Requirements* (page 268)

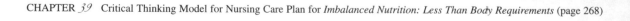

KNOWLEDGE

- Physiology of fluid balance
- Anatomy and physiology of normal urine production and urination
- Pathophysiology of selected urinary alterations
- Factors affecting urination
- Principles of communication used to address issues related to self-concept and sexuality

EXPERIENCE

- Caring for clients with alterations in urinary elimination
- Caring for clients at risk for urinary infection
- Personal experience with changes in urinary elimination

Assessment

- Gather health history of the urination pattern, symptoms, and factors affecting urination
- Conduct a physical assessment of body systems potentially affected by urinary change
- Assess the characteristics of urine
- Assess Mrs. Grayson's perception of urinary problems as it affects self-concept

STANDARDS

- Maintain Mrs. Grayson's privacy and dignity
- Apply intellectual standards to ensure history and assessment are complete and in depth
- Apply professional standards of care from professional organizations such as CNA and the Canadian Continence Foundation

ATTITUDES

- Display humility in recognizing limitations in knowledge
- Establish trust with Mrs. Grayson to reveal full picture of this potentially sensitive topic

CHAPTER 40 Critical Thinking Model for Nursing Care Plan for *Functional Urinary Incontinence* (page 278)

KNOWLEDGE

- Role of the other health care professionals in returning the client's bowel elimination pattern to normal
- Impact of specific therapeutic diets and medication on bowel elimination patterns
- Expected results of cathartics, laxatives, and enemas on bowel elimination

EXPERIENCE

- Previous client response to planned nursing therapies for improving bowel elimination (what worked and what did not)

Planning

- Javier needs to select nursing interventions to promote normal bowel elimination
- Consult with nurtitionists
- Involve Larry and his family in designing nursing interventions

STANDARDS

- Individualize therapies to Larry's bowel elimination needs
- Select therapies consistent within wound and ostomy professional practice standards

ATTITUDES

- Javier needs to be creative when planning interventions for Larry to achieve normal bowel elimination patterns
- Display independence when integrating interventions from other disciplines in Larry's plan of care
- Act responsibly by ensuring that interventions are consistent within standards

CHAPTER 41 Critical Thinking Model for Nursing Care Plan for *Constipation* (page 287)

KNOWLEDGE

- Characteristics of improved mobility status on all physiological systems and the client's psychosocial and developmental status

EXPERIENCE

- Previous client responses to planned mobility interventions.

Evaluation

- Reassess Ms. Adams for signs and symptoms of improved or decreasd mobility status
- Ask for Ms. Adam's perception of mobility status after intervention
- Ask if Ms. Adam's expectations of care have been met

STANDARDS

- Use established expected outcomes for Ms. Adam's plan of care (lung fields remain clear) to evaluate her response to care

ATTITUDES

- Display humility when identifying those interventions that were not successful
- Use creativity when redesigning interventions to improve Ms. Adam's mobility status

CHAPTER 42 Critical Thinking Model for Nursing Care Plan for *Impaired Physical Mobility* (page 297)

KNOWLEDGE

- Pathogenesis of pressure ulcers
- Factors contributing to pressure ulcer formation or poor wound healing
- Factors contributing to wound healing
- Impact of underlying disease process on skin integrity
- Impact of medication on skin integrity and wound healing

EXPERIENCE

- Caring for clients with impaired skin integrity or wounds
- Observation of normal wound healing

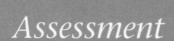

Assessment

- Identify Mrs. Stein's risk for developing impaired skin integrity
- Identify signs and symptoms associated with impaired skin integrity or poor wound healing
- Examine Mrs. Stein's skin for actual impairment in skin integrity

STANDARDS

- Apply intellectual standards of accuracy, relevance, completeness, and precision when obtaining health history regarding skin integrity and wound management
- Apply agency and professional standards for prevention and management of pressure ulcers (eg., AHCPR, RNAO)

ATTITUDES

- Use discipline to obtain complete and correct assessment data regarding Mrs. Stein's skin and/or wound integrity
- Demonstrate responsibility for collecting appropriate specimens for diagnostic and laboratory tests related to wound management

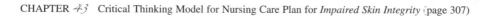

CHAPTER 43   Critical Thinking Model for Nursing Care Plan for *Impaired Skin Integrity* (page 307)

602   Answers to Critical Thinking Models

KNOWLEDGE

- Understand how a sensory deficit can affect Judy's functional status
- Role other health professionals might have in sensory function management
- Services of community resources
- Adult learning principles to apply when educating Judy and her family

EXPERIENCE

- Previous client responses to planned nursing interventions to promote sensory function

Planning

- Select strategies that assist Judy to remain functional in her home
- Adapt therapies based on short- or long-term sensory deficit
- Involve the family in helping Judy adjust to her limitations
- Refer Judy to an appropriate health care professional and/or community agency

STANDARDS

- Individualize therapies that allow Judy to adapt to sensory loss in any setting
- Apply standards of safety

ATTITUDES

- Use creativity to find interventions that help Judy adapt to the home environment

CHAPTER 44   Critical Thinking Model for Nursing Care Plan for *Disturbed Sensory Perception* (page 314)

KNOWLEDGE

- Behaviours that demonstrate learning
- Characteristics of anxiety and/or fear
- Signs and symptoms or conditions that contraindicate surgery

EXPERIENCE

- Previous client responses to planned preoperative care
- Any personal experience Joe has had with surgery

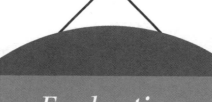

Evaluation

- Evaluate Mrs. Campana's knowledge of surgical procedure and planned postoperative care
- Have Mrs. Campana demonstrate post-operative exercises
- Observe behaviours or non-verbal expressions of anxiety or fear
- Ask if client's expectation are being met

STANDARDS

- Use established expected outcomes to evaluate Mrs. Campana's plan of care (eg., ability to perform post-operative exercises)

ATTITUDES

- Demonstrate perseverance when Mrs. Campana has difficulty performing post-operative exercises

CHAPTER *45* Critical Thinking Model for Nursing Care Plan for *Deficient Knowledge Regarding Preoperative and Post-operative Care Requirements* (page 325)